Essentials of Fitness

Harold B. Falls, Ph.D.

Southwest Missouri State University
Springfield, Missouri

Ann M. Baylor, Ph.D.

The University of Texas
Austin, Texas

Rod K. Dishman, Ph.D.

Southwest Missouri State University
Springfield, Missouri

SAUNDERS COLLEGE
Philadelphia

Saunders College
West Washington Square
Philadelphia, PA 19105

Essentials of Fitness

ISBN 0-03-056777-7

2 3 4   026   9 8 7 6 5 4

Preface

Over 100 years ago, physical education (physical training) gained a niche in some of our institutions of higher learning because it was believed to be important as a form of preventive medicine. During the first 50 to 60 years of this century, the preventive medicine aspects of physical activity in college and university general education courses gradually eroded. The courses for the general college student became almost totally sports-oriented. Most of those courses that did deal with conditioning and personal fitness were usually nothing more than a "work-out period." Emphasis was on the techniques—the how of exercise—rather than on the rationale, the why. The student was provided with very little basis for making intelligent future decisions in regard to his personal exercise habits and program.

Fortunately for the college-age public, that situation began to change about 15 years ago. Since 1965, there has been a resurgence in the emphasis on the role of physical activity in human well-being. A large volume of research has demonstrated that vigorous physical activity can be instrumental in the prevention and/or alleviation of many "hypokinetic" disease problems—both physical and emotional in nature. There is a whole new awareness of physical activity as preventive medicine, and many institutions of higher learning have established courses for the express purpose of "educating" their students in regard to the techniques of exercise, the reasons for exercise, and the scientific base that supports it. The emphasis on "training" the student in techniques and "working up a sweat" is outmoded. The new emphasis is on establishing regular physical activity as a part of one's lifestyle, something that has always been one of man's basic needs.

Personal fitness has become a major interest in our society. One need only look at the number of running clubs, tennis and racquetball facilities, and swimming pools, and the fact that exercise books now rival in sales those on sex, to realize this.

The renewed interest in exercise for personal fitness has created a demand for up-to-date, authoritative materials to support learning in this most important area. In order adequately to supply that, a book first of all must establish a rationale for exercise (the why). It must then provide readers with a plan (the techniques). Finally, it must present the basic scientific facts and other technical material that support various philosophies and forms of exercise (the base). The latter is very important in helping readers to understand the techniques. It is also important in equipping them with knowledge for making future intelligent decisions in regard to exercise. This material should also help them achieve optimal benefits from a fitness program in relation to time, money, and effort devoted. The major shortcoming of most textbooks in this area is that they provide too little "base." A text must also be practical. Even though scientific basis and rationale are adequately covered, practicality and application must be the major thrust.

We believe this book meets the above criteria. Chapter 1—Introduction—identifies the components of health-related fitness and explains the importance of each. Further elaboration on the "why" of exercise is provided in both Chapter 3—Cardiovascular Disease Risk Factors—and Chapter 7 on the psychological aspects of exercise. Chapter 2 provides an introduction and/or basic review of important anatomical and physiological topics, and is intended to aid the reader in comprehending terminology of exercise and understanding some of the phenomena associated with form and function in the human during movement. We believe that a study of Chapter 2 will enhance learning within all the concept areas covered in the book. However, the other chapters could be utilized more or less independently of Chapter 2, with only occasional references to it.

Chapters 4 through 8 contain significant sections on the techniques of exercise. Specific exercises, well illustrated, are presented. Suggestions are made for obtaining optimal benefits from strength, endurance, cardiovascular function, flexibility, and weight control programs. The impact of environmental conditions and psychological factors is covered in detail. In Chapter 8, specific dietary practices for the control of obesity, blood fats, and cholesterol are presented. Chapter 3 also touches somewhat on this topic. The techniques are always discussed in the context of the "base." However, even though a great deal of scientific and technical material is presented, a concerted effort has been made to present it in as simple and straightforward language as possible. The book has been written for *students,* not for our research peers or the teacher. It is intended as an aid to learning.

At the end of each chapter 20 to 60 learning objectives have been provided, selected to highlight the major concepts of each chapter. They are written in modified behavioral objective form and indicate to students what they should be able to do after completing a study of the chapter. We believe that if students study these objectives conscientiously, they will have no difficulty in mastering the chapter materials. The learning objectives also may provide a basis for examination questions prepared by the instructor.

An important feature of the text is the Appendix sections. Twenty-three different appendices have been provided, and are intended primarily for use as laboratory exercises. In other words, they ask students to *do* something of a cognitive nature in addition to the physical activity that will be associated with the text materials. The appendices supplement material in Chapters 3 through 8. Specific cross-references from chapters to appendices are provided.

An extensive list of references is provided at the end of each chapter, and a few specific references are provided within the chapters and appendices. They have been carefully chosen and will provide good supplementary reading on the various topics should it be desired and/or needed.

Readers will be encountering certain terminology for the first time. In recognition of the fact that many words will be unfamiliar, a glossary is provided at the end of the book to aid readers' comprehension and help them to master the concepts presented.

Another important feature of the book is the chapter on the psychological aspects of exercise. The material presented therein is authoritative and up-to-date, and in a very readable format. We are strongly convinced that this chapter provides the best coverage of this area available in any similar textbook on the market.

A final important feature is the illustrations, which we have attempted to provide for most of the major and/or difficult concepts. In addition, there are over 100 photographs of specific exercises. The book, therefore, provides coverage from both a visual and a narrative perspective.

Acknowledgments. The authors wish to acknowledge the following individuals who aided materially in the completion of the manuscript: Mr. John Butler, Ms. Juliana Kremer, Ms. Susan Loring, and Mr. John Snyder of the W.B. Saunders Co., who were especially patient, helpful, and encouraging during the extended interval when the manuscript was in preparation; Dr. George Simpson of Southwest Missouri State University, who provided helpful comments in regard to certain sections of the manuscript draft; Ms. Carla Diemer, Ms. LeaAnn Fuson, Ms. JoAnn Twibell, and Ms. Cherie Wenninger, who, along with Dr. Rod Dishman, enhanced the visual appeal by posing for the photographs; and Ms. Arlene Eickler, Ms. Toni Meyer, and Ms. Shirley Minger, who assisted in the final preparation of the manuscript. Special thanks also go to Dr. Dennis Humphrey who did the photographic work.

HAROLD B. FALLS

ANN M. BAYLOR

ROD K. DISHMAN

Contents

Chapter 6
FLEXIBILITY ———————————————————— 166

Chapter 1

Introduction

THIS THING CALLED FITNESS

This is a book about health. It deals with exercise and diet as a form of preventive and rehabilitative medicine. Within its covers we hope to be able to present in a logical and understandable manner the "why" as well as the "how" of exercise. The emphasis is on basic concepts related to personal fitness. To us, personal fitness means a form of self-motivated, systematic participation in exercise that is geared toward improvement in one's quality of living.

Fitness is certainly a problem of national concern for everyone, from the President's Council on Physical Fitness and Sports down to the individual who notices the stairs getting steeper and the waistline getting larger. Current estimates reveal the general population not only below reasonable fitness standards but also obese. The problem is widespread and is not confined to any one component of fitness.

Figure 1–1 illustrates one aspect of the fitness problem in the young adult segment of our society. It is constructed from data appearing in a 1971 study that compared Austrian Army members with similar personnel in the United States Air Force. The test criterion used for comparison was the distance that could be covered by running and/or walking in a 12-minute time period. This has become a popular, practical test of circulatory fitness over the past few years (see Chapter 5). One and one-half miles covered in the 12-minute period represents a reasonable standard for a good fitness classification on the test. As can be seen from the illustration, only about 65 per cent of U.S. Air Force personnel aged 19 years could achieve the good fitness classification, compared with 85 per cent of the Austrians. Beyond age 19, there is a steady decline in the percentage of Americans achieving the 1.5 mile standard until, at age 29, only 25 per cent can do so. There is some decline between ages 19 and 29 in the percentage of Austrians reaching the good classification, but even at age 29, 70 per cent could do so—a better performance than the U.S. military personnel ten years younger.

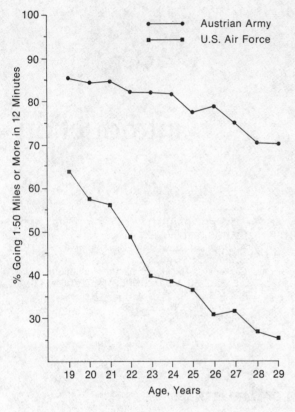

Figure 1–1. Results of 12-Minute Run Performance Test in U.S. Air Force and Austrian Army Personnel Age 19 to 29. (Adapted from data presented by Cooper, K. H., and Zechner, A.: Physical fitness in U.S. and Austrian military personnel: a comparative study. J.A.M.A. *215*:931, 1971.)

FITNESS DEFINED: THE COMPONENTS OF FITNESS

The term "fitness" has been rather vaguely defined in most cases. The concept thus has developed into one that is somewhat confusing, especially to those who are not experts in the area. For those desiring to improve their fitness levels, the problem is often even more confusing than the concept. They probably experience great difficulty in evaluating their current level of fitness, and the question of what to do to improve the state is doubly perplexing. Not only are they confronted with a large array of published programs emphasizing various components of fitness, but also with advertisements of various groups and clubs making all sorts of conflicting claims.

This book is predicated on our belief that there are certain basic principles or foundations on which every personal fitness program should be based, and that participants who follow these principles will be successful in elevating their level of fitness to one that will make a significant contribution to an improved lifestyle. Alternatively, if a reasonably high level of fitness already exists, they will be able to maintain it throughout their lifetime. In this regard, we have attempted to substructure the components of fitness into those that are health-related as opposed to those that are performance-related.

Health-related and Performance-related Fitness

Health-related fitness refers to those aspects of physiological and psychological functioning which are believed to offer some protection against degenerative type diseases such as coronary heart disease, obesity, and various musculoskeletal disorders.

These afflictions have been referred to as "hypokinetic diseases" by physicians Hans Kraus and Wilhelm Raab because they often are associated with low levels of energy expenditure common to the sedentary person. Surely this type of fitness should be of primary concern to every individual within our society. Performance-related fitness, on the other hand, includes those qualities of function that provide the individual with the wherewithal to participate in sport activities with greater power, strength, endurance, skill, etc., than otherwise would be the case. The ultimate example of a person with this type of fitness is the outstanding professional or Olympic athlete.

Our emphasis in this book is on health-related fitness—fitness important to everyone. We have referred to these components as the "Essentials of Fitness." However, the basic components of health-related fitness are also important components of performance-related fitness in many sports, and the basic principles of development and maintenance of the components are common to the two areas. The major differences lie in the *degree* to which each component must be developed. For example, Olympic marathon champions must have a heart and circulatory system functioning at an extremely high level in order to be able to deliver enough oxygen to the muscles to sustain the level of energy metabolism demanded by their sport. The average individual, on the other hand, can have a system functioning at 60 to 70 per cent of the marathoner's capacity and still receive optimal levels of protection from the development of circulatory disease. This will be explained more fully in later sections of this book. It should be noted at this juncture that an individual may be high in certain components of performance-related fitness but low in health-related fitness. An example is provided by baseball players who train only for their sport. Although these athletes are often very strong, usually exhibit high levels of skill in throwing, catching, and batting, and may possess exceptional sprinting speed, they are not necessarily high in other components of fitness. In a study comparing several men's athletic teams at the University of Minnesota, the baseball team was shown to be lowest on maximal oxygen consumption (a measure of cardiorespiratory fitness) and highest on percentage body fat. The oxygen consumption capacity of the baseball players was only about 11 per cent higher than that of nonathlete college students and soldiers of the same age, and their body fat percentages were approximately equal to the nonathletes. As we shall see later, both maximal oxygen consumption and percentage body fat are important components of health-related fitness.

The reason for the relatively low standing of baseball players on certain components of health-related fitness is that their sport is one that does not demand the kind of activity that would develop cardiorespiratory fitness and low percentage of body fat. Baseball is a low-energy sport requiring only about 5 kilocalories per minute of energy expenditure— less than one-half the energy cost of handball. In the report from another study on heart rates during Little League baseball competition, it was stated that "the exercise involved in the ½ to 2 hours of a Little League baseball game, excluding defensive positions of pitching and catching, is minimal. So minimal, in fact, that it should not be considered as a major contributing factor to the development of cardiovascular-respiratory fitness. Children in this age group need vigorous large-muscle activity to promote their optimal growth and development. It is to be hoped that they are given an opportunity to gain these advantages elsewhere rather than expecting baseball to provide the experience."[10] Baseball, therefore, does not place a very high stress on the circulatory system, and does not burn up many extra calories. It is a sport requiring speed, skill, and strength. The longest continuous run a player would be expected to make is for an inside-the-park home run, a distance of 120 yards! Football is another popular sport that emphasizes strength, speed, and skill, and analyses of fitness components in football players show them to be very similar to nonathletes on tests of body composition and cardiorespiratory function.

The foregoing is often difficult for even many physicians, physical educators, and athletic coaches to understand. When a 40- to 50-year-old ex-athlete from *any* sport dies of a heart attack, it nearly always evokes great surprise along with the question, "How could this happen? He was an athlete and exercised a lot." What often is not apparent on the surface is that he may have been an athlete from baseball, football, or a similar sport in which the exercise demands were mostly strength, power, and speed, with little emphasis on exercise requiring great activity by the heart. The heart, therefore, was not really trained to the extent of other parts of the body, even during the teen and young adult years of high school, college, and professional competition. In addition, the athlete may have discontinued even the forms of exercise within his sport after his competitive days were over. As a result, he may really have been no different from the average sedentary person as far as the essential components of fitness are concerned.

Table 5–5 (Chapter 5) should help to illustrate the preceding discussion. In it, two well-known Ohio State University exercise physiologists, Edward L. Fox and Donald K. Mathews, have analyzed various sport activities and classified them according to the relative contribution of the body's energy systems. The ATP (adenosine triphosphate), PC (phosphocreatine), and LA (lactic acid) systems represent sources of energy to support speed and power activities. The O_2 system represents a source of energy to support oxidation of food, and depends on a high level of functioning within the circulatory system. Those activites showing this system contributing a high proportion of the total energy yield are the ones that would be expected to provide a significant cardiovascular conditioning effect from participation in them. Chapters 2 and 5 will discuss the interaction among the body's energy systems in more detail. Chapter 5 will also discuss factors involved in the choice of activities from Table 5–5 to use in the development of health-related components of fitness.

The Components of Health-related Fitness

The basic components of health-related fitness are cardiovascular function, body composition, strength, and flexibility. These are also basic components in the performance-related fitness area. Again, it should be emphasized that the major differences lie in the *degree* to which each component must be developed within the two areas.

Cardiovascular Function

Cardiovascular function is the most important component in the health-related fitness area. The leading cause of death among the adult populations of most industrialized societies throughout the world is circulatory disease of various kinds. The United States leads the world in this gruesome statistic (Fig. 1–2), and the percentage of total adult deaths attributable to circulatory problems has only recently begun to decline in spite of greater emphasis on their etiology, prevention, and/or cure. *It now stands at slightly over 50 per cent.* An alarming aspect of this is the prevalence of heart disease among younger adults, which accounts for 16 and 33 per cent, respectively, of all male deaths in the age ranges 25 to 35 and 36 to 45 years. And the problem is not confined to adults. In two recent studies of boys and girls 7 to 12 years of age, it was noted that 60 per cent exhibited at least one of the risk factors associated with increased coronary heart disease in adult populations (obesity, high serum cholesterol and/or triglycerides, elevated blood pressure, low work capacity). Fourteen per cent in one study and 36 per cent in the other exhibited at least two or more of these factors. Twenty per cent of the children in one of the studies had three or more risk factors.

Figure 1–2. Mortality Rates from Atherosclerosis and Degenerative Heart Disease from Certain Selected Countries. (Based on data from Demographic Year-book, 1967, New York, 1968, Statistical Office of the United Nations. From Hockey, R. V.: *Physical Fitness: The Pathway to Healthful Living*. 3rd ed. St. Louis, The C. V. Mosby Co., 1977.)

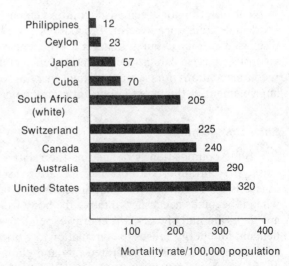

Mortality rate/100,000 population

Although the evidence accumulated thus far is not unequivocal, many cardiologists, physiologists, physical educators, and other health professionals are convinced that physical activity at levels sufficiently high enough to promote improved cardiovascular function is a potent factor in either preventing circulatory disease altogether or reducing its effect if it does occur. One study that effectively illustrates the effect of sedentary habits on the risk of development of heart disease is the Health Insurance Plan study in New York. This was a very large survey that examined the development and prognosis of certain clinical manifestations of coronary heart disease in a defined population of 110,000 adult men and women in New York City. Some of the results are summarized in Table 1–1, in which the incidence of myocardial infarction (heart attack) and the death rate therefrom are compared in men classified according to their level of habitual physical activity. It is clearly evident that sedentary individuals have a much higher incidence of myocardial infarction, and also that the fatality rate is higher in those who are not very physically active.

Another recent study of 3000 adult men revealed that there is an inverse relationship between the level of cardiovascular fitness and the degree to which an individual exhibits certain cardiovascular disease risk factors. Specifically, this means that the higher the level of cardiovascular fitness, the lower the levels of serum cholesterol, serum tri-glycerides (blood fats), serum glucose, serum uric acid, blood pressure, and body fat percentage. Elevated levels of all the above have been implicated in one or more epidemiological studies as being positively related to increased incidence of cardiovascular disease.

Table 1–1. AGE-ADJUSTED MYOCARDIAL INFARCTION (MI) AMONG MEN AGED 25–64: INCIDENCE AND EARLY MORTALITY IN RELATION TO PHYSICAL ACTIVITY.

	No. of 1st MIs per 1000 Men at Risk per Year	% of Men Dying with First MI	No. of Deaths per 1000 Men at Risk per Year
Least Active	6.26	52.6	3.29
Intermediate Active	3.78	26.7	1.01
Most Active	3.81	19.6	0.75

Adapted from Frank, C. W., Weinblatt, F., Shapiro, S., and Sager, R. V.: Myocardial infarction in men: role of physical activity and smoking in incidence and mortality. J.A.M.A. *198*:1241, 1966.

The criterion for cardiovascular fitness is the relative level of functioning within the heart and circulatory system. Procedures for evaluating that level of functioning are discussed in some detail in Chapter 5, which also covers the specific effects that regular vigorous exercise can have on cardiovascular function, along with general and specific recommendations for setting up and carrying out an exercise program for personal improvement in this most important component of fitness.

Body Composition

Body composition is defined as the relative percentages of fat and fat-free body mass. It is an important correlate to cardiovascular function as far as health-related fitness is concerned. Excess amounts of body fat take the form of "excess baggage" when it becomes necessary to move the body from one place to another. Therefore, for any given amount of work, the energy expenditure is increased in the obese. The greater demand for energy causes the circulation to work harder. Also, an obese person usually consumes a diet high in saturated fats and cholesterol. The resulting greater levels of circulating blood fats increase the probability of developing atherosclerosis—an important precursor to coronary heart disease. Figure 1–3, constructed from data gathered in the Framingham, MA, epidemiological study of heart disease, illustrates the effect that overweight and obesity have on coronary heart disease mortality. It is readily seen that men who are 20 per cent or more overweight for their height and build have a mortality rate from coronary heart disease 2.28 times that expected, and a rate 2.62 times greater than those persons exhibiting average or below average relative weight.

The problem of obesity in the United States is widespread. The American Medical Association has estimated that over 50 per cent of all adults can be considered overweight, and surveys among schoolchildren indicate that a similar situation exists for at least 40 per cent of that population. Retention of body fat at any age is a health problem of considerable concern, but it is especially significant in children and adolescents because obese individuals in those age ranges are much more likely to be fat adults than their non-fat peers. The major causes of obesity appear to be:

1. a higher standard of living;
2. increased mechanization;
3. more leisure time;

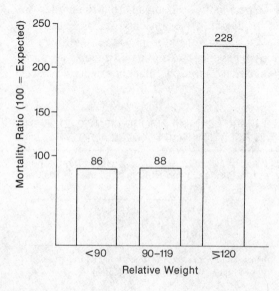

Figure 1–3. Risk of Fatal Coronary Attacks (16 Years) According to Relative Weight. Men 30 to 62 at entry: Framingham, Massachusetts Epidemiological Study. Relative weight is actual weight/predicted weight × 100. Predicted weight is based on skeletal body build (see Appendix A–16). Values under 100 mean actual weight less than predicted, and values over 100 are actual weight greater than predicted. (Adapted from Kannel, W. B.: Medical Evaluation for Physical Exercise Programs. *In* R. L. Morse (ed.) *Exercise and the Heart,* 1972. Courtesy of Charles C Thomas, Publisher, Springfield, Ill.

4. low physical activity;

5. insufficient knowledge about weight control; and

6. lack of motivation with regard to weight control.[12]

In addition to an increased incidence of coronary heart disease among obese persons, certain other health problems are manifest. These include greater risk of developing and suffering from hypertension, diabetes mellitus, gallbladder disease, degenerative arthritis, kidney disease, adverse postural changes, delayed puberty in children, and decreased endurance and work capacity. It has been estimated that if all deaths from cancer were eliminated, two years would be added to the human life span, and if all the deaths related to obesity were removed, the life span would increase 7 years! Indeed, most medical authorities recommend that one of the best personal preventive and rehabilitative health practices available to an individual is reduction or prevention of excess body fat.

Strength

A third important component of health-related fitness is muscular strength. Strength usually is defined as the relative capacity of a muscle or muscle group for exerting force against some external resistance. The importance of strength to high level performance in sport activities is rather obvious to most persons. Everything else being equal, higher levels of strength usually enable the possessor to jump higher, throw farther, push harder, and resist the efforts of an opponent to a greater degree. The importance of strength in general health is perhaps less readily apparent. However, stronger muscles better protect the joints which they cross. As a result, the individual is less susceptible to strains, sprains, and pulls that sometimes occur when participating in physical activity. In addition, better tone in the muscles of the trunk helps to prevent some of the more common postural problems that plague us (e.g., sagging abdominal organs, round shoulders, low back pain, etc.).

In addition to such protection, those possessing optimal levels of strength development are likely to derive more satisfaction from recreational sports participation. They should be more successful in the execution of sport skills and less susceptible to fatigue. Because of this success, they are more likely to engage in recreational sport activities and derive the major benefits of cardiovascular conditioning, weight control, and tension relief.

Flexibility

The fourth important component of health-related fitness is flexibility. In the physical education and sport context, flexibility refers to the degree to which a joint may move through its maximal possible normal range of motion. The determining factor in joint range of motion is the extensibility of the associated connective tissue in and around the joint (tendons and ligaments). Any restriction in the normal extensibility of a joint's connective tissue defines a flexibility problem. From a health standpoint, loss of joint flexibility often contributes to postural difficulties. These usually result from the adaptive shortening of connective tissue on one side of a joint concurrent with a loss of tone in the muscles on the opposite side of the joint. Examples are: (1) the condition of round shoulders in which shortened tendons and ligaments in the upper chest area allow the associated muscles to draw the shoulders forward; and (2) the common adult inability to bend forward and touch the toes with the hands while keeping the knees fully extended. A primary cause of the latter problem is adaptive shortening of the connective tissue in the lower back and posterior thigh areas.

In the lower back as well as in certain other areas of the body, a dense connective tissue known as fascia has the function of reinforcement of active muscle contraction. This holding action of connective tissue "spells off" the antigravity muscles of the back and serves as an energy-conserving mechanism. When the antigravity muscles fatigue, and their burden is borne completely by the heavy connective tissue of the back, the fascia may become adapted to the stress of bearing the weight. A body position that is sustained, as in an increased lower back curve, often results in shortening of these tissues. Once adaptive shortening has occurred, the need for flexibility becomes evident.

Loss of flexibility in the average individual may result in misalignment of body structures, crowding of internal organs, and/or low back pain. These are all common in the adult population, and recent studies have shown that the most frequent underlying cause is lack of proper exercise. One study of 5000 patients with back pain revealed that only 20 per cent had some underlying organic problem such as damaged vertebrae, ruptured intervertebral discs, or arthritis. The remainder were diagnosed as being caused by either inelastic or weak muscles. The implications for adequate levels of both flexibility and strength in the prevention of back problems are obvious.

Adequate flexibility is also an important factor in the performance of many sport skills—both recreational and at higher competitive levels. If individuals suffer from a loss of flexibility, even very high levels of development in other fitness components such as strength and endurance may be of decreased benefit. If there is decreased range of motion in a joint, a person will be less effective in expressing whatever strength quality is present within the muscles acting over that joint. Also, the reduced range of motion may prevent him from observing proper mechanical principles in the execution of a skilled movement, lowering the level of performance. Any resulting misalignment of body segments and/or compensations within other joints can increase the possibility of joint or muscle injury.

OTHER BENEFITS OF EXERCISE AND HAZARDS OF INACTIVITY

Physical Growth and Development

It is important for the adult to be concerned about a well-conditioned body, but perhaps more important is the need for physical activity in the growth process of children. Vigorous physical activity is essential in order that the child's physical potential may be realized. Available evidence suggests that a childhood devoted to heavy muscular activity tends to accentuate lateral growth, i.e., increase in breadth and girth measures, with little noticeable effect on height. Those who lead an active and vigorous childhood have firmer, stronger, and more supple muscles, with sturdier physiques and less adipose tissue than those who are sedentary.

The growth of bone has received extensive study since the middle of the 19th century. One of the earliest and perhaps most important results of these efforts was the formulation of Wolff's law, which states in essence that the internal architecture and the external shape of bones are altered by stresses applied to them. Research on the relationship between pressure and bone growth has shown that slight continuous pressure often causes atrophy. On the other hand, pressures that are intermittent, including those that are just short of causing trauma, appear to stimulate bone growth. In regard to the concept of structure and function as it relates to growth of muscles and bones, it has been postulated that the kinetic stimulus is indispensable for life and that lack of this stimulus results in underdevelopment. Other, more recent reviews have presented considerable evidence favoring physical activity as a means of optimally stimulating bone growth and metabolism.

The contribution of exercise to prevention and correction of body misalignments as a factor in normal growth and development cannot be overemphasized. Marked deviations in body alignment during the growth years may become more pronounced, persist even into adulthood, and become irreversible. Since a child's malleable bones can be malformed in shape and structure in accordance with Wolff's law, proper alignment is essential. It is during childhood that corrective measures must be taken. The value of good posture is important from both physiological and aesthetic viewpoints. Aesthetic standards of posture demand an upright, alert, active-looking appearance. Because posture is often the result of mental state, a well-conditioned body does not always assure desirable alignment. When individuals' attitudes are optimistic and they are well, an erect posture is usually evident. In contrast, when they are depressed, dissatisfied, or ill, the characteristics of poor posture are often seen. Consequently, the solution of postural problems does not depend on exercise alone. Attitude and inherited bone structure impose limitations that exercise alone cannot overcome. However, exercise can serve as a valuable therapeutic adjunct, especially in the relief of chronic fatigue conditions that often contribute to postural difficulties.

Injury Prevention

There are several ways in which conditioning serves to lessen the incidence of injury. Factors involved in the prevention of bodily injury are strength, endurance, flexibility, and skill. The development of an optimal level of these qualities tends to provide a more efficient and skillful function when an injury situation is imminent. In an extensive study dealing with head and neck injuries received in high school football, it was reported that fewer injuries occurred where schools had longer preseason conditioning programs. Most of the reports of contact injuries during sports participation tend to show that the ankle, knee, and shoulder joints are the most frequent sites for injuries causing disablement and loss of participation time. Strengthening of the muscles that support these joints is one way that increased stability can be attained. In addition, optimal levels of muscular endurance provide the ability to sustain activity for a longer period, thereby delaying the onset of fatigue. In a fatigued state individuals are more susceptible to injury because they are apt to react more slowly and less vigorously in situations in which injury might occur than would be the case if fatigue were not present. Improved endurance will reduce the number of instances in which individuals must participate in exercise while in an overly fatigued state. Furthermore, the stronger the ligaments and tendons, the greater will be joint stability. Recent scientific studies indicate that habitual exercise is sufficient to cause a significant increase in the strength of ligaments and tendons surrounding and protecting various joints in the body.

Increased flexibility plays a part in the prevention of injury by allowing a greater range of motion before stretching or tearing of muscle and connective tissue occurs.

Improved skill of movement is also an adjunct to the avoidance of injury. In hazardous situations, it appears likely that the more skilled individual would be less accident-prone. Thus, the development of skill through muscular activity not only is important for the performance of the physical activity, but also provides other benefits, less obvious, perhaps, than those directly related to the activity being performed.

Another injury preventing outcome of muscular activity, especially in males, is hypertrophy, or increased girth of muscle. In some vulnerable areas of the body, this thickened tissue may serve as a form of padding and thereby offer a deterrent to traumatic injury to underlying structures. One who is well-muscled thus has the advantage of being less susceptible to injury in contact sports. Of particular importance is the need for muscular development of the trunk and upper limbs. In almost all reports concerning the incidence of injury in sports, a plea is made for emphasis on the development of the upper body. It should be noted here that increase in size and toughness of muscle tissue is *not a significant factor in females* because the male sex hormone, testosterone, is a major factor in hypertrophy of muscle. Females normally possess low levels of this hormone, and their muscles, therefore, will not hypertrophy to the extent of those of the male. Physical training *will* aid the female in developing significantly higher strength levels, and this will help to protect her body segments from injury. She need have no fear, however, that she will develop large, bulky muscles that detract from her "aesthetic" appearance.

Tension Relief and Mental Well-being

One of the significant problems facing the individual in today's society is mental and emotional stress and the associated anxiety that it often produces (see Chapter 7). The adverse mental states often associated with anxiety are usually referred to as tension. Many persons use physical activity as a means of release from tension. Emotions are best dissipated in the form of diversionary activity. Sports and other forms of exercise supply outlets for the expression of emotions, and it has been claimed by mental hygienists that the outward expression of emotion in approved activities tends to provide a release from strain and to promote mental health.

There are several ways in which exercise can offer emotional outlets. These include providing opportunities for creative expression, development of self-confidence, and achievement. Furthermore, physical activity as a form of diversion in which the participant becomes "lost" in the activity can supply tension-releasing intervals for many individuals. Those who have experienced a mild state of physical fatigue after a pleasant, vigorous bout of exercise can attest to the benefits of "natural" relaxation during and after the ensuing recovery period. Too often, this value of exercise is overlooked.

The principle of mind–body unity is a sound one, and there is a close relationship between organic health and adequate adjustment. To the extent that it can be demonstrated that exercise and sports contribute positively to the attainment and maintenance of organic health, it may be concluded that they also will help prevent poor mental health.

EXERCISE AND PROPER NUTRITION AS A LIFETIME GOAL

Although definite benefits will accrue to the person who begins a rational exercise and nutrition program at any age, optimal benefits will be derived by those who engage in regular, vigorous physical activity with controlled dietary practices at an early age, and who continue to do so throughout their lifetime. The generalized curve of the relationship between age and most biological functions is approximately as shown in Figure 1–4. In general, there is an increase in function from infancy through childhood and adolescence into the young adult years, where a plateau is noticeable for several years. Thereafter, the functions gradually decline into old age. A major concern is accelerating the rising part of the curve for most functions during childhood and adolescence, thereby reaching a higher plateau of function for the young adult years, and decelerating the rate of decrease usually seen in function throughout the later adult years. Proper exercise and nutritional practices can be a definite aid in the achievement of this goal.

In terms of cardiovascular function, the childhood years are especially important.

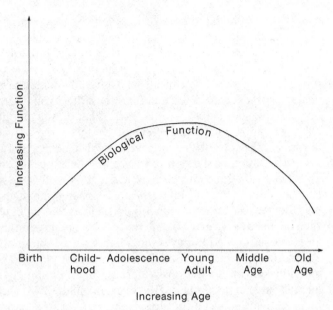

Figure 1–4. Generalized Biological Function Curve in Relation to Age. Most biological functions show an increase through the growth years, a plateau in young adulthood, and a gradual decline as aging progresses. For a look at aging curves for specific organs and functions, see Shock, N. W.: The Physiology of Aging. Sci. Am. *206*:100, 1962.

Although the ultimate level to which the function of the cardiovascular system may be developed is largely hereditary, endurance exercise during the growth and development years will enhance whatever hereditary potential an individual may possess. The most effective type of training in terms of retention of the effects by the organism is that which is carried out over a number of years. Those who exercise regularly during the growth years reach young adulthood already in a trained state, and therefore their bodies may need little, if any, "remedial" work to bring them to an optimal state of function. Also, the body is more "trainable" at younger, as opposed to older, age levels. In other words, a given amount and type of exercise is more likely to effect changes in bodily functions, and to a greater degree, when applied at young ages rather than at later stages in life (see Chapter 5, Fig. 5–23). Furthermore, there is evidence to indicate that if individuals are ever to achieve their ultimate physical potential, some training must occur before full growth and development have been reached. This is probably an obvious concept in the case of the potential champion athlete, but it is also a very important consideration in regard to those who inherit the potential for an average or below-average cardiovascular function. These latter are already functioning under a biological disadvantage, and any further limitations placed on their ultimate physiological development can be very damaging to their adult physical fitness levels.

A person's I.Q. (Intelligence Quotient) and ultimate mental development is an analogous type of situation. Some are born with a brain that makes them "basically bright" whereas others, less fortunate, have a brain that makes them "basically dull." Most of us are somewhere in between the two extremes. However, regardless of our potential position on the continuum of mental capacity, where we eventually end up is strongly influenced by environmental factors. These include, among other things, whether we have parents who place a high value on learning, whether learning is encouraged from an early age, whether materials to enhance learning are available in the home, the quality of elementary and secondary school experiences, the college or university we attend, and our friends, relatives, and acquaintances. Similar factors are operative in regard to biological development. The growth and development years are thus a very critical time for physical, as well as mental and emotional, development.

Once the individual has reached adulthood, the problem shifts from one of development to one of maintenance, or to redevelopment if original function has been lost. The goal thus should be to maintain physical fitness functions as close to the person's best young adult levels as possible. This is not as difficult to accomplish as many might assume. It can be achieved through regular, *moderate* exercise. It is quite common for *nonathletes* 50 to 70 years of age who have maintained a regular exercise regimen over the years to possess cardiovascular function equal to or greater than that of the average 18- to 30-year-old (see Chapter 5, Fig. 5–4). What these individuals have done through regular exercise is to reduce the effect of aging on the cardiovascular system. They have decreased the rate of decline in the right-hand portion of the curve in Figure 1–4.

In body composition, too, we see the same type of critical age relationship emerging. Here, instead of one curve, there are two—one for body fat percentage and another for lean body mass. For the latter, the curve is similar to that shown in Figure 1–4. Lean body mass increases during childhood and adolescence, levels off in young adulthood, and then declines as we grow older. Body fat percentage exhibits a different pattern. There is an increase during infancy, coinciding with a rapid increase in number and size of fat cells. After the first year of life, the body fat percentage will decrease in the average individual owing to a slower increase in the number of fat cells and a concomitant increase in lean body mass. However, in children who are developing obesity, the body fat percentage may continue to increase as a result of poor dietary practices and/or lack of physical activity.

During the adolescent growth spurt there is another increase in body fat percentage, again coinciding with an increase in the number of fat cells. What happens after this spurt varies between the two sexes. The female shows a gradual increase in body fat percentage throughout her lifetime. In the male there is usually a decrease in fat percentage for a few years and then a gradual increase throughout the adult years, just as in the case of the female (Fig. 1–5). The increase in fat percentage during the adult years in both sexes is a function of increases in fat cell size as well as a decrease in lean body mass. Fat cells do not increase in number after adulthood is reached.

Proper diet and exercise are important at all ages for the control of body fat percentages below critical levels and for the development and maintenance of an optimal lean body mass. However, there are several critical periods when major consideration should be given to body composition. It appears that the only times during a lifetime when fat cells increase in number are the last trimester of pregnancy, the first year of life, and during the adolescent growth spurt. During pregnancy, the mother must make an effort to control her own weight so as not to contribute to an increase in number of fat cells in the

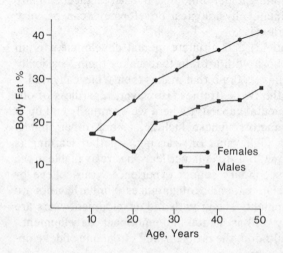

Figure 1–5. Typical Body Fat Percentages in Males and Females from Ages 10 to 50. (Adapted from Rarick, G. L., Montoye, H. J., and Seefeldt, V.: Growth, Development, and Body Composition. *In* H. J. Montoye (ed.) *An Introduction to Measurement in Physical Education,* Vol. 2. Indianapolis, Phi Epsilon Kappa, 1970.)

developing fetus. During the first year of her infant's life, she must exercise control of his diet to avoid the common mistake of developing a fat baby. It is a common misconception that fat babies are healthier than lean babies, but this most assuredly is not true! Fat babies become fat adults! When the adolescent growth spurt begins, parents must be alert to prevent their children from consuming an excess of calories in their food intake, which could lead to a further increase in the number of fat cells.

One reason why it is so important to hold fat cell numbers as low as possible is that obesity that begins in childhood is the most resistant to correction, and occurs primarily as a result of development of a large number of fat cells. Obesity that is due to an increase in size of existing fat cells is corrected much more easily if these cells are at a reasonable number to begin with.

Once children become adults, their exercise and dietary practices should be directed toward preventing the above-noted increase in the size of fat cells, and exercise can be used specifically to counteract the general decrease that occurs in lean body mass with aging. Between ages 25 and 70, males and females lose lean body mass at the rate of about 0.30 and 0.20 kg/year, respectively. Just what accounts for the decrease is not yet known, but it is a fact of life. However, research has shown that vigorous physical activity may counteract most, if not all, of the normal decline in lean body mass with aging.

Improved cardiovascular function and more optimal body composition are but two benefits to be derived from a lifetime emphasis on vigorous exercise and dietary control as part of a person's lifestyle. The whole area of aging has many implications. Aging is characterized by a reduction in the ability to adapt to and recover from physiological and psychological stress. Regular exercise improves the body's ability to counteract those stresses. It seems possible, then, that some degenerative changes in various organs and systems of the body that previously were attributed to aging may, in fact, be the result of a reduction in certain physiological functions such as circulatory supply. This may be more a reflection of sedentary living than an effect of aging per se.

This text is aimed primarily at identifying and illuminating the potential hazards of sedentary living. Further, it goes into some detail in discussing lifestyle practices that can be used by the individual to counteract sedentary living habits and/or their effects. Also, procedures for optimizing these lifestyle practices are covered. In the remaining sections of the text, one full chapter is devoted to detailed discussion of each major component of health-related fitness. Another chapter is provided to enhance the student's understanding of basic human biology. There is also a chapter specifically identifying each of the major cardiovascular disease risk factors and indicating the magnitude of risk associated with each. Finally, an important chapter illuminates some of the known psychological aspects of exercise participation. Appropriate supplementary materials for each chapter are provided in the appendix. There is also a glossary in which many words that may prove unfamiliar to the student are defined. The student is encouraged to supplement the glossary with a good general dictionary and/or medical dictionary. An important feature of the text is the listing of learning objectives at the end of each chapter. The authors have attempted to structure the major knowledge to be gained from each chapter into these objectives. Properly used, they should prove a valuable learning aid for the student.

LEARNING OBJECTIVES

After completing a study of Chapter 1, students should be able to:

1. Define hypokinetic disease and identify several such diseases prevalent in our society.

2. Distinguish between health-related and performance-related fitness.

3. Identify the basic components of health-related fitness.

4. Explain why many athletes such as football and baseball players may be fit for participation in their sport, but may score low on components of health-related fitness.

5. Define cardiovascular function as a component of health-related fitness and explain why it is important.

6. Explain why cardiovascular disease is described by many physicians as a "pediatric problem."

7. Define body composition and explain its importance as a component of fitness.

8. Define atherosclerosis and explain why obesity may be a contributing factor in its development.

9. Demonstrate a knowledge of the magnitude of the obesity problem in the U.S. by citing statistics on the incidence of obesity and the degree to which it increases the risk of heart disease.

10. Define strength and explain its relationship to optimal health.

11. Define flexibility and explain its importance to the general health of the individual.

12. Demonstrate a knowledge of the manner in which physical conditioning may aid in injury prevention.

13. Explain why regular vigorous physical activity may be beneficial to mental health.

14. Demonstrate a knowlege of the general shape of biological function curves in relation to age. Explain what effect regular vigorous exercise may have on the level of the curve at various ages.

15. Identify the most critical periods in a person's life span for the development of increased numbers of fat cells.

16. Explain what general steps may be taken at various ages to prevent development of obesity.

17. Explain the general trends in percentage lean body mass and percentage fat as one ages. Indicate how regular vigorous physical activity may affect those trends.

18. Demonstrate a knowledge of the cardiovascular disease mortality rate of the U.S. compared with that of other countries.

19. Demonstrate a knowledge of the effect that regular vigorous physical activity appears to have on the incidence of cardiovascular disease.

20. Explain in what way(s) regular physical activity may affect growth and development.

REFERENCES

1. Allsen, P. E., Harrison, J. M., and Vance, B.: *Fitness for Life: An Individualized Approach*. Dubuque, Iowa, Wm. C. Brown Co., 1976.
2. Banister, E. W., and Brown, S. R.: The Relative Energy Requirements of Physical Activity. *In* H. B. Falls (ed.) *Exercise Physiology*. New York, Academic Press, 1968.
3. Booth, F. W., and Gould, E. W.: Effects of Training and Disuse on Connective Tissue. *In* J. H. Wilmore, and J. F. Keogh (eds.) *Exercise and Sport Science Reviews, Vol 3*. New York, Academic Press, 1975.
4. Cooper, K. H., Pollock, M. L., Martin, R. P., White, S. R., Linnerud, A. C., and Jackson, A.: Physical fitness levels vs. selected coronary risk factors: a cross-sectional study. J.A.M.A. *236*:166, 1976.
5. Dempsey, J. A.: Relationship between obesity and treadmill performance in sedentary and active young men. Res. Q. Am. Assoc. Health Phys. Educ. *35*:288, 1964.
6. Falls, H. B., Wallis, E. L., and Logan, G. A.: *Foundations of Conditioning*. New York, Academic Press, 1970.
7. Forbes, G. B.: The adult decline in lean body mass. Hum. Biol. *48*:161, 1976.

8. Frank, C. W., Weinblatt, E., Shapiro, S., and Sager, R. V.: Myocardial infarction in men: role of physical activity and smoking in incidence and mortality. J.A.M.A. *198*:1241, 1966.
9. Gilliam, J. B., Katch, V. L., Thorland, W., and Weltman, A.: Prevalence of coronary heart disease risk factors in active children, 7 to 12 years of age. Med. Sci. Sports *9*:21, 1977.
10. Hanson, D. L.: Cardiac response to participation in Little League baseball competition as determined by telemetry. Res. Q. Am. Assoc. Health Phys. Educ. *38*:384, 1967.
11. Hartung, G. H.: Physical activity and coronary heart disease risk—a review. Am. Correct. Ther. J. *31*:110, 1977.
12. Hockey, R. V.: *Physical Fitness: The Pathway to Healthful Living*. St. Louis, C. V. Mosby Co., 1977.
13. Katch, F. I., and McArdle, W. D.: *Nutrition, Weight Control, and Exercise*. Boston, Houghton Mifflin Co., 1977.
14. Knipping, H. W., and Valentin, H.: Sports in Medicine. *In* S. Licht (ed.) *Therapeutic Exercise*. New Haven, Conn., Elizabeth Licht, 1961.
15. Kollias, J., Buskirk, E. R., Howley, E. T., and Loomis, J. L.: Cardio-respiratory and body composition measurements of a select group of high school football players. Res. Q. Am. Assoc. Health Phys. Educ. *43*:472, 1972.
16. Kraus, H., and Raab, W.: *Hypokinetic Disease*. Springfield, Ill., Charles C Thomas, 1961.
17. Lamb, D. R.: Influence of Exercise on Bone Growth and Metabolism. *In Kinesiology Review 1968*. Washington, D.C., American Alliance for Health, Physical Education, and Recreation, 1968.
18. Larson, R. L.: Physical Activity and the Growth and Development of Bone and Joint Structures. *In* G. L. Rarick (ed.) *Physical Activity: Human Growth and Development*. New York, Academic Press, 1973.
19. Layman, E. M.: Contributions of Exercise and Sports to Mental Health and Social Adjustment. *In* W. R. Johnson, and E. R. Buskirk (eds.) *Science and Medicine of Exercise and Sports*. New York, Harper and Row, 1974.
20. Mainland, D.: *Anatomy as a Basis for Medical and Dental Practice*. New York, Harper and Row, 1945.
21. Mayer, J.: *Overweight: Causes, Cost, and Control*. Englewood Cliffs, N.J., Prentice-Hall, 1968.
22. Novak, L. P., Hyatt, R. E., and Alexander, J. F.: Body composition and physiologic function of athletes. J.A.M.A. *205*:764, 1968.
23. Rarick, G. L.: Human Growth and Development. *In* H. J. Montoye (ed.) *An Introduction to Measurement in Physical Education*. Indianapolis, Phi Epsilon Kappa, 1970.
24. Rarick, G. L. (ed.): *Physical Activity: Human Growth and Development*. New York, Academic Press, 1973.
25. Rarick, G. L.: Exercise and Growth. *In* W. R. Johnson, and E. R. Buskirk (eds.) *Science and Medicine of Exercise and Sports*. New York, Harper and Row, 1974.
26. Skinner, J. S.: Age and Performance. *In* J. Keul (ed.) *Limiting Factors of Physical Performance*. Stuttgart, Germany, Georg Thieme, 1973.
27. Steindler, A.: *Kinesiology of the Human Body*. Springfield, Ill., Charles C Thomas, 1955.
28. Williams, G., III: Your aching back. Family Health *9(3)*:26, 1977.
29. Wilmore, J. H., and Haskell, W. L.: Body composition and endurance capacity of professional football players. J. Appl. Physiol. *33*:564, 1972.
30. Wilmore, J. H., and McNamara, J. J.: Prevalence of coronary heart disease risk factors in boys, 8 to 12 years of age. J. Pediatr. *84*:527, 1974.

Chapter 2

Body Chemistry: The Biology of Human Physical Activity

INTRODUCTION

Anatomy is the science of the structure of animals and plants; physiology is the science dealing with the functions of these organisms or their integral parts. In order to fully understand the concepts of physical fitness outlined in this text, or any other text for that matter, it is desirable that the student have a basic understanding of those aspects of human anatomy and physiology that are most important to physical fitness. Exercise, both acute and chronic, has the potential to alter body structures and functions. Basic knowledge in regard to human anatomy and physiology should accelerate and reinforce comprehension of the components of physical fitness and other exercise-related topics.

The purpose of this chapter is to present briefly some very basic general and specific details of human anatomy and physiology. Emphasis is only on those structures and functions that are most important to human movement in general, and strength, flexibility, cardiovascular fitness, and body composition in particular. Even then, only the most basic anatomy and physiology is covered—just enough to give the student some working knowledge. The student who previously has had good course work (or other study forms) in biology, personal health, and/or physical education should find much of the material in the chapter quite familiar, supplying a basic review. For the student who has not engaged in previous study of these topics, the chapter should provide a base on which to build additional and stronger knowledge in regard to fitness.

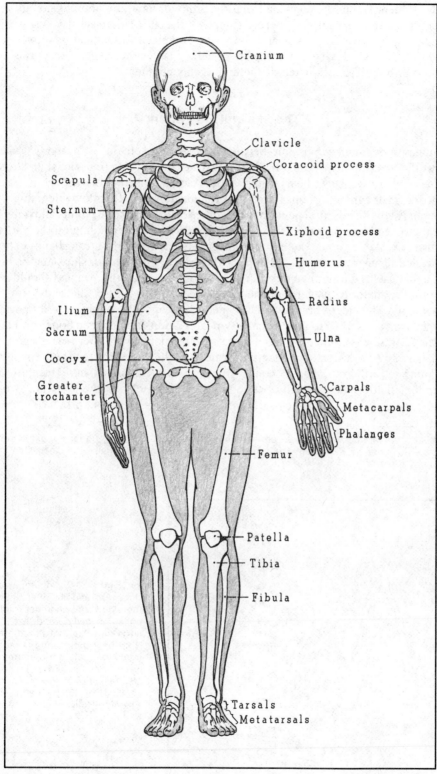

Figure 2–1. The Skeletal System of the Human Body—Anterior View. Major bones are identified. (From Jacob, S. W., Francone, C. A., and Lossow, W. J.: *Structure and Function in Man,* 4th ed. Philadelphia, W. B. Saunders Co., 1978, p. 93.)

The student should be cognizant that the study of anatomy and physiology in this chapter is not an end in itself, but merely a means to the end of increased knowledge about human physical fitness and physical activity. It by no means offers an in-depth coverage of the topic. If more detailed or complete coverage is desired or necessary, the reader should note the references listed at the end of this chapter.

The Skeletal Framework

Human movement is possible because of the arrangement of the body's skeletal framework into segments (Fig. 2–1). The soft tissues of the body (muscle, skin, stomach, intestines, blood vessels, heart, lungs, etc.) are supported on the bony skeletal framework. The segments of this framework (hands, forearm, foot, lower leg, thigh, etc.) are coupled at their ends by articulatory processes called joints. The joints allow the bony segments to bend and turn in various directions and ways, depending on the particular joint structure. At the joints, bones are connected to each other by strong bands of fibrous tissue called ligaments. Figure 2–2 depicts the typical interrelationships among bones, joints, and muscles within the body. The illustration presents the arm and shoulder area of the human anatomy. Several of the large bones in this part of the body are shown schematically. The biceps brachii and brachialis, large muscles on the anterior portion of the upper arm, are shown to illustrate the typical relationship between bones, joints, and muscles. A muscle is connected either directly to the bone by its fibers (upper portion of brachialis) or by extension of connective tissue from the fibers (the tendon). The tendons cross joints and attach to adjacent bones. One of the muscles shown here (biceps brachii) has tendons that cross two joints. Although several muscles in the body are two-joint muscles, usually a muscle crosses only one joint. When the muscle contracts (shortens),*

---

*This occurs in what is known as an isotonic concentric contraction. Under certain conditions, the muscle does not shorten (isometric and eccentric contractions). See also the discussion of contraction in Chapter 4.

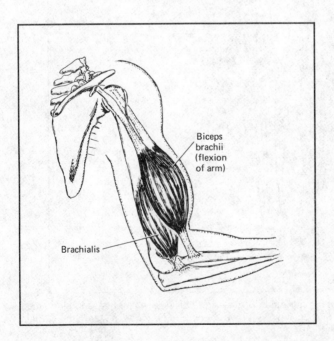

Biceps
brachii
(flexion
of arm)

Brachialis

Figure 2–2. Anatomy of the Upper Arm and Shoulder. Shown are the elbow and shoulder joints, the bones involved, and two of the large muscles that flex the elbow. Note how their tendons cross the joints to create a force arm for the lever systems. (From Easton, D.: *Mechanisms of Body Functions.* © 1963, p. 46. By permission of Prentice-Hall, Englewood Cliffs, N. J.)

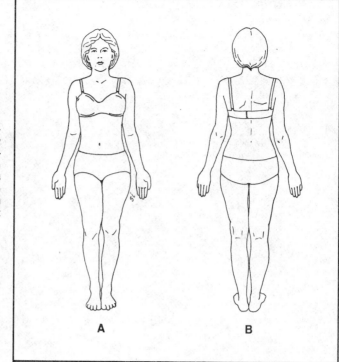

Figure 2-3. The Anatomical Position: anterior view *(a)*; posterior view *(b)*. All movements are described in relation to this position; therefore, it is important to remember it. Note that the thumbs are away from the body, with the head and feet pointing straight forward.

A   B

pull is applied to the adjacent bone through the tendon. This causes the bone to rotate around its pivotal point at the joint. Thus, a body segment moves.

Basic Movements

The position illustrated in Figure 2-3 is known as *anatomical position* and is important to an understanding of movements, all of which are described as beginning from and returning to this position. Although most everyday movements are really combinations of basic movements occurring in many body segments at once, it is possible to understand movement by looking at the movement of each body part at each joint. Movements in the sagittal or anteroposterior plane are flexion and extension (Fig. 2-4). *Flexion* is a movement in which the joint angle becomes smaller, usually where the body part is moving toward the front. An exception to the latter rule of thumb is flexion of the lower leg at the knee. Examples of flexion are tilting the head forward; curling the fingers, hand, or forearm; moving the trunk forward, the lower leg backward, the upper leg forward, etc. *Extension* is the return movement from flexion back to anatomical position. In most extension movements, the body part is moving toward the back of the body, except in extension of the lower leg. Extension-type movements beyond the point of anatomical position, or which are not preceded by flexion, are called *hyperextension*. Movements similar to flexion and extension in the side plane are abduction and adduction (Fig. 2-4). Abduction is analogous to flexion and is a movement away from the midline of the body, such as moving the arms to the side or spreading the feet shoulder width apart. *Adduction* is the return movement from abduction back toward the midline to anatomical position.

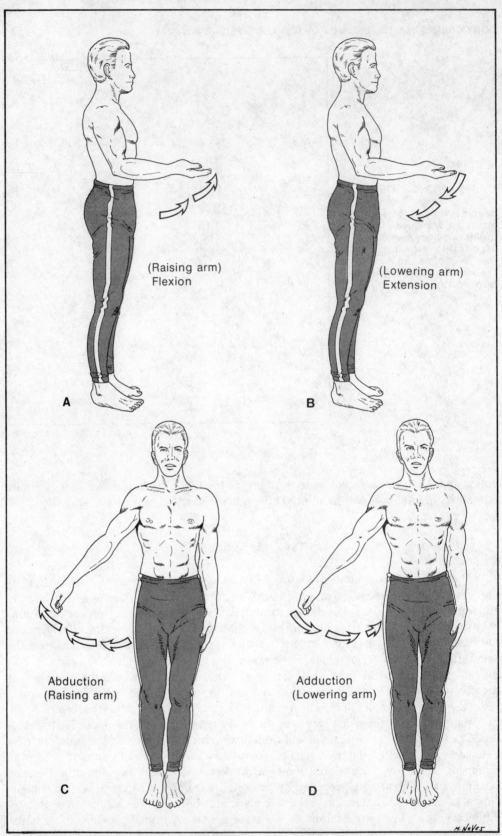

Figure 2–4. Basic Movements. *A, Flexion* of the forearm at the elbow involves a movement away from the anatomical position in which the joint angle becomes smaller. *B, Extension* involves the return movement from flexion. *C, Abduction* is a movement away from the anatomical position in the side plane. D, *Adduction* is the return movement back toward the anatomical position.

THE MUSCLES

Types of Muscle Action

All muscles function by developing or releasing tension. However, the same muscle may vary from time to time in its specific role, depending on the type of action desired in various body segments. There are four basic roles that a muscle or muscle group may perform. The specific role depends on the requirements of the situation: (1) the muscle or muscles most directly responsible for executing the desired movement are called *agonists, movers,* or *muscles most involved;* (2) the muscles located on the opposite side of the joint or body part from the movers or agonists are responsible for the opposite joint action, and are called *antagonist* muscles; (3) muscles that are located on either side of the muscles most involved and help to eliminate unwanted extraneous movements are known as *guiding muscles, neutralizers,* or *synergists;* (4) muscles that fixate or hold a joint or a body part so that other joints or body parts can move are known as *fixators* or *stabilizing* muscles.

One of the basic principles governing muscle activity in the above is that of *reciprocal innervation.* This is a *hard-wired neural circuit* intended automatically to relax the antagonist muscle as the agonist muscle is commanded to contract. This circuit minimizes the co-contraction of agonist and antagonist muscle groups. It is best illustrated with an example involving agonist and antagonist muscles. In Figure 2–2, the pictured muscles would be classified as agonist muscles for the movement shown (elbow flexion). The triceps brachii, which is located on the posterior upper arm, is the antagonist muscle during the movement. In elbow extension against resistance (opposite movement to flexion), the triceps brachii would become the agonist, and the biceps brachii and brachialis the antagonist muscles. When the biceps brachii and brachialis are stimulated to contract during elbow flexion, the triceps brachii is reciprocally innervated to relax. If elbow extension were involved, the triceps brachii would be stimulated to contract, and the biceps brachii and brachialis would be reciprocally innervated to relax. Reciprocal innervation basically means that, when a stimulus for contraction is sent to a muscle or muscle group, relaxation is sent to the antagonist muscle. The neural mechanism involved will be discussed later in this chapter.

The Antigravity Musculature

The muscles shown in Figure 2–5b are classified as the anteroposterior antigravity muscles. This subgrouping contains most of the large muscles in the body. They are important to each of the basic components of physical fitness. Their strength and flexibility determines to a great extent whether proper alignment is maintained in the anatomical structures of the trunk and hip. During vigorous exercise, they are used quite constantly and forcefully. Therefore, they help to determine a large portion of our energy (oxygen consumption) needs, and their leanness has a great deal to do with our basic body composition. These muscles must not be ignored in any fitness program.

The antigravity musculature is of major importance because our muscles must be such that we can resist adequately the pull of gravity to maintain an erect posture. Since the skeletal framework of the body has a tendency to collapse with the force of gravity (Fig. 2–5a), a great deal of energy is spent throughout the day in combating that force through the use of muscles that maintain an upright posture. In other words, we are almost constantly making an effort to extend the body. Those muscles that maintain

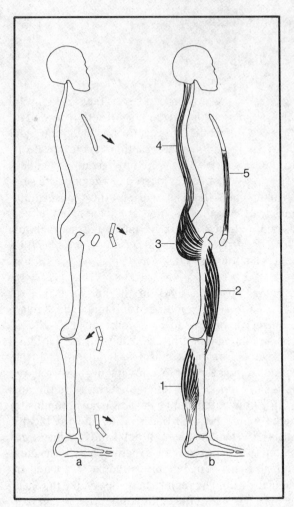

Figure 2–5. Anteroposterior Antigravity Musculature of the Body. *(a),* Force of gravity results in a tendency for the skeleton to collapse at points shown by arrows. *(b),* Antigravity muscle groups resist the effect of gravity and help hold the body in upright posture. The muscle groups are: *(1)* Triceps surae; *(2)* Quadriceps femoris; *(3)* Gluteus maximus; *(4)* Erector spinae; and *(5)* Abdominals. (From Wallis, E. L., and Logan, G. A.: *Figure Improvement and Body Conditioning through Exercise.* © 1964, p. 11. By permission of Prentice-Hall, Englewood Cliffs, N. J.)

extension, the antigravity muscles, tend to become fatigued from constant activity as one reaches the end of the day. If these muscles are not well-conditioned, they are not equipped to withstand for many hours the stresses imposed on them by gravity.

The downward pressure of gravity applied to the bones of the skeleton tends to cause it to buckle at three principal points: the ankle, knee, and hip. Since the weight of the body is largely in front of the spinal column, the body tends to fall forward. In order to counteract these tendencies toward buckling, a minimum of five muscles or muscle groups must be activated. The muscles involved in the lower limb are the soleus and gastrocnemius (triceps surae) at the ankle, the quadriceps femoris at the knee, and the gluteus maximus at the hip. The trunk is held upright by the erector spinae muscles running from the sacrum to the base of the skull. If these muscles should pull equally from both ends, the trunk would tend to move backward. Therefore, a fifth muscle group, the abdominals, serves as reflex antigravity muscles by maintaining the proper relationship between the rib cage and pelvis in the front. Exercises for these antigravity muscles are fundamental to any general conditioning exercise program. In fact, the design of any well-rounded exercise program might well begin with a consideration of this minimally essential musculature.

The Contractile Process in Muscle

An English physiologist, H. E. Huxley, and his co-workers have been mainly responsible for developing the currently prevailing theory of muscle contraction. Their experiments, which led to what is described as the "sliding filament" model of muscle contraction, are considered classics in the field of muscle physiology.

Micrographs made with the aid of the very powerful electron microscope show what appear to be tiny filaments within each muscle fiber. During contraction, the filaments appear to slide past each other in opposite directions. Figure 2–6 is a schematic representation of the manner in which the filaments are arranged in the intact muscle. Figure 2–6e and f shows the basic unit of contraction, the sarcomere. In f the sarcomere is more highly magnified so that the filaments are readily discernible. It can be seen in Figure 2–6d that the sarcomeres are arranged in series along the entire length of the fiber. Figure 2–7 schematically demonstrates the behavior of a single sarcomere during contraction. Shortening of the sarcomeres occurs along the entire length of the fiber, thereby also shortening the fiber itself. The shortening of several fibers simultaneously causes the muscle to contract, and results in a joint movement, as illustrated in Figure 2–2.

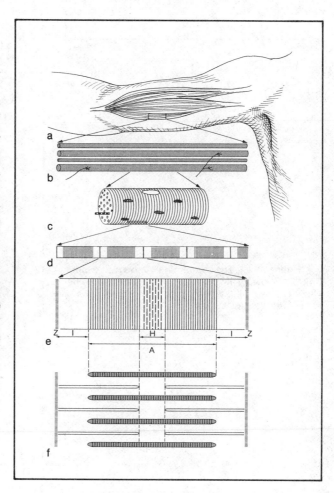

Figure 2–6. Skeletal Muscle is Dissected in these Schematic Drawings. A muscle (a) is made up of muscle fibers (b) which appear striated in the light microscope. The small branching structures at the surface of the fibers are the "endplates" of motor nerves which signal the fibers to contract. A single muscle fiber (c) is made up of myofibrils. In a single myofibril (d) the striations are resolved into a repeating pattern of light and dark bands. A single unit of this pattern (e) consists of a "Z-line," then an "I-band," then an "A-band" which is interrupted by an "H-zone," then the next "I-band," and finally the next "Z-line." Electron micrographs have shown that the repeating band pattern is due to the overlapping of thick and thin filaments (f) (Adapted from Huxley, H. E.: The Contraction of Muscle. Sci. Am. 199(5):67. Copyright © November 1958 by Scientific American, Inc. All rights reserved.)

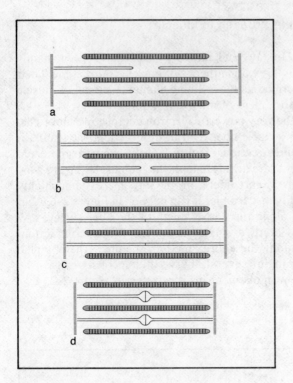

Figure 2–7. Sliding Filament Model of Muscle Contraction. Changes in length of the muscle change the arrangements of the filaments. In *(a)* the muscle is stretched; in *(b)* it is at its resting length; in *(c)* and *(d)* it is contracted. (Adapted from Huxley, H. E.: The Contraction of Muscle. Sci. Am. *199(5)*:67. Copyright © November 1958 by Scientific American, Inc. All rights reserved.)

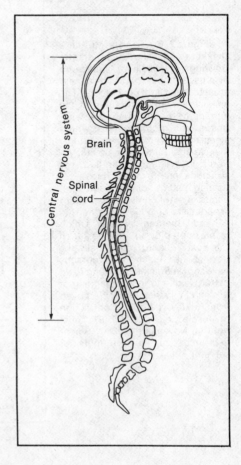

Figure 2–8. The Skull and Vertebral (Spinal) Column, Showing the Brain and Spinal Cord Contained Therein. The brain and spinal cord together make up the central nervous system.

THE NERVOUS SYSTEM—THE CONTROLLER OF MOVEMENT

Muscles receive their commands to contract through the central nervous system (CNS), which consists of the brain and spinal cord housed in the skull and vertebral column, respectively (Fig. 2–8), and through the peripheral nervous system, which includes the cranial and spinal nerves (Fig. 2–9). The peripheral nerves are pathways of sensory information from the various receptors entering the CNS and of motor information going from the CNS to muscles and glands. The basic functional cell in the nervous system is the neuron, of which there are in excess of 10 billion. Neurons, which are specialized in receiving and transmitting neural impulses (messages), are highly specialized in different parts of the nervous system.

The Sensory Neurons

Most neurons receive neural impulses from other neurons on their cell bodies and dendrites, which are branch-like projections of the cell body enlarging the reception area. Impulses from a neuron are transmitted to another neuron or structure over the axon,

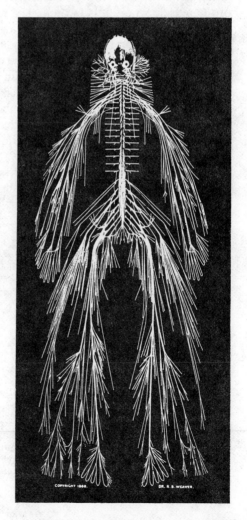

Figure 2–9. Model of the Peripheral Nerves of the Body. Harriet Cole, a scrubwoman at Hahnemann Medical College, willed her body to Anatomy Professor Rufus B. Weaver. The doctor used it for what is probably the only preserved dissection of the human nervous system. The brain was removed, but the spinal cord and peripheral nerves are shown. (From Rasch, P. J., and Burke, R. K.: *Kinesiology and Applied Anatomy.* Philadelphia, Lea and Febiger Co., 1971, p. 101.)

which is a long, cable-like structure, and finally the neuron makes functional contact with the next structure at the synapse. These areas are illustrated for a neuron in Figure 2–10. The motor neuron, a special type that innervates muscle, is an example of this type of neuron; however, the primary sensory neurons located in the body are different. These have a specialized receptor functioning as the *receiving area*, i.e., they change one form of energy into a neural message. The energy may be pressure, stretch, warmth, cold, etc., but the process is the same. The term *somatosensory* refers to sensory information from the body, and the sensory receptors are located in the skin, muscles, tendons, joints, and vestibular structure of the inner ear. Neuroscientists have divided these receptors into two basic categories: (1) cutaneous receptors, of which various types give information about touch-pressure, heat, cold, and pain; and (2) proprioceptors, which specifically give us movement information. The four classes of proprioceptors are muscle spindles, Golgi tendon organs, joint receptors, and the vestibular apparatus.

The muscle spindle is a complex stretch receptor located in muscles. It acts as a fine tuner of muscle force. The receptor has six to eight small intrafusal muscle fibers inside a spindle-shaped capsule connected to regular muscle fibers (Fig. 2–11). Two types of sensory endings which respond to stretch are wrapped around the intrafusal fibers, so that contraction of these intrafusal fibers shortens the length and makes the spindle endings more sensitive. The spindle receptor, as illustrated in Figure 2–12, has a direct reflex connection into the spinal cord which, when stretched, causes a reflex contraction of the muscle where it is located. The nervous system actually stimulates these small intrafusal muscles in the spindle as it causes the muscles to contract. During contraction these spindles compare the length of their shortening intrafusal muscle fibers with that of the contracting muscle fibers. When the contraction is too fast and forceful, the spindles are relaxed and fire less information into the spinal cord, making the contraction less forceful; when the contraction is weak and slow, the spindles fire heavily, causing a reflexive recruitment of more muscle fibers, and thus a more forceful contraction. This process is termed *alpha-gamma coactivation*. The spindle is responsible for a reflexive fine tuning of muscle force and for sending valuable information about muscle stretch into the CNS.

Feedback from the muscle spindle is also part of the neural mechanism for reciprocal innervation discussed earlier in the chapter. As the agonist muscle contracts and spindle

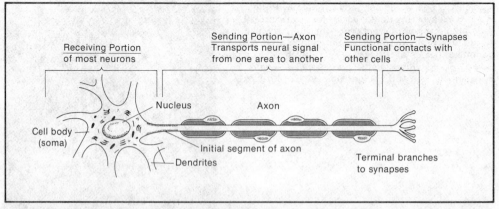

Figure 2–10. Neuron. A neuron has a soma or cell body and dendrites (branch-like enlargements of the cell body) which receive synapses from other neurons. The sending portion consists of the axon, which is a long, cable-like projection that transmits the neural messages from the cell body to another neuron or muscle, and the synapse portion, which consists of all the neuron's functional contacts with other neurons or muscles.

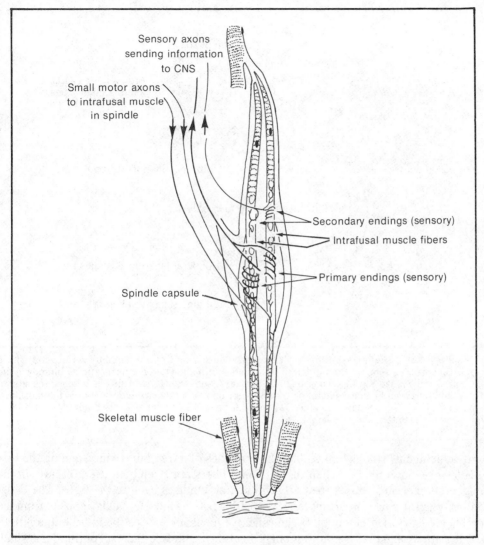

Sensory axons sending information to CNS

Small motor axons to intrafusal muscle in spindle

Secondary endings (sensory)

Intrafusal muscle fibers

Primary endings (sensory)

Spindle capsule

Skeletal muscle fiber

Figure 2–11. Muscle Spindle. Spindles are important stretch receptors located in muscles. A spindle is a small, spindle-shaped capsule containing 6 to 8 small intrafusal muscle fibers which can shorten to make the spindle more sensitive to muscle stretch. Its primary sensory receptor is illustrated as a coil-like wrapping around the center portion. When the spindle is stretched, this ending is displaced and reports the stretch to the central nervous system. To avoid losing spindle feedback in shortening contractions of the muscle, the small intrafusal muscle fibers are coactivated with the extrafusal or large muscle fibers. Thus, as the shortening of the muscle fibers relieves the stretch on the spindle, the spindle is gradually shortening its length to remain sensitive to small amounts of muscle stretch. (Adapted from Gardner, E.: *Fundamentals of Neurology*. Philadelphia, W. B. Saunders Co., 1975.)

feedback comes into the spinal cord, one branch carries information to higher centers, another branch carries excitatory information back to the agonist muscle motor pool, and still another branch synapses with an inhibitory interneuron (Ia) and sends inhibition or relaxation information to the antagonist motor pool. This feedback loop for reciprocal innervation is combined with reciprocally organized voluntary commands from higher brain centers acting on the same (Ia) inhibitory neuron.

Another movement-related receptor is the Golgi tendon organ. This also responds to stretch, but is a less complicated receptor located in tendons between the muscle and

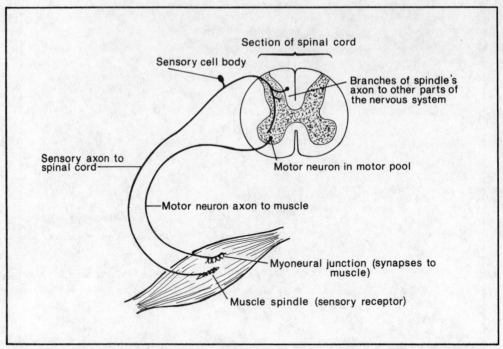

Figure 2-12. A Reflex Arc Showing Complete Sensory and Motor Circuitry Associated with a Muscle Spindle. The sensory axon (afferent) transmits information about muscle stretch directly to the motor pool of the muscle in which it is located. Its reflex feedback to its own muscle is called the stretch or myotatic reflex, and causes excitation of the motor pool and reflexive contraction of the muscle. It is this excitatory feedback loop which allows the muscle spindle to act as a fine tuner of muscle force and aid in the maintenance of posture.

bony attachment. It looks much like the branches of a tree intertwined among the tiny bundles of tendon fibers. When these tendon fibers are stretched, the pressure on the Golgi tendon organs causes them to send neural impulses back to the CNS. The Golgi tendon organ also has important reflexive feedback to its muscle, but is opposite from the spindle feedback. Golgi tendon organ reflexive feedback causes the muscle to contract with less force, and thus is important in protecting the muscle against contractions which are so forceful that they would tend to damage the muscle or its tendon attachment. The Golgi tendon organ also sends important information about the force of the muscle contraction to higher brain centers. Both the muscle spindle and Golgi tendon organ are very important in the proper application of stretching exercises for flexibility development (Chapter 6).

The third classification of proprioceptors consists of the joint receptors, of which there are four different types. Three are specialized to give information about position, pressure, speed, acceleration, and direction of joint movements, and the fourth is believed to report joint pain. These receptors traditionally have been considered a primary source of body position information.

The final class of proprioceptors consists of the vestibular apparatus which, instead of being associated with muscles, joints, or tendons, is housed in the inner ear next to the hearing apparatus. Three different types of vestibular receptors report information about acceleration/deceleration of head movements in all planes and when the head is not aligned properly with gravity. These receptors commonly have been called our balance receptors because they report important information concerning balance to motor areas in the brain, and because they contribute to many balance or righting reflexes.

Sensory information from the various cutaneous and proprioceptive receptors, as well as information from vision, hearing, and smell, is conveyed to brain structures that will receive and interpret these neural messages into information about the environment. From a movement sense, it is important to know the initial body position before the movement can be planned or performed.

The Motor Unit

Voluntary control of movement is caused by neural impulses that originate in the motor centers in the brain and are sent to the spinal cord motor pools for the various muscles, and then on to the specific muscles needed for the movements. Each muscle has a motor pool which is the group of motor neurons controlling the motor units for that particular muscle. Neural impulses sent from the brain and from various reflexes in the spinal cord are collected and integrated on the cell bodies of the motor neurons. These neural messages coming to the motor pool are either excitatory, telling the motor neurons to start firing or to fire more rapidly and in greater numbers, or inhibitory, telling the motor neurons to stop firing or to fire more slowly. Muscle relaxation is the absence of activity in the motor unit, and thus of contraction in the muscle. Muscles contract when more excitatory than inhibitory impulses are collected in the motor pool and are sent to the muscles via the motor units.

Three motor units are illustrated in Figure 2–13. One moter unit consists of the motor neuron plus all the muscle fibers (cells) which are innervated (supplied) by that one neuron. Thus, each motor neuron has its cell body in the motor pool of the spinal cord, with a long neural process (axon) which lies in a nerve with many other axons. These axons carry the contraction message from the motor pools in the spinal cord to the various muscles. At the muscle, each axon branches many times and makes functional

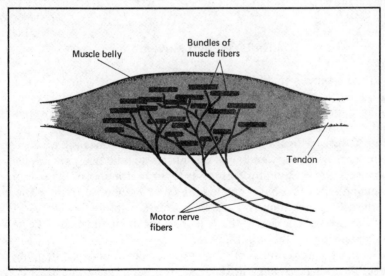

Figure 2–13. Motor Units. This schematic drawing of a muscle shows the distribution of nerve fibers supplying three motor units. One motor neuron and all the muscle fibers connected to it constitute one motor unit, which is the functional unit of muscle contraction. Stronger muscle contractions are made by exciting more motor units in the muscle and by causing those already firing to fire faster. The only time the muscle fibers of a particular unit contract is when their motor neuron sends them a neural message for contraction. The motor unit works on an "all or none principle," i.e., all fibers in the unit contract as a unit. (From Guyton, A. C.: *Function of the Human Body.* Philadelphia, W. B. Saunders Co., 1974, p. 245.)

contacts *(synapses)* with a large number of muscle fibers. Some large powerful muscles have motor units containing a large number of muscle fibers. These muscles are well designed for fast, forceful contractions. Other, smaller muscles with fewer muscle fibers per motor unit are better designed for finely controlled movements. The number of muscle fibers per motor unit is reflected by what is called the *innervation ratio*, i.e., the number of muscle fibers to one neuron. Large innervation ratios occur in muscles of force such as the gastrocnemius (1500 muscle fibers to one motor neuron), whereas small innervation ratios occur in the small muscles of the hand and eye (ten to one), which are designed for finely controlled movements involving little force. Most other muscles, e.g., the biceps brachii (200 to one) in the anterior upper arm, have innervation ratios between these extremes.

In addition to their innervation ratios, muscles also differ in the types of muscle fibers which are contained in motor units. Small motor units (small innervation ratios) usually fire more easily than larger units in the same muscle. Thus, smaller units are used more often than larger units, and their muscle enzyme systems reflect this property. Small units that fire more often are more fatigue-resistant, are better supplied by capillaries (blood) in the muscle, and basically use aerobic or oxygen-dependent energy systems. Larger units are added when the muscle needs more force. These larger units, which are quick to fatigue, have anaerobic energy systems, but add larger increments of force per unit. Muscles appear to have a continuum of motor unit sizes reflected in their primary use, and within each muscle there appears to be a smaller continuum of small to large.

The motor unit is the basic element of contraction and operates on the "all or none" concept. The only time the particular muscle fibers in a motor unit contract is when they receive a neural message from their controlling motor neuron. Thus, in lifting a heavy weight or making a very rapid movement, more muscular force is achieved by sending more neural impulses over more and larger motor units supplying the muscle. For slower movements without weights, fewer motor neurons send fewer impulses, so that fewer muscle fibers contract.

Reflexes and Movement

The two main sources of impulses coming into motor pools, and thus to muscles, are reflex and voluntary activity. Reflexes are hard-wired neural circuits in which a known stimulus will produce a predictable movement. For example, the simplest is the stretch reflex, which can be illustrated by tapping someone on the tendon just below the patella (kneecap), as shown in Figure 2–14. This tendon tap stretches the quadriceps femoris muscle group, and the primary ending of the muscle spindle, which is a sensitive stretch receptor in muscle, sends excitatory impulses to the motor pool of the stretched muscle. Another common reflex that has a much more complex neural circuit is the withdrawal reflex, i.e., the reflexive withdrawal of a limb from a painful stimulus. As illustrated in Figure 2–15, this involves flexion of the body part receiving the pain—the *flexion reflex*, and usually extension of the contralateral limb—the *crossed extension reflex*. The importance of this reflex is apparent when you consider someone stepping on a sharp object. The leg receiving the pain is flexed, and the other leg is extended for body support. Touching a hot stove with the hand will show the same movement pattern in the arms.

These are two obvious examples of a complex set of many reflexes that continually operate in an individual. Although the various reflexes are not always seen in an adult who has learned to voluntarily control many hard-wired reflexes, their effects are present in the motor pools of the muscles. We simply learn to use or inhibit these impulses in our daily movements, but reflexes play an important role in organizing movements.

Figure 2-14. Stretch Reflex or Myotatic Reflex. The stretch reflex to the tendon tap is shown. As the tendon to the quadriceps femoris muscle group is tapped, the tendon is stretched, which in turn stretches the muscle, and some of its muscle spindle receptors are excited. Their sensory axons transport this information directly to the motor pool as shown in the stretched muscle in Figure 2-12. A few motor units in the muscle are excited and send contraction signals to their muscle fibers. A reflex contraction of the stretched muscle results. This reflex may be easily demonstrated on yourself. (Reprinted with permission of Macmillan Publishing Co., Inc., from *The Human Body: Its Structure and Physiology* by Sigmund Grollman. Copyright © 1978 by Sigmund Grollman.)

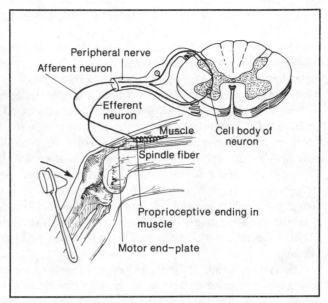

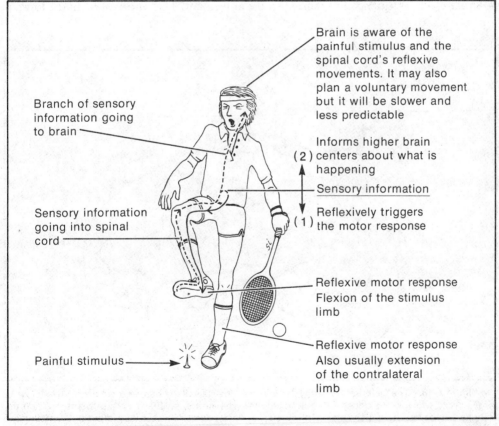

Figure 2-15. Withdrawal Reflex. The withdrawal reflex is a more complex reflex than the stretch reflex and involves a painful stimulus to one of the arms or legs. As the pain information enters the spinal cord, it synapses with appropriate motor pools to get the following reflex actions: *(1)* flexion of the stimulus limb from the painful stimulus, which usually is accompanied by *(2)* crossed extension reflex, i.e., the extension of the contralateral limb not receiving the pain.

Voluntary Movement

The other primary source of input to the motor pools consists of impulses for voluntary movement from higher centers in the brain. Unlike reflexes, voluntary movements are not hard-wired. Sensory information is taken into the brain from the many sensory receptors. This information is perceived and associated with memory, and a movement is planned. Although scientists interested in motor control do not fully understand the way the brain produces the movement commands, they know that three brain structures appear to play key roles in planning, initiating, and controlling movements: the motor cortex; the basal ganglia; and the cerebellum. Figure 2–16 is a close-up view of the cortex, with the motor areas just anterior to the central sulcus and the sensory areas just posterior to it. The motor cells in this area have long axons to the motor pools in the spinal cord, and the sensory areas receive a great deal of information from the somatic senses. The relation of the cortex to the other primary motor areas of the brain is illustrated in Figure 2–17, in which the basal ganglia and cerebellum also are shown.

Evarts, who has studied the brains of alert monkeys during voluntary movement, has given a general summary of the roles of these brain structures in movement. It appears as if the motor cortex formulates an intent to move, which is sent to the cerebellum and/or basal ganglia for additional planning of which muscles are needed to contract in what sequence to accomplish the movement. This information in the form of

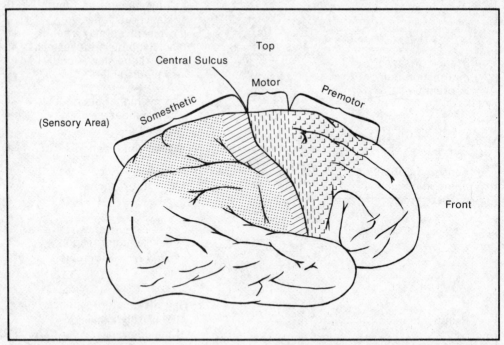

Figure 2–16. The Cerebral Cortex of the Brain. A side view of the human brain is drawn to show its large cortex, which is the upper and outermost part. The central sulcus is a deep fissure dividing the front part of the cortex from the back. The area around the central sulcus is very important to movement because a large part of voluntary movement comes through large pathways (the pyramidal tracts, also called the corticospinal tracts) beginning in the motor areas and ending in the motor pools in the spinal cord. The somesthetic area is the sensory cortex whereby various receptors from the body report sensory information to the brain. (Adapted from Guyton, A. C.: *Textbook of Medical Physiology.* Philadelphia, W. B. Saunders Co., 1966, p. 802.)

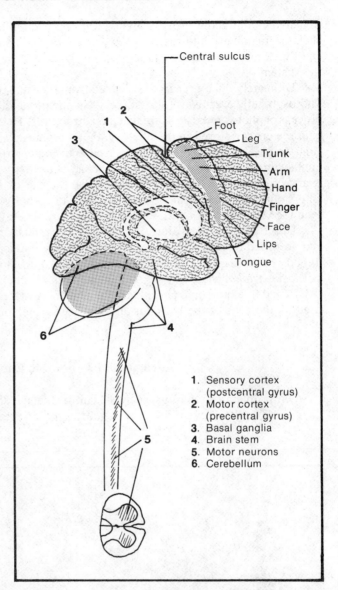

Figure 2–17. Primary Motor Areas of the Brain. In addition to the cortex illustrated in Figure 2–16, the other major motor centers in the brain are shown: the basal ganglia in the midportion and the cerebellum at the base of the brain behind the brain stem. The basal ganglia are several nuclei (groups of cell bodies) which are important to planning and initiating movement. The cerebellum is also important in planning and controlling movement. The motor cortex, basal ganglia, and cerebellum send motor messages to the motor neurons in the motor pools of the spinal cord over nerve tracts that originate in the motor cortex and end in the spinal cord (pyramidal tracts), and over tracts from nuclei in the brain stem areas that also connect to the spinal motor pools (extrapyramidal tracts). (Adapted from Ganong, W. F.: *The Nervous System.* Los Altos, CA, Lange Medical Publications, 1977, p. 163.)

1. Sensory cortex (postcentral gyrus)
2. Motor cortex (precentral gyrus)
3. Basal ganglia
4. Brain stem
5. Motor neurons
6. Cerebellum

neural messages is then sent back through the motor cortex for finishing touches, and on to the appropriate motor pools for the various muscles. The planning, execution, and feedback of complex movements are not at all well understood, but these problems are currently being studied by a number of outstanding neuroscientists and physical educators.

THE MOTOR FOR HUMAN MOVEMENT: ENERGY TRANSFORMATION

Even though the skeletal framework is arranged very effectively to make movement possible, it should be quite obvious that, in order for any movement to occur on that framework, a force must be applied through muscular contraction. To enable the muscle to apply that force, an energy transformation must take place within the individual cells to trigger the contractile process involved in the sliding filament model. In a sense, the skeletal framework and the muscles can be viewed as a mechanical system, and the energy-storing and liberating processes within the muscle cell as the "motor" that drives the system.

Ultimately, all our energy is derived from the sun—radiated to the earth's surface. Photosynthetic organisms (plants) receive some of the radiated energy and, through the process of photosynthesis, store it in their structures. Heterotrophic organisms (animals) gain the energy stored in the photosynthetic organisms by consuming them in the diet (Fig. 2–18). The energy thus is transferred to the body structures of these organisms. The human organism (heterotrophic) has a dietary consumption including both photosynthetic and other heterotrophic organisms. Thus, the energy sent to earth by the sun finally enters our bodies bound in the chemical form of carbohydrates, fats, and proteins in our food (see Chapter 8 for further discussion of the energy value of these foods).

Unfortunately, even after the carbohydrates, fats, and proteins have been digested and absorbed by the cells of the body, the energy that is bound in them cannot be used directly by those cells. It must first be transferred onto another molecular structure called *adenosine triphosphate (ATP)*. ATP is then split chemically into adenosine diphosphate (ADP) and free inorganic phosphate (P). The energy released in that splitting process is used by the cells of the body for all their needs, including muscle contraction.

Aerobic and Anaerobic Energy

One problem with ATP usage by the body is that it is stored in very small quantities in the cells. Therefore, we must be constantly synthesizing it, or our cells would have to

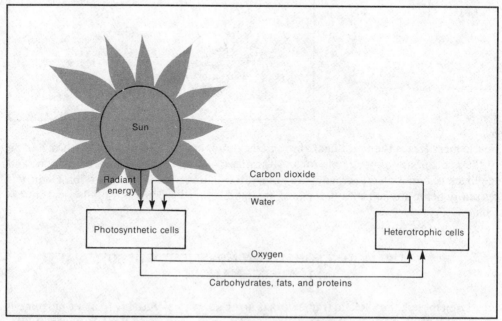

Figure 2–18.   The Cycling of Carbon and Oxygen Through the Plant and Animal Worlds. (Adapted from Lehninger, A. L.: *Bioenergetics: The Molecular Basis of Biological Energy Transformations,* 1971, p. 10, by permission of the Benjamin Cummings Publishing Co., Menlo Park, CA.)

Figure 2–19. The Relative Role of Anaerobic and Aerobic Energy Metabolism in Supplying the Total Energy Needed for Best Effort Runs of Defined Time Intervals. The unshaded area represents the proportion of total energy requirements that must be supplied anaerobically for runs of various duration. (From Balke, B.: A Simple Field Test for the Assessment of Physical Fitness. Oklahoma City, Civil Aeromedical Research Institute, Report 63-6, 1963.)

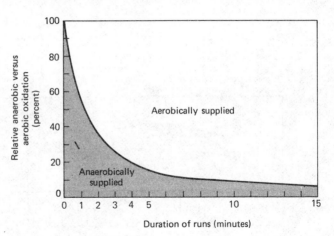

shut down operations. The synthesis is made by rejoining the ADP and P, using the energy bound in the carbohydrates, fats, and proteins. Carbohydrate can provide the energy in two ways:

(1) A small quantity of it is stored in cells in the form of *glycogen*. Under conditions of high energy needs, the glycogen can break down to lactic acid and release energy for ATP synthesis.

(2) It also can be "burned" (oxidized) in combination with oxygen. This process releases large quantities of energy for synthesis of ATP.

The breakdown of glycogen to lactic acid is what is known as *anaerobic* energy release. No oxygen is used in the process. The oxidation of carbohydrate with oxygen is an *aerobic* process.

In contrast to carbohydrate, energy from fats and proteins can be released only by oxidation. *They do not provide an anaerobic source of energy.*

During exercise, the electrical impulse from the nervous system can trigger the breakdown of ATP in the muscle cell, and the secretion of the hormone *epinephrine* from the adrenal glands can cause glycogen to break down to lactic acid, in turn releasing its energy. Both of these provide a powerful anaerobic energy source for use in short bursts of activity, such as sprinting. However, because both ATP and glycogen are in short supply in the muscle, exercise cannot continue at such intensity for very long. Continuous, endurance-type exercise must depend on the supplying of oxygen at a relatively high rate for the oxidation of carbohydrates and fats.* The supply of oxygen at a high level depends on its transport by the circulatory system, primarily the pumping capability of the heart. This serves to emphasize the importance of maximum oxygen consumption in the assessment of functional circulatory capacity (cardiovascular fitness), as discussed in Chapter 5. Figure 2–19 shows graphically the aerobic–anaerobic relationship for best effort runs of various time intervals. It is readily apparent that, as the length of running increases, a larger and larger percentage of the work is done aerobically, giving a truer picture of the functioning of the oxygen transport mechanisms.

Because anaerobic exercises do not depend on an oxygen supply, they do not tax the circulatory system to any significant extent. Therefore, they are not useful in developing cardiovascular fitness. In Chapter 5 an emphasis is placed on duration of exercise as a key

---

*Proteins are not oxidized as an energy source unless both the intake and storage amounts of carbohydrates and fats are completely inadequate—a condition rarely found except in a starvation diet.

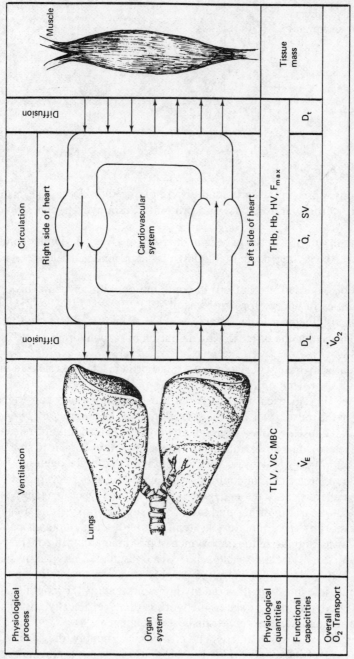

Figure 2–20. Schematic Illustration of the Oxygen Transport System with Measures of Quantities and Functional Capacities of the Important Components. Arrows pointing right indicate direction of O_2 diffusion, and arrows pointing left the direction of CO_2 diffusion. TLV is total lung volume; VC is vital capacity; MBC is maximum breathing capacity; THb is total circulating hemoglobin; Hb is hemoglobin concentration; HV is heart volume; F_{max} is maximum heart rate; $\dot{V}_E$ is minute volume of ventilation; D_L is lung diffusing capacity; Q is cardiac output; SV is stroke volume of the heart; D_t is tissue diffusing capacity; $\dot{V}_{O_2}$ is maximum oxygen uptake. (Adapted from Holmgren, A.: Cardiorespiratory Determinants of Cardiovascular Fitness. Can. Med. Assoc. J. 96:697, 1967.)

criterion in the development of cardiovascular fitness. Only those exercises depending on oxygen usage in oxidizing carbohydrates and fats can be continued for a long enough time to provide a significant training effect (for further discussion of this topic, see Chapter 5, Section IV, C, 2, and Table 5-5).

Oxygen Transport

Figure 2-20 is a schematic representation of what is commonly referred to in exercise physiology as the oxygen transport mechanism. Two physiological systems, respiratory and circulatory, combine to deliver oxygen (O_2) to a third system, the muscular. Concomitant with the delivery of oxygen is the removal of the major waste product of metabolism, carbon dioxide (CO_2).

Respiration and circulation, modified by nervous and chemical mechanisms, are the primary functions involved in insuring an adequate supply of oxygen to the working muscles. Atmospheric air contains approximately 21 per cent O_2, and this is the source from which, ultimately, muscles and other body cells are supplied. Virtually all the remaining atmospheric air is nitrogen (N_2). Carbon dioxide and other gases account for less than 1 per cent of the total mixture. The total pressure exerted by this gaseous mixture is 760 millimeters (mm) of mercury (Hg) at sea level. This is referred to as atmospheric or barometric pressure. Since O_2 makes up 21 per cent of the total pressure, or 160 mm Hg, this fraction of the total pressure is called the partial pressure of oxygen (P_{O_2}).

The lungs are responsible for supplying the body with fresh O_2, and also for removing excess CO_2 and H_2O. Air is brought into the lungs by action of the diaphragm and the mechanical deformation of the rib cage by the external intercostal muscles. Contraction of these muscles increases the size of the chest cavity. This decreases the pressure of the gas in the lungs, according to Boyle's law, causing it to drop below that of the atmospheric pressure outside the body. Air then rushes into the lungs owing to the difference in pressure (pressure gradient) (see Fig. 2-21).

By the time the oxygen reaches the air sacs (alveoli) of the lungs, its partial pressure has been reduced to approximately 100 mm Hg as a result of mixing with air having lower O_2 concentrations. The lung-capillary membrane is only three cells in thickness, and O_2 diffuses easily into the blood steam, again because of a pressure gradient (see Figs. 2-22 and 2-23). Oxygen partial pressure in the venous blood returning to the lungs from the body is approximately 40 mm Hg. This blood picks up enough new oxygen in the lungs so that it has a P_{O_2} equal to approximately 100 mm Hg when it leaves them. From the lungs the blood returns to the left side of the heart, from which it is pumped to all parts of the body. A schematic representation of circulation is presented in Figure 2-24.

The heart itself has four chambers: two upper chambers, the atria, that receive blood from the systemic (right side) and pulmonary (left side) circuits; and two lower chambers, the ventricles, which pump the blood into the systemic (left ventricle) and pulmonary (right ventricle) circuits. The atria and ventricles are separated by valves, the atrioventricular valves, which have a primary purpose of preventing backflow of blood into the atria when the ventricles pump. An additional set of heart valves are found where the aorta and pulmonary arteries exit from the left and right ventricles, respectively. These are the aortic and pulmonary valves, and in the normal heart they prevent backflow of blood after it has been pumped from the ventricles.

As with other tissues of the body, the heart muscle must have its own blood supply. This is provided by the coronary arteries, which branch off from the aorta just after it exits from the left ventricle. These vessels are illustrated in Figure 5-18. They

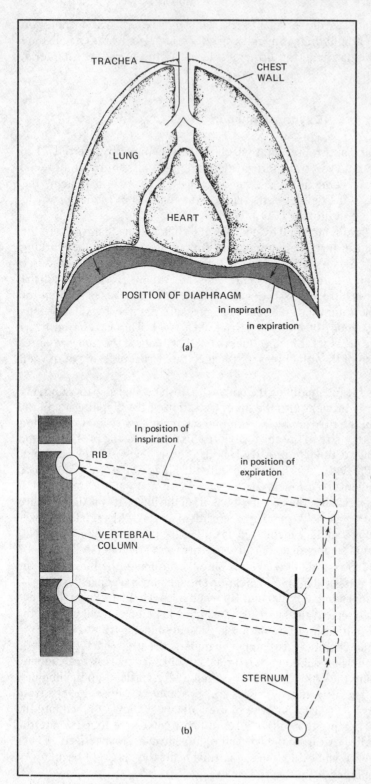

TRACHEA

CHEST WALL

LUNG

HEART

POSITION OF DIAPHRAGM

in inspiration

in expiration

(a)

In position of inspiration

RIB

in position of expiration

VERTEBRAL COLUMN

STERNUM

(b)

Figure 2–21. Lung Space Changes During Respiration. *(a)* shows that the contraction of the diaphragm during inspiration causes it to descend. The resultant increase in chest volume is indicated by the darker shaded area. *(b)* shows the elevation of the front ends of the ribs, or of the sternum to which the ribs are attached. This causes an increase in the front-back diameter of the chest. Both the above movements allow air to rush into the lungs. The reverse occurs during expiration. (From Carlson, A. J., and Johnson, V.: *The Machinery of the Body.* Chicago, University of Chicago Press, p. 231. © Copyright 1948 by the University of Chicago Press. All rights reserved.)

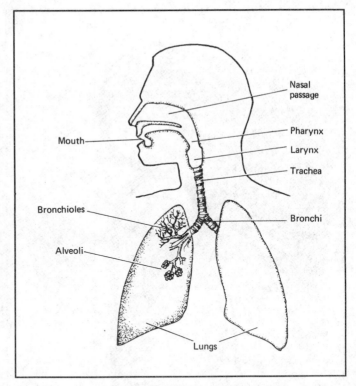

Figure 2–22. Schematic Representation of the Respiratory Passageways. Oxygen enters the mouth and nose, and passes through the trachea to the lungs, where it diffuses from the alveoli into the blood stream. Carbon dioxide diffusion follows a reverse path. (From Mathews, D. K., Stacy, R. W., and Hoover, G. N.: *Physiology of Muscular Activity and Exercise.* New York, Ronald Press. Copyright © 1964, p. 214. Reprinted by permission of John Wiley and Sons, Inc.)

are very important in circulatory health because they provide the heart with its only blood supply. A very common form of heart disease occurs when one or more of these vessels becomes wholly or partially blocked by fat deposits.

Most of the oxygen entering the blood stream from the lungs combines with hemoglobin, a protein found in the red blood cell. The circulation of the red blood cell serves as the major O_2 transporting mechanism. Owing to the oxygen used in oxidizing carbohy-

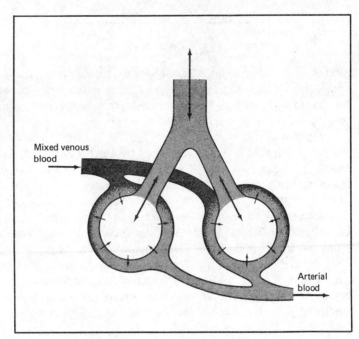

Figure 2–23. Schematic of the Pulmonary Circulation of the Lungs. The rounded areas represent the alveoli; the shaded tubes leading to them represent all of the conducting airways. Mixed venous blood *(dark)* flows through vessels in intimate contact with ventilated alveoli and becomes arterial blood *(light)* as it picks up oxygen. The fine arrows represent the transfer of O_2 and CO_2 between gas and blood. (Reproduced with permission from Comroe, J. H., Jr.: *Physiology of Respiration,* an Introductory Text, 2nd edition. Copyright © 1974 by Year Book Medical Publishers, Inc., Chicago.)

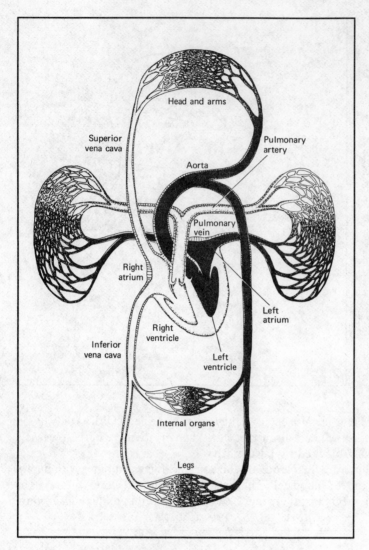

Figure 2–24. Schematic of Heart and Circulation. Lighter shaded areas represent mixed venous blood. Darker areas show parts containing arterial (oxygenated) blood. (From Wiggers, C. J.: The Heart. Sci. Am. *196(5):* 74, 1957. Copyright © by Scientific American, Inc. All rights reserved.)

drates, fats, and proteins in the cell, as discussed earlier in the chapter, P_{O_2} in the muscle cells is low. This creates a pressure gradient between the blood in the capillaries and the muscle tissues, causing hemoglobin to release oxygen, which then diffuses into the muscle cells (Fig. 2–20).

Carbon dioxide produced through the oxidation processes must be removed from the body. This, too, is accomplished by simple diffusion. The partial pressure of CO_2 builds up to approximately 48 mm Hg in the muscle tissue owing to oxidation. The partial pressure in the blood coming from the heart is only about 40 mm Hg. This pressure gradient results in diffusion of CO_2 into the blood as it passes through the capillaries. It then is transported through the right side of the heart to the lungs. Because P_{CO_2} in the lung alveoli is only 40 mm Hg, the excess diffuses from the blood into the alveoli, where it is removed from the body by exhalation from the lungs.

Exhalation is accomplished by relaxation of the diaphragm and external intercostals plus contraction of the internal intercostals, abdominal muscles, and some shoulder muscles. These actions decrease the size of the chest cavity, thereby compressing the enclosed gas and raising its pressure above that of atmospheric air (Boyle's law). This causes a pressure gradient toward the outside of the body, and air rushes out of the lungs (Fig. 2–21).

Maximal Oxygen Consumption and Its Importance to Cardiovascular Fitness

During normal resting activities, the processes illustrated in Figure 2–20 supply approximately 225 milliliters* of oxygen per minute, and they remove the accumulated CO_2. In order to exercise intensely, O_2 delivery and CO_2 removal must be speeded greatly. These increased demands are met primarily by greater release of oxygen from hemoglobin at the tissue level, and a speed-up of circulation and respiration.

At rest, hemoglobin releases at the tissues approximately 25 per cent of the oxygen bound to it. During strenous exercise, as much as 75 to 80 per cent of the O_2 is released. This response is dependent on the partial pressure decrease that occurs in muscle when the metabolism is increased. The increased release from hemoglobin can triple the oxygen supply to the muscles. The cardiac output (volume of blood pumped by the heart in 1 minute) at rest is approximately 4000 to 5000 ml. Strenuous exercise can cause this output to reach 20,000 to 25,000 ml, five times the resting level. The cardiac output is increased by raising the heart rate from approximately 70 per minute at rest to a maximum of 190† per minute, and by increasing the stroke volume (amount of blood pumped per heart beat) from approximately 70 to 130 ml. (See Chapter 5, Section III, A for a discussion of the interaction between stroke volume and heart rate in determining cardiac output.)

The combined mechanisms—greater release of O_2 by hemoglobin and increased cardiac output—can provide a 15-fold increase in O_2 delivery to the tissues. The oxygen supply thus may increase from 225 to 3375 ml per minute; the higher figure approximates the average maximal oxygen consumption for a young adult male. In the female, maximal oxygen consumption is smaller owing to a somewhat smaller maximal cardiac output and lower hemoglobin concentration in the blood (see Chapter 5, which also provides a more detailed discussion of maximal oxygen consumption as a measure of cardiovascular fitness).

EFFECTING ANATOMICAL AND PHYSIOLOGICAL CHANGES BY EXERCISE: THE *SAID* PRINCIPLE

As Steggerda [13] most aptly put it, "I am fit to do things that you cannot do because of the type of physical activities I have forced my nervous system to adjust to." The body responds rather specifically to demands placed on it. This is a unifying principle that applies to any of the characteristics that comprise physical fitness. The concept is called the *SAID* principle. The word has been coined from the first letter of each word in the phrase: "*S*pecific *A*daptations to *I*mposed *D*emands."[14] This principle provides a general guide to the design of an exercise program, and its application leads to an efficient application of exercise stresses. The SAID principle is justified in theory and supported by much research and other careful observation. In order to obtain results from an

---

*A milliliter (ml) is 1/1000 of a liter, and a liter is slightly larger than a quart by volume. Therefore, 225 ml is approximately ¼ quart by volume.

†Average maximal heart rate for young adults. Note from Table 5–4 that maximal heart rate decreases in the older age groups. In children, it is somewhat over 200 beats per minute.

exercise program, *the demands must be sufficient to force adaptation,* and the adaptation that occurs will be specific to the type of training performed. It is hypothesized that much of the training adaptation comes from a learning effect of the central nervous system, and more efficient neural processing as a basis of improvement with repeated use. A number of learning theories implicate changes in neurons with repeated use. Such changes as increased area on the cell body for synaptic connections, larger and more efficient synapses, the establishment of new neural connections, and changes in protein synthesis have all been hypothesized as basic changes accompanying improvements with repeated use.

In addition to hypothesized changes in the CNS with repeated exercise, changes in the broader physiological "bases" also occur as in the circulatory system, the muscles, and their connective tissues. For example, the improvement in strength with a training program is partly because the nervous system has learned the movement better, and partly because of changes in the muscle and its connective tissue. Enzymes necessary for breaking down carbohydrates and fats as food stuffs increase, so that the muscle has a greater supply of energy. More oxygen is delivered through an improved circulatory system, and muscle fibers increase in size, thus becoming stronger.

The development of endurance involves a similar neurological basis to that of strength development. Some types of localized endurances result from the continued facilitation of the same mechanisms already described. In addition, endurance involves the elevation of the general base—greater output of the heart muscle, the opening of more capillaries, improved oxygen-carrying capacity of the blood, and other related training effects which are basic adaptations.

An increase in the range of motion of the joints of the body also has a basis in neurological function. Flexibility results from stretching the muscles, the membranes that surround muscles, and tendons and other tissues that limit the movement of the joint.

In order to stretch the muscles and their connective tissue, it is necessary that the muscles being stretched remain relaxed. When the muscles contract, their contraction elements slide together and shorten; thus, their connective sheaths also are shortened. Their connective sheaths can maintain their flexibility by periodic stretching of the relaxed muscles. The nervous system plays an important role in keeping muscles relaxed during the flexibility exercises, and many techniques have been developed for using basic neural circuits for maintaining relaxation. These concepts are more fully explained in Chapter 6, but basically involve the use of slow static stretches to avoid evoking a reflex contraction of the stretching muscle via excitation of the muscle spindle. The hard wiring for reciprocal innervation can be used by contracting the muscle antagonistic to the one being stretched; thus, inhibition is sent to the stretching muscle from the contraction of its opposite group. The Golgi tendon organ inhibition has also been used by preceding the stretch with a maximal isometric contraction, so that the motor pool is reflexively inhibited at the beginning of the stretch.

The demands placed on the organism by exercise must be sufficient to force adaptation. Therefore, exercise that is too mild is nearly valueless and a waste of time from a conditioning standpoint. The same applies to the wrong type of exercise. The one major principle, SAID, through which improvement of fitness, bodily function, and form may be achieved, involves placing the body under stresses of varying intensity and duration. By attempting to overcome these stresses, the body adapts rather specifically to these imposed demands and, as a result, elevates the tolerance for further activity of greater intensity and duration. Since individual tolerance for exercise varies, it becomes necessary to have gradation or progression in the intensity or severity of the exercise. This principle of pushing systems to force their development of cardiovascular function, flexibility, strength, and desirable body composition is the theme of this book. We go a step further in attempting to provide the reader with a background for understanding the physiology, psychology, and anatomy of adaptations that are made in response to the imposed demands.

LEARNING OBJECTIVES

After completing a study of Chapter 2, students should be able to:

1. Demonstrate a general knowledge of respiratory anatomy by drawing a schematic diagram of the lungs and respiratory passageways, showing (with labels) all significant parts related to respiration.

2. Explain the importance of a pressure gradient in the partial pressure of oxygen for diffusion to occur at the lungs and at the muscle tissue.

3. Explain how oxygen is transported from the lungs to the tissues of the body so that they can use it for metabolism.

4. Identify the parts of the circulatory system and explain the function(s) of each.

5. Draw a schematic diagram of the heart and label the parts.

6. Draw a schematic diagram of the complete circulatory system, label all parts, and show the direction of blood flow.

7. Identify and explain the functions of each of the heart's chambers.

8. Explain the coronary circulation of the heart.

9. Define the SAID principle and give examples of how it would operate for conditioning on cardiovascular function, strength, flexibility, and body composition.

10. Explain the differences between aerobic and anaerobic exercise (metabolism), and indicate why one or the other may be more important in cardiovascular conditioning.

11. Explain the function of the red blood cell in delivery of oxygen to the tissues (cells) of the body.

12. Explain in what ways the antigravity musculature is important in cardiovascular conditioning.

13. Write out a general definition of the terms *anatomy* and *physiology*.

14. Define the terms *joint, ligaments,* and *tendons* as they relate to human movement.

15. Define the term *contraction* as it relates to skeletal muscle.

16. Identify and demonstrate the *anatomical position* as a basis for describing human movement.

17. Define and demonstrate each of the following movement terms: *flexion, extension, hyperextension, abduction, adduction.*

18. Explain reciprocal innervation.

19. Identify and explain each of the four roles in which a muscle may act within the body.

20. Identify the antigravity musculature of the human body.

21. Explain why the antigravity musculature should be a major focus in any conditioning program.

22. Explain Huxley's "sliding filament" model of muscle contraction.

23. Identify the major parts of the nervous system and list the general functions of each.

24. Define a neuron, draw a schematic diagram of it, label the important parts, and explain the function of each.

25. List the body's four proprioceptive mechanisms and give a general indication of the function(s) of each.

26. Define the term *motor unit* as it relates to a muscle.

27. Explain the "all or none" concept in muscle contraction.

28. Demonstrate a knowledge of neuromuscular reflexes by explaining both the "knee-jerk" and withdrawal reflexes.

29. Identify the areas of the brain controlling voluntary movement.

30. Explain the process whereby energy from the sun is ultimately stored for use in the human body.

31. Explain the function of the atrioventricular, aortic, and pulmonary valves of the heart.

32. Explain the interaction between hemoglobin release of oxygen and increased cardiac output during exercise in increasing oxygen delivery to the tissues of the body. Indicate which has the greatest effect on oxygen delivery.

33. Explain the effect of the Golgi tendon organ on its motor pool (the muscle spindle reflexively excites its motor pool).

34. Explain a motor pool within the nervous system.

35. Explain why differences may exist in motor units.

36. Describe how reflex and voluntary movements differ.

37. Give an example of a reflex.

38. Give an example of a voluntary movement.

REFERENCES

1. deVries, H. A.: *Physiology of Exercise for Physical Education and Athletics*. Dubuque, Iowa, Wm. C. Brown Co., 1974.
2. Easton, D. M.: *Mechanisms of Body Functions*. Englewood Cliffs, N. J., Prentice-Hall, 1974.
3. Edington, D. W., and Edgerton, V. R.: *The Biology of Physical Activity*. Boston, Houghton Mifflin Co., 1976.
4. Evarts, E. V.: Brain mechanisms in movement. Sci. Am. *229*:96, 1973.
5. Fox, E. L.: *Sports Physiology*. Philadelphia, W. B. Saunders Co., 1979.
6. Guyton, A. C.: *Textbook of Medical Physiology*. Philadelphia, W. B. Saunders Co., 1976.
7. Guyton, A. C.: *Physiology of the Human Body*. Philadelphia, W. B. Saunders Co., 1979.
8. Logan, G. A., and McKinney, W. C.: *Anatomic Kinesiology*. Dubuque, Iowa, Wm. C. Brown Co., 1977.
9. Mathews, D. K., and Fox, E. L.: *The Physiological Basis of Physical Education and Athletics*. Philadelphia, W. B. Saunders Co., 1976.
10. Sage, G. H.: *Introduction to Motor Behavior: A Neuropsychological Approach*. Reading, MA, Addison-Wesley Co., 1977.
11. Schmidt, R. F. (ed.): *Fundamentals of Neurophysiology*. New York, Springer-Verlag, 1976.
12. Singer, R. N.: *Motor Learning and Human Performance*. New York, Macmillan Co., 1968.
13. Steggerda, F. R.: The Role of the Nervous System in Fitness. In *Exercise and Fitness*. Chicago, The Athletic Institute, 1960.
14. Wallis, E. L., and Logan, G. A.: *Figure Improvement and Body Conditioning through Exercise*. Englewood Cliffs, N.J., Prentice-Hall, 1964.
15. Wells, K. F., and Luttgens, K.: *Kinesiology: Scientific Basis of Human Motion*. Philadelphia, W. B. Saunders Co., 1976.

Chapter 3

Cardiovascular Disease Risk Factors

INTRODUCTION

Premature death from coronary heart disease among both men and women in their productive years is probably *the* major health problem in the United States. In many instances, apparently healthy middle-aged persons die from coronary artery disease. About one-half of these deaths are sudden and unexpected. Coronary heart disease, which comprises the major portion of mortality due to cardiovascular diseases in most technologically advanced societies, is the leading cause of death in the U.S. In Figure 3–1 the astonishing 54 per cent of deaths due to cardiovascular diseases is illustrated in proportion to other causes of death in this country. Coronary heart disease is believed to account for about 75 per cent of total cardiovascular disease deaths. It is not just a problem of older persons; between the years of 1951 and 1961, the average death rate among 35- to 54-year-old men increased by 50 per cent. Figure 3–2 shows the disease rate at various ages.

Coronary heart disease is believed to be associated with atherosclerosis of the coronary arteries—a process by which the artery is gradually narrowed by the deposition of materials along the arterial walls. As a larger portion of the artery is narrowed by the obstruction (see Fig. 5–19), an inadequate supply of blood gets to the heart, a muscle that must work continually and thus must receive adequate oxygen.

Although scientists have not been able to pinpoint the exact cause(s) of atherosclerosis, they have established factors in an individual's heredity or lifestyle that seem to predispose to the disease. Epidemiological studies of large population groups have identified various so-called *risk factors* for coronary heart disease. Those who develop

45

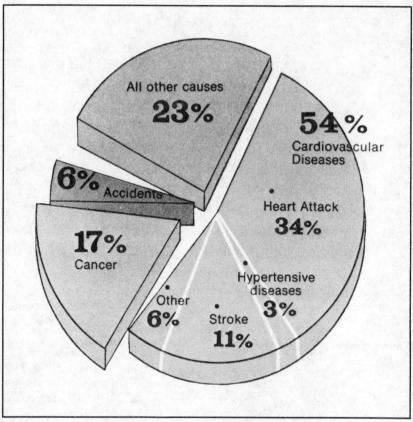

Figure 3–1.   Leading Causes of Death in the United States. Deaths from cardiovascular disease and related coronary problems represent major health problems in this country. (From Borhani, N. O.: Epidemiology of Coronary Heart Disease. *In* E. A. Amsterdam, J. H. Wilmore, and A. N. DeMaria (eds.) *Exercise in Cardiovascular Health and Disease.* New York, Yorke Medical Books, 1977, p. 2.)

coronary heart disease have many factors in common, and scientists have developed predictions concerning the chances of developing coronary heart disease in persons having various levels of these identified risk factors. Available evidence suggests that the most powerful predictors of coronary heart disease are age, sex, blood pressure, level of serum cholesterol and/or blood fat, cigarette smoking, and physical inactivity. Other factors include a family history of coronary heart disease; diabetes or elevated levels of blood sugar; and stress or tension. Current preventive efforts are aimed at making individuals more aware of the risk factors that appear to predispose them to coronary heart disease. It is hoped that increased knowledge will improve health practices concerning these factors. Age, heredity, and sex are difficult to alter, but the others are more subject to individual control. All persons should attempt to analyse their risk factors and determine if they are generally at low, medium, or high risk. For convenience in doing this, a widely-used heart disease risk index is provided in Appendix A–1. This index is not meant as a substitute for regular medical checks, but is intended to give a general analysis of high, medium, or low risk. Complete the exercise in Appendix A–1 to determine where you fall in the risk category.

Often, the realization that a person is high in one factor will necessitate more careful attention to other factors. The major purposes of education concerning these factors are to identify those who, because of multiple risk factors, are very likely to develop coronary heart disease, and to encourage them to develop healthier lifestyles in regard to

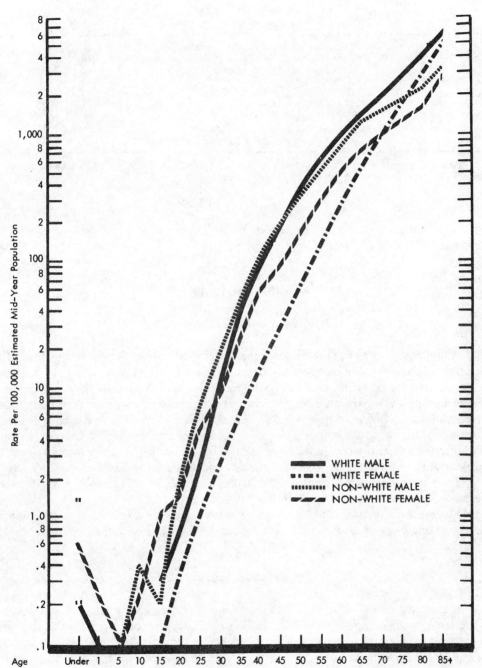

Figure 3–2. Death Rate in the United States from Coronary Heart Disease by Five-Year Age-group, Sex, and Race. Coronary heart disease is not strictly a disease of the elderly. Data in this Figure illustrate that young adults also should be concerned with this disease. (From Borhani, N. O.: Epidemiology of Coronary Heart Disease. *In* E. A. Amsterdam, J. H. Wilmore, and A. N. DeMaria (eds.) *Exercise in Cardiovascular Health and Disease.* New York, Yorke Medical Books, 1977, p. 5.)

Table 3–1. RECOMMENDATIONS OF THE AMERICAN HEART ASSOCIATION FOR REDUCING RISK OF CORONARY HEART DISEASE*

Why Risk Heart Attack?
How to Guard Your Heart

1. Reduce saturated fat and cholesterol in the diet
2. Count your calories and avoid excess weight
3. Control high blood pressure
4. Don't smoke
5. Exercise regularly
6. Avoid unnecessary tension
7. Enjoy leisure activities
8. Have regular medical checks
9. Follow your doctor's advice

*Based on the pamphlets TEM 414, "Why Risk Heart Attack," and TEM 517, "Heart Attack: How To Reduce Your Risk." American Heart Association, Texas Affiliate, Inc.

each of these factors. Table 3–1 is a guide for use in accomplishing a reduction in cardiovascular disease risk.

RISK FACTORS

Age, Sex, and Family History

Although age, sex, and heredity are risk factors we cannot modify, it is beneficial to understand their relation to coronary heart disease. As illustrated in Figure 3–2, the incidence of coronary heart disease rapidly increases in both sexes with increasing age. Women often develop the concept that, owing to the greater incidence of coronary heart disease in males, it is no problem for the female. It is true that the prevalence is much greater in young men than in young women by about six times; however, in older persons the difference is minimized until it disappears in the elderly. Many women develop coronary heart disease, and it should not be considered a "male" disease.

Since we do not select our parents, another risk factor that cannot be modified is heredity. Those who have a family history of coronary heart disease are about twice as likely to develop the disease as those who do not. A positive family history in combination with one or more of the other risk factors appears to be even more unfavorable.

High Blood Pressure

It is estimated that 15 per cent of the entire U.S. population suffers from definite hypertension (high blood pressure), and an additional 15 per cent from borderline hypertension. Estimates for adults are even higher, as illustrated in Figure 3–3. Below the age of 50 years, instances of hypertension are more frequent for men than for women; however, past this age, women experience greater hypertensive problems than do men. Mortality rates associated with insurance data show the optimal blood pressures for longevity are those below 110 mm Hg systolic and 70 mm Hg diastolic. The higher the blood pressures, the greater is the risk for coronary heart disease and many other related diseases. It is highly recommended that blood pressures be checked regularly, so that hypertension can be detected early, and in most cases successfully treated with antihypertensive therapy.

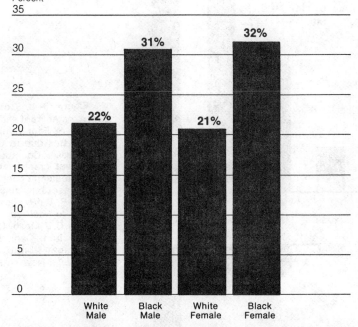

Hypertension Prevalence by Sex and Race
U.S. Adults Age 18 and over: 1976 Estimate

Figure 3–3. High Blood Pressure. Adults, both men and women, often experience problems with high blood pressure. (From *Heart Facts 1979*. Dallas, Texas, by permission of American Heart Association, Inc., #55-005-C, 1978, p. 2.)

Diet

The role of dietary excess is especially important in coronary heart disease, because two factors are closely linked to diet: (1) the level of saturated fat and cholesterol; and (2) the amount of excess calories or body fat. *Hyperlipidemia* is a term describing high levels of serum cholesterol and triglycerides. Dietary foods that are high in saturated fat and cholesterol tend to increase cholesterol levels, whereas diets low in saturated fats but high in polyunsaturated fats tend to lower the level of blood cholesterol (Fig. 3–4). Scientists who wish to develop atherosclerosis in laboratory animals recognize that a diet high in saturated fat, leading to increased serum cholesterol, is necessary. These data, like those from the population studies illustrated in Figure 3–5 in which higher occurrences of coronary heart disease are associated with higher levels of saturated fat in the diet, indicate that high serum cholesterol is an important precursor to the disease. One should become familiar with foods that are high in saturated fat and cholesterol and with sources of polyunsaturated fats.

Table 3–2 will help the student become familiar with some common sources; more detailed information is contained in Appendix A–19. The idea is to omit many of the cholesterol-rich foods, and substitute polyunsaturated fats for many of the saturated fats. The American Heart Association has developed the leaflet "The Way to a Man's Heart" (EM 455) and its companion booklet "Recipes" (EM 455A) to help people to accomplish this goal.* Additionally, the Select Committee on Nutrition and Human Needs of the

---

*These may be obtained from local American Heart Association offices.

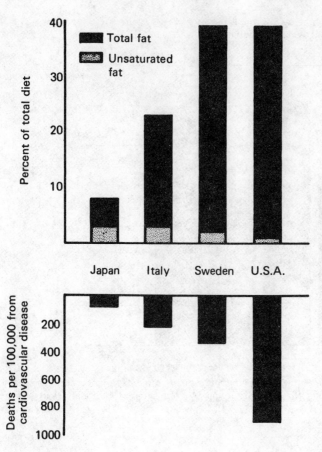

Figure 3-4. Comparison between the Amount and Type of Fat in the Diet of Four Countries and the Death Rates due to Cardiovascular Heart Disease. Countries whose populations eat greater amounts of fat have a greater number of deaths from cardiovascular diseases. (From Hockey, R. V.: *Physical Fitness: The Pathway to Healthful Living.* 3rd ed. St. Louis, C. V. Mosby Co., 1977, p. 28. Adapted from Cant, G.: What you must know about diet. *In The Healthy Life.* New York, Time, Inc.)

Figure 3-5. Cholesterol. The incidence of coronary heart disease is higher among individuals with high levels of blood cholesterol. (From Loviglio, L.: What's Your Risk: A Layman's Guide to Cardiovascular Disease. Bostonia (Boston University Alumni Magazine) *52*:1, Winter 1978, p. 6.)

TWENTY-TWO YEAR INCIDENCE OF CORONARY HEART DISEASE/CHOLESTEROL LEVEL IN MEN AGED 30-39

INCIDENCE OF CORONARY HEART DISEASE PER 1,000

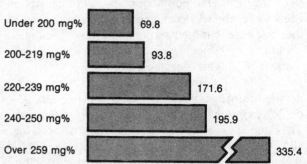

Under 200 mg%	69.8
200-219 mg%	93.8
220-239 mg%	171.6
240-250 mg%	195.9
Over 259 mg%	335.4

Graph illustrates increase in numbers of cases of coronary heart disease with increases in serum (blood) cholesterol levels.

Table 3-2.   CLASSIFICATION OF SOME FOODS ACCORDING TO PRUDENT DIET STATUS*

Class	Characteristics	Recommended Usage	Foods	
I	Low fat; low saturated fat; little or no cholesterol	Normal	Fish (boiled or broiled); chicken (without skin); fruits or fruit juices; vegetables, bread, cereals	
II	High fats; low in saturated fats; no cholesterol	Moderate	Olives, olive oil, avocados, cashew nuts	
III	High fat; high in polyunsaturated fats; little or no cholesterol	Encouraged	Corn oil, cottonseed oil, soybean oil, margarines containing above in liquid form	
IV	High fat; high in saturated fat; moderately high in cholesterol	Limited or consumed in modified form	*Normal form:*	*Modified form:*
			Milk	Skim or 99% fat-free
			Cheeses	Made from skim milk
			Ice cream	99% fat-free or ices
			Butter	Margarine
			Beef, pork lamb	Lean meat only
			Pastries	Made with appoved oils or margarines
V	High in cholesterol	Severely limited or consumed in modified form	Eggs	
			Organs	Brain, liver, kidney

*Adapted from Livingston, G. E.: The prudent diet: what? why? how? Preventive Med., 2:321, 1973.

U.S. Senate (Sen. George McGovern, chairman) has issued a report with the following specific recommendations.

U.S. Dietary Goals*

1. Increase carbohydrate consumption to account for 55 to 60 per cent of the energy (caloric) intake.
2. Reduce over-all fat consumption from approximately 40 to 30 per cent of energy intake.
3. Reduce saturated fat consumption to account for about 10 per cent of total energy intake; and balance that with polyunsaturated and monounsaturated fats, which should account for about 10 per cent of energy intake each.
4. Reduce cholesterol consumption to about 300 mg a day.
5. Reduce sugar consumption by about 40 per cent to account for about 15 per cent of total energy intake.
6. Reduce salt consumption by about 50 to 85 per cent to approximately 3 gm a day.

The goals suggest the following changes in food selection and preparation.

1. Increase consumption of fruits and vegetables and whole grains.
2. Decrease consumption of meat and increase consumption of poultry and fish.
3. Decrease consumption of foods high in fat, and partially substitute polyunsaturated fat for saturated fat.
4. Substitute nonfat milk for whole milk.
5. Decrease consumption of butterfat, eggs, and other high cholesterol sources.
6. Decrease consumption of sugar and foods high in sugar content.
7. Decrease consumption of salt and foods high in salt content.

*See Figure 3-6 for a graphic representation.

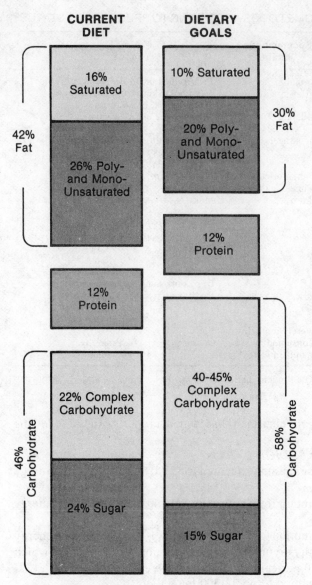

Figure 3–6. Graphic Representation of Current Diet and Dietary Goals Recommended by the U.S. Senate Select Committee on Nutrition and Human Needs. (From Loviglio, L.: What's Your Risk: A Layman's Guide to Cardiovascular Disease. Bostonia (Boston University Alumni Magazine) 52:1, Winter 1978, p. 9.)

Calories are the other dietary consideration. Avoid excess fat. If you are currently overweight, seek a sensible reducing diet. Study Chapter 8 on exercise and weight control carefully for the role of exercise in maintaining ideal weight.

Cigarette Smoking

Another very important coronary risk factor is cigarette smoking. The heart attack death rate is 50 to 200 per cent higher for men who are heavy cigarette smokers, compared with nonsmoking men (Fig. 3–7). Although the dangers of cigarette smoking have been highly publicized in regard to lung cancer, the excess mortality among smokers due to coronary heart disease is almost twice that due to lung cancer (19 per cent lung cancer, 37 per cent coronary heart disease). Another unfortunate set of data indicate that the increased death rate from coronary heart disease among young women has almost paralleled the rate of increase in women's cigarette smoking. Smoking is a risk factor in which the association with coronary heart disease is strong, but also one that can be readily controlled by never developing the habit, or stopping if it has already begun. For smokers who give up the habit, the risk returns almost to nonsmokers' levels. For the young person who has never been involved with long years of a well-established smoking habit, the path is clear—do not smoke. The prognosis for young smokers who desire to break the habit is excellent, both in terms of continued abstinence and for their risk returning to near-normal levels.

Stress*

Scientists have identified two basic behavior patterns based on various factors of behavior. The *Type A* behavior profile is associated with increased risk of coronary heart disease, and is characterized by a strong sense of time urgency and high levels of aggressive and competitive behavior. Type A individuals have been described as intensely ambitious persons who drive themselves against the clock. In a more recent paper, Type A coronary-prone behavior pattern was defined as "an overt behavior syndrome or style of living characterized by excesses of competitiveness, striving for achievement, aggressiveness (sometimes stringently repressed), time urgency, acceleration of common activities, restlessness, hostility, hyperalertness, explosiveness of speech, amplitude, tenseness of facial musculature, and feelings of struggle against the limitations of time and the insensitivity of the environment." *Type B* individuals, who are equally capable, are more easy-going and do not appear constantly to "race the clock."

*The reader should complete the questionnaire in Appendix A–2 before reading this section.

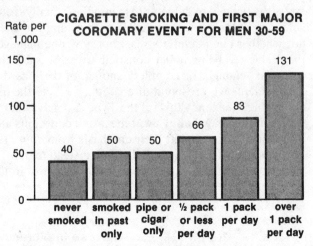

CIGARETTE SMOKING AND FIRST MAJOR CORONARY EVENT* FOR MEN 30-59

Rate per 1,000

Figure 3–7. Smoking. The incidence of coronary events, which is greater among smokers than non-smokers, is even greater among those who smoke heavily. (From Loviglio, L.: What's Your Risk: A Layman's Guide to Cardiovascular Disease. Bostonia (Boston University Alumni Magazine) 52:1, Winter 1978, p. 9.)

Graph illustrates the varying rates of coronary events* depending upon smoking habits. For example, those men who never smoked had a rate of 40 coronary events per 1,000 individuals, while those smoking over a pack a day had a rate of 131 events per 1,000 individuals.

*A coronary event is defined as any clinically significant manifestation of coronary artery disease, such as heart attack or angina.

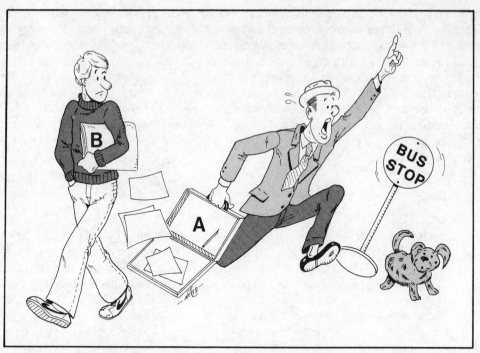

Figure 3–8. Type A and B Behavior Patterns. The time conscious, goal oriented, rushed Type A behavior has been linked with greater incidence of cardiovascular disease. The less hurried Type B behavior is less likely to result in disease.

Obviously most people are not entirely "A" or "B," but have combined behavioral patterns of both. One is not automatically Type A if one's life contains a large amount of stress, as defined by a high-pressure job or family troubles. Everyone is under pressure sometimes. Most people struggle with it, and it usually passes. The important thing is not whether one is under stress, but how one manages it. Type A individuals think of themselves as being under constant stress because they can never get where they are going fast enough, or complete enough of the jobs they set themselves.

Students who respond often with "yes" to the questions in Appendix A–2 should realize their tendency toward the Type A behavioral profile. These individuals can alter this pattern somewhat by awareness and conscious attention to these behavioral traits. They might want to shift their emphasis from *doing* to *being*, to stop judging worth on how much they produce each day, but instead to think about the kind of person they are. This would mean a shift of concern for quantity in life to its quality.

Glucose Intolerance

The glucose tolerance test is a screening test for diabetes, a very significant coronary risk factor. Premature atherosclerosis commonly has been a complication of diabetes. Coronary risk increases parallel the severity of the intolerance for glucose as indicated by the glucose tolerance test..All persons, especially those with a family history of diabetes, should have regular medical checks for this disease.

Inactivity

Does Exercise Offer Protection?

Many studies indicate that active persons are less susceptible to coronary heart disease. Although these investigations do not offer conclusive "proof" that increasing the activity level will lower the coronary risk, this assumption certainly is strongly supported in the various findings. Generally, populations who are more physically active have lower incidences of coronary heart disease. For example, Morris and his colleagues, who compared the incidence of heart disease among inactive English bus drivers to that in the more active bus conductors who walk up and down the double-decker buses, reported that drivers had twice the incidence of heart disease as had the conductors. These data were supported in studies of postal workers in whom the incidence of coronary heart disease was significantly less in active mail carriers than in inactive clerical workers. It also was shown to be less in active farmers and in more active railroad workers. These findings were confirmed again in a study of communal settlements in Israel, where the incidence of heart disease and mortality rate was about three times greater in the inactive group, which had a similar lifestyle except for level of activity.

Another interesting confirmation study involved pairs of Irish brothers both of whom were born in Ireland; one brother remained there and the other emigrated to the Boston, MA, area. The Irish brothers had healthier hearts than their U.S. counterparts. Their smoking and drinking habits were comparable. Despite the fact that the homeland Irish brothers ate more total calories per day and more animal fat, their blood pressure was lower, they weighed less, and they had less body fat and lower serum cholesterol levels than their U.S. brothers. The researchers emphasized the difference between the groups in terms of level of activity. The Irish brothers generally were physically active, whereas the Americans were generally sedentary. The higher risk associated with the American sedentary way of life has also been validated by studies comparing more active lifestyles such as those of the Bushmen, Eskimos, and Masai to that of western societies.

Paffenbarger, who addressed questions concerning the "protection or selection" interpretation of these data, attempted to minimize those problems in a population study of 3686 San Francisco longshoremen for a 22-year follow-up study period. He argued that the above-mentioned investigations from which we infer "protection" afforded by activity could possibly be "selection," i.e., workers in the active groups had selected themselves into it because of a "rugged constitution." In the longshoreman study, no differences in coronary risk factors existed between men in heavy work and those in light work, except that heavy workers smoked less and weighed less, both of which were attributed to their higher level of activity. From the findings, it was concluded that neither of these factors could account for the 80 per cent excess risk of fatal heart attack among the lighter workers.

How Does Exercise Protect Against Coronary Heart Disease?

Discussions on this topic center around two basic concepts: (1) exercise favorably affects other risk factors; and (2) other mechanisms for the protection afforded by exercise have been proposed. Exercise has been reported to favorably affect hypertension, hyperlipidemia, obesity, stress, or tension.

Bonanno summarized findings relating to exercise and blood pressure, and reported that exercise probably does not affect normal blood pressure levels (either systolic or diastolic), and does not affect high levels for diastolic, but probably does reduce hypertensive systolic pressure. This is discussed in more detail in Chapter 5. The favorable effects of exercise on obesity are covered in Chapter 8.

The other diet-related risk factors also may be influenced by exercise. Evidence indicates that triglycerides are reduced following vigorous exercise bouts, and gradually return to their baseline value approximately 48 to 72 hours after the exercise. Thus, the habit of regular work-outs every two or three days is a definite help in maintaining reduced triglyceride levels (see Chapter 5). Serum cholesterol levels have not shown such consistent changes. Studies are contradictory, and it is doubtful whether exercise alone, without accompanying weight reduction, will reduce these levels.

In addition to the above exercise-related reductions in risk factor levels, there are also significant psychological factors to be considered. The general feeling of increased well-being normally associated with chronic exercise apparently applies to psychological as well as physiological factors. Exercise has been shown to reduce anxiety, depression, and hostility, and to improve sleep (see Chapter 7 for further discussion of the psychological effects).

Besides reduction in risk factor levels, other mechanisms by which chronic activity reduces the occurrence or severity of coronary heart disease include many of the benefits to the cardiovascular system outlined in Chapter 5. Although these mechanisms vary slightly from one author to the next, the list presented in Table 3–3 is a good representation. Most of these changes center around increased efficiency of the heart, where the stronger heart muscle pumps more blood per stroke so that, during rest or any given submaximal workload, the heart rate is lower. The blood enters a "fit" vascular system in which increased coronary collateral vascularization has been shown (at least in laboratory animals); larger vessel size has been demonstrated; the blood is distributed in an increased arterial network, and venous return is efficient. The blood itself has good characteristics for volume, numbers of red blood cells to transport oxygen, and clotting ability. In addition to these changes, increased hormone production and function have been reported.

In summary, multiple coronary heart disease risk factors have been identified and briefly discussed. Exercise has been examined as a risk factor in itself and in combination with the reductions of other risk factors. The concept of multiple risk factors interacting to produce greater risks for coronary heart disease is an important one, and is illustrated for three of the most important in Figure 3–9. When the three most-studied risk factors (serum cholesterol, blood pressure, and smoking) are all elevated in the same individual,

Table 3–3. MECHANISMS BY WHICH PHYSICAL ACTIVITY MAY REDUCE THE OCCURRENCE OR SEVERITY OF CORONARY HEART DISEASE*

Increases	Decreases
Coronary collateral vascularization	Serum lipid levels
Vessel size	Triglycerides
Myocardial efficiency	Cholesterol
Efficiency of peripheral blood distribution and return	Glucose intolerance
Electron transport capacity	Obesity-adiposity
Fibrinolytic capability	Platelet stickiness
Thyroid function	Arterial blood pressure
Growth hormone production	Heart rate
Tolerance to stress	Vulnerability to dysrhythmias
Prudent living habits	Neurohormonal over-reaction
"Joie de vivre"	"Strain" associated with psychic "stress"

*Adapted from Pollock, M. L., Wilmore, J. H., and Fox, S. M., III: *Health and Fitness Through Physical Activity*. Reprinted with permission of John Wiley & Sons, Inc., New York, 1978.

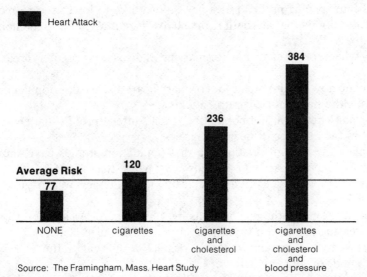

**The Danger of Heart Attack
Increases with the Number of Risk
Factors Present**

(example: 45 year old male)

■ Heart Attack

Source: The Framingham, Mass. Heart Study

Figure 3–9. Combining the Risk Factors. Persons with combinations of risk factors have experienced even more problems with coronary artery disease than those with fewer numbers. How risk factors are combined is a very important consideration. (From *Heart Facts 1979,* Dallas, Texas, by permission of American Heart Association, Inc. #55-005-C, 1978, p. 16.)

the risk is five times higher than if there are no risk factors and three times higher than if just one exists. Thus, one isolated risk factor is not nearly so important as are combinations of factors. We constantly hear about a heart attack in someone who has never smoked; in a slim and trim person; in someone with low blood cholesterol levels; in the individual with no family history of heart disease; or even in someone who ran 5 miles per day, Certainly, low values in any one risk factor cannot be considered "protective," but the implications are that the optimal combination of low risk levels for any one individual reduces that person's chances for coronary heart disease.

LEARNING OBJECTIVES

After completing a study of Chapter 3, students should be able to:
1. Indicate the relative rank of coronary heart disease as a cause of adult deaths in the U.S., and list the proportion of all deaths attributable to this disease.
2. Explain why so much attention is given by the medical profession to risk factors for coronary heart disease.
3. Calculate how they rate on the coronary risk index, and pinpoint individual factors of greatest risk.
4. Explain the risk factors for coronary heart disease over which the individual has little control.
5. Identify the risk factors that can be modified.

6. Explain procedures that can be followed to reduce the modifiable risk factors.

7. Explain the Type A and Type B behavior patterns discussed in the chapter.

8. List the adjectives that best describe the Type A behavior pattern.

9. Indicate which of the two behavior patterns seems to be most related to the development of coronary heart disease.

10. Explain the over-all objective in reducing serum cholesterol.

11. Indicate specific procedures a person can take to lower serum cholesterol.

12. Identify foods that are both high and low in saturated fats and cholesterol (see also Appendix A–19).

13. Say whether lung cancer or coronary heart disease is a greater threat to cigarette smokers.

14. Explain how the prognosis for coronary heart disease development may change if one "breaks the habit" of cigarette smoking.

15. Explain whether or not population studies offer "proof" that chronic physical activity lowers the chances of heart disease.

16. Explain the kind of relationship that population studies have shown to exist between chronic physical activity and coronary heart disease.

17. Say whether or not exercise affects other risk factors. Which ones? How? (See also Chapter 5.)

18. Indicate some of the mechanisms by which exercise has been supported as a factor in increasing protection from heart disease. (See also Chapter 5.)

19. Explain how a person who runs 5 miles a day can suffer a heart attack if "exercise is good for you."

20. Summarize the ways in which individuals can lower their levels of coronary disease risk factors.

REFERENCES

1. American Heart Association.: Risk Factors and Coronary Disease: A Statement for Physicians. Booklet EM 451, released by the Central Committee for Medical and Community Program of the American Heart Association, December, 1967.
2. American Heart Association, Texas Affiliate, Inc.: Why Risk Heart Attack? Leaflet TEM 414, 1968.
3. Barboriak, J. J., et al.: Coronary artery occlusion and blood lipids. Am. Heart J. *87*:716, 1974.
4. Bonanno, J. A.: Coronary Risk Factor Modification by Chronic Physical Exercise. *In* E. A. Amsterdam, J. H. Wilmore, and A. N. DeMaria (eds.) *Exercise in Cardiovascular Health and Disease*. New York, Yorke Medical Books, 1977.
5. Borhani, N. O.: Epidemiology of Coronary Heart Disease. *In* E. A. Amsterdam, J. H. Wilmore, and A. N. DeMaria (eds.) *Exercise in Cardiovascular Health and Disease*. New York, Yorke Medical Books, 1977.
6. Breslow, L., and Buell, P.: Mortality from coronary heart disease and physical activity of work in California. J. Chronic Dis. *11*:421, 1960.
7. Brunner, D., Manelis, G., Modan, M., et al.: Physical activity at work and the incidence of myocardial infarction, angina pectoris, and death due to ischemic heart disease: an epidemiological study in Israeli collective settlements (kibbutzim). J. Chronic Dis. *27*:217, 1974.
8. Cassel, J., Heyden, S., Bartel, A. G., et al.: Occupation and physical activity and coronary heart disease. Arch. Intern. Med. *128*:920, 1971.
9. Edington, D. W., and Edgerton, V. R.: *The Biology of Physical Activity*. Boston, Houghton Mifflin Co., 1976.
10. Epstein, F. H.: Coronary heart disease epidemiology revisited: clinical and community aspects. Circulation *48*:185, 1973.
11. Falsetti, H. L., Schnatz, J. D., Greene, D. G., and Bunnell, I. L.: Lipid and carbohydrate studies in coronary artery disease. Circulation *37*:184, 1968.
12. Fox, S. M., III, and Paul, O.: Controversies in cardiology: physical activity and coronary heart disease. Am. J. Cardiol. *23*:298, 1969.
13. Fox, S. M., III, and Skinner, J. S.: Physical activity and cardiovascular health. Am. J. Cardiol. *14*:731, 1964.

14. Frank, C. W., Weinblatt, E., and Shapiro, S.: Physical inactivity as a lethal factor in myocardial infarction among men. Circulation *34*:1022, 1966.
15. Friedman, M., and Rosenman, R. H.: Association of specific overt behavior pattern with blood and cardiovascular findings. J.A.M.A. *169*:1286, 1959.
16. Froelicher, V. F.: Animal studies of effect of chronic exercise on the heart and atherosclerosis: a review. Am. Heart J. *84*:496, 1972.
17. Hatch, F. T.: Interactions between nutrition and heredity in coronary heart disease. Am. J. Clin. Nutr. *27*:80, 1974.
18. Jenkins, C. D., Rosenman, R. H., and Zyzanski, S. J.: Prediction of clinical coronary heart disease by a test for the coronary-prone behavior pattern. N. Engl. J. Med. *290*:1271, 1974.
19. Kahn, H. A.: The relationship of reported coronary heart disease mortality to physical activity of work. Am. J. Public Health *53*:1058, 1963.
20. Lew, E. A.: High blood pressure, other risk factors and longevity: the insurance viewpoint. Am. J. Med. *55*:281, 1973.
21. Loviglio, L.: What's your risk? Boston University Alumni Magazine *52*:1, Winter, 1978.
22. Mann, G. V., Shaffer, R. D., Anderson, R. S., et al.: Cardiovascular disease in the Masai. J. Atherosclerosis Res. *4*:289, 1964.
23. Morris, J. H.: Occupation and coronary heart disease. Arch. Intern. Med. *104*:903, 1959.
24. Morris, J. N., Heady, J. A., Raffle, P. A., Roberts, C., and Parks, J.: Coronary heart disease and physical activity of work. Lancet *2*:1053, 1953.
25. Paffenbarger, R. S., Jr.: Physical Activity and Fatal Heart Attack: Protection or Selection? *In* E. A. Amsterdam, J. H. Wilmore, and A. N. DeMaria (eds.) *Exercise in Cardiovascular Health and Disease*. New York, Yorke Medical Books, 1977.
26. Phillips, R. L., Lilienfeld, A. M., Diamond, E. L., and Kagan, A.: Frequency of coronary heart disease and cerebrovascular accidents in parents and sons of coronary heart disease index cases and controls. Am. J. Epidemiol. *100*:87, 1974.
27. Pollock, M. L., Wilmore, J. H., and Fox, S. M., III: *Health and Fitness Through Physical Activity*. New York, John Wiley & Sons, 1978.
28. Schaefer, O.: Vigorous exercise and coronary heart disease. Lancet *1*:840, 1973.
29. Taylor, H. L., et al.: Death rates among physically active and sedentary employees of the railroad industry. Am. J. Public Health *52*:1697, 1962.
30. Zukel, W. J., Lewis, R. H., Enterline, P. E., et al.: A short-term community study of the epidemiology of coronary heart disease: a preliminary report on the North Dakota study. Am. J. Public Health *49*:1630, 1959.

Chapter 4

Strength and Muscular Endurance

INTRODUCTION

Muscle strength and muscle endurance, although different components of fitness, are highly related in many activities. Although the methods for best development of each differ, as do the specific changes evoked with training, the two are very interrelated in many exercise programs. Strictly speaking, muscle strength is concerned with the ability of a muscle group to contract against a resistance, as in the amount of weight moved or in breaking strength in holding against a resistance. It usually is determined by a single maximal contraction. The emphasis is on the amount of resistance overcome. Muscle endurance, on the other hand, is the ability of the same muscle group to make repeated contractions against a defined resistance, or to sustain a defined muscular contraction. The emphasis is on the number of repetitions performed or the time of continued contraction. Thus, it is entirely possible for any one calisthenic exercise, e.g., push-ups, to be a heavy strength involvement for one individual, a good muscular endurance exercise for another, and perhaps neither for a third. Asking each person in an exercise program to perform 20 push-ups may require vastly different work loads for different individuals within the group.

Muscle size and muscle strength are related. Throughout history, references are made to the size, strength, and abilities of warriors and sportsmen. Men have known for thousands of years that hard work and vigorous training increase muscle strength and bulk (hypertrophy). Females traditionally have not shared the male enthusiasm for strength development, and only recently have begun to understand its importance to performance, health, and appearance. Many women share the misconception that a weight-training program will have them qualifying as a football fullback in a few months; many men wish it could be accomplished that easily. It appears that the amount of strength and muscle hypertrophy that can be expected from an optimal strength development program varies both within the same person from muscle to muscle, and from individual to individual. Differences in muscle strength between individuals and between the sexes can be partially explained by combinations of the following three influences: (1) amount of muscle tissue; (2) amount of androgens available (primarily testosterone); and (3) cultural or social influences.

Individuals are born with different numbers of muscle cells (fibers), and in the adult these numbers are not likely to change. Although there is some evidence of longitudinal splitting of muscle cells in experimental animals, hypertrophy via an increase in myofibrils is the usual response. Women on the average have fewer muscle fibers than the average man; however, there is considerable variation in both men and women.

Variations in muscle tissue are evidenced by various attempts such as W. H. Sheldon's somatotype system, used to quantify the amount of different body components. He recognized three components: linearity; muscularity; and roundness or soft tissue. Within each of these components, he rated persons on a scale of one to seven for the amount of each component. Certainly a slight person with a muscularity (mesomorphic) rating of "one" would not have the strength potential of a "seven" with a maximal muscularity rating. Individuals differ in the number of muscle fibers (cells) within a muscle, and muscles within an individual differ in their number of fibers. Later modifications of the somatotype system by Barbara Heath and J. E. L. Carter rely heavily on muscle size measurements in assessing the strength of the mesomorphic rating.

The trainability of adult male muscle appears greater than that of the young adult female. It has been estimated that women on the average have about two-thirds the strength of men, and that this difference is primarily due to an over-all difference in total muscle mass, not to differences in muscle force exerted in kilograms per square centimeter of muscle tissue. Although muscle strength per cross-sectional area is similar for males and females (3 to 4 kg/cm^2), the total muscle mass in males may be as much as 50 per cent greater than that in females. In addition, the number of nuclei in the skeletal muscle of males begins to exceed the number in female muscle at the time of puberty, and this difference continues to increase into young adulthood. Since the nucleus is involved in protein production, it has been hypothesized that the difference is related to the increased strength trainability for male muscle.

Another very important influence in strength development is the presence of the male sex hormones (androgens, primarily testosterone from the testes), which vary greatly between the sexes and also somewhat within the sexes. It has been reported that only testosterone and androstenedione are present in sufficient quantity to have strong influences on muscle trainability. In adult males the secretion rates are 5 to 10 mg/day for testosterone and 1 to 2 mg/day for androstenedione; the corresponding rates for women are less then 0.1 mg testosterone and 2 to 4 mg androstenedione. Testosterone is approximately five times more powerful than androstenedione, and therefore appears to be the primary influence for the male. However, for the female, androstenedione may be more important. These hormones are primarily secreted by the gonads, but androstenedione is also secreted by the adrenal glands. Blood serum testosterone levels in adult males range from 333.7 to 848.1 ng/dl and in adult females from 32.8 to 121.5 ng/dl. Lower levels have been noted in high school students.

Other sex differences appear at least related to, if not caused by, higher levels of anabolic hormones in males vs. lower levels in females. A greater percentage of fat is found in females. In the average young adult, the male usually exhibits 10 to 15 per cent of his body weight as fat, whereas in the female the corresponding value is 20 to 25 per cent. In addition, the over-all body size of the female is less, which in itself is a significant performance factor. Females appear to have a better tolerance for low environmental temperatures, but begin sweating at lower body temperatures, and do not appear to tolerate high environmental temperature as well as males. Higher muscle glycogen levels are reported in animals with greater testosterone. Other sex differences occur in the oxygen transport systems, and these are discussed in Chapter 5.

Because testosterone is known to stimulate the protein-synthesizing apparatus, whereas estrogen has a slight atrophying effect, the increase in muscle bulk and lean body mass traditionally has been associated with puberty in males, or more specifically, with greater amounts of testosterone from the testes. When prepubertal boys and girls are observed, differences in strength are small. However, postpubertal differences are quite large, approximately 33 per cent. Although some of this influence has been attributed to cultural patterns, much has been associated with androgens.

The influence of cultural expectations, aided by some misconceptions about muscle hypertrophy, probably has had a significant effect on the strength-developing activities of women. Perhaps we can improve on the very narrow sex roles traditionally accepted. "Girls wear pink, like dolls and other indoor activities, are allowed to cry, do not like sports, and are not strong!" "Boys, on the other hand, wear blue, enjoy outdoor activities and sports, do not enjoy cooking or sewing, and are strong!" Although these roles have become much less limiting, many cultural influences still affect the activity patterns of both males and females. The unfortunate and usual effect for the female has been to make her less physically fit.

Although men's athletic records in almost all cases are better than women's, and few if any women are able to compete realistically in athletic contests on an equal basis with young adult male athletes, even in other cultures, there are some examples of physically demanding tasks in which women have excelled. Two of these have been reported by Edington and Edgerton. One is a group of women divers off the coast of Korea and Japan, especially Cheju Island, who are better able to tolerate the particular set of conditions: depths of 20 meters, long dive times, and winter temperatures near 0°C in air and 10°C in water. The other example concerns the tea pluckers of Sri Lanka, who reportedly carry baskets of picked tea leaves that weigh approximately 40 per cent of the body weight on steep mountainsides at elevations exceeding 5000 feet. The men of this culture are involved in less demanding tasks of general maintenance of the tea plantations.

Another factor that affects the amount of strength gain to be expected by an individual depends partly on the level of strength at the onset of the program. Those who have no previous participation in a strength development program can anticipate rather large percentage increases, whereas those with high-level strength at the beginning can expect very small increases. However, it should be noted that animal studies have shown large increases of 30 to 50 per cent within six days in the rat soleus muscle after the tendon of the synergistic gastrocnemius muscle was cut. This increase in muscle size reflected an increase in muscle protein through greater protein synthesis and reduced protein breakdown. The work-induced muscle hypertrophy in this experimentally contrived overload condition appeared to be independent of the growth, insulin, testosterone, and thyroid hormones. The increase in size was also demonstrated in fasting animals who generally were losing over-all muscle tissue. These animal studies seem to indicate that skeletal and cardiac muscle may not have as limited a growth capacity as traditionally has been accepted.

Even though strength gain differences do exist, diligently applied effort according to the methods suggested in this text will produce significant gains in most persons. Generally, significant strength gains in the beginner can be noted after three or four weeks of training, five periods per week. In other words, 15 to 20 exercise periods usually produce noticeable gains. Beyond that point, gains tend to accrue less dramatically, and eventually level off, with relatively smaller weekly increases.

Many fitness programs have concentrated solely on the development of strength because of its very significant contribution to general body tone and appearance. Obviously, such programs are shortsighted, but strength is an important prerequisite to some other fitness qualities. Sufficient strength and endurance of the antigravity musculature is the foundation for proper posture. Strengthening the musculature surrounding joints is also important to the prevention of injury. The joints and connective tissue also respond to a strength and muscle endurance program by becoming stronger; at least, this effect has been demonstrated in the male. An active person can expect stronger ligaments connecting bones within the joints and stronger muscle attachments to bone through tendons.

The amount of strength desired varies greatly from the weight-lifter and various other athletes to the individual mainly concerned about body posture and appearance. Many women entering a conditioning program express a desire to lose weight and firm their bodies, and are not interested in a strength program. However, through proper instruction and/or experience with a strength program, they generally are quite satisfied with the body contour and firmness resulting from such a program. Weight control is another issue. The best procedure for avoiding ''flabby'' body areas is strength exercise. The specific requirements for various sport activities vary with the type of activity and specific musculature involved. Therefore, a general strength program is suggested here.

The development of strength is highly specific. If strength is desired in a particular muscle, that particular muscle must be exercised (SAID principle). Although there is a tendency for a person with a large number of muscle fibers in one muscle to have a large number in another, the training effect is specific to the muscle group involved and type of training. The body responds specifically to metabolic needs by selective hypertrophy of muscles needed for specific purposes, and by atrophy of inactive tissues that are metabolically expensive and physiologically unnecessary.

Although most individuals will want to adapt a strength program to their particular needs and interests, several muscle groups not generally used in everyday activities should receive special attention in most programs. The antigravity muscles also must receive emphasis because of their major role in general movement and body configuration. Therefore, we can conclude that most programs must strengthen the posterior upper

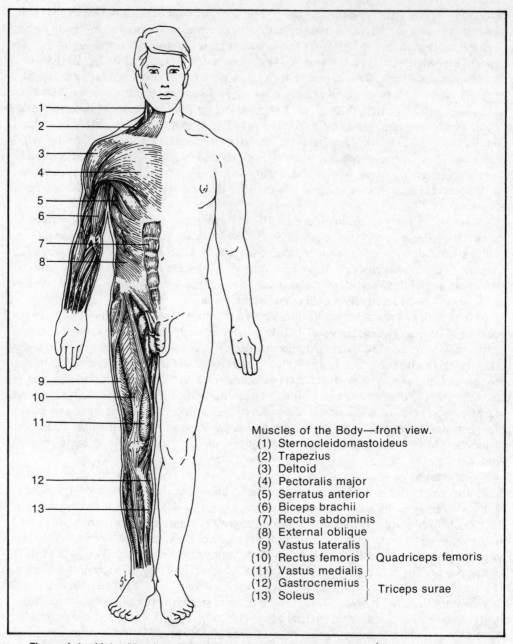

Figure 4–1. Major Muscles of the Human Body—Front View. The gastrocnemius and soleus muscles comprise the antigravity group known as the triceps surae, and the rectus femoris, vastus lateralis, and vastus medialis are part of the quadriceps femoris group. The vastus intermedius, also part of the quadriceps femoris group, lies directly underneath the rectus femoris.

arm, the upper back muscles, the middle and lower back muscles, the abdominals and lateral trunk muscles, the posterior thigh muscles, the posterior hip, and the anterior thigh. (See Figs. 4–1, 4–2, and 4–9ff for locations and specific names of the major skeletal muscles. See also Fig. 2–5 for specific identification of the antigravity muscles.)

All of these except the posterior upper arm, lateral trunk muscles, and posterior thigh muscles are included in the grouping known as the antigravity muscles. Their

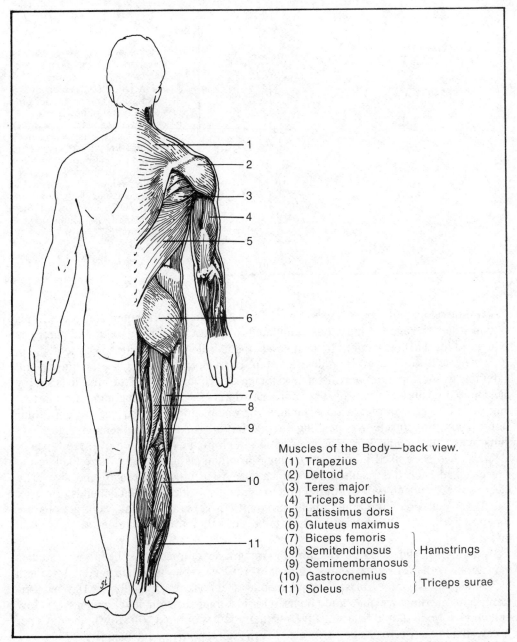

Muscles of the Body—back view.
(1) Trapezius
(2) Deltoid
(3) Teres major
(4) Triceps brachii
(5) Latissimus dorsi
(6) Gluteus maximus
(7) Biceps femoris
(8) Semitendinosus   } Hamstrings
(9) Semimembranosus
(10) Gastrocnemius   } Triceps surae
(11) Soleus

Figure 4–2. Major Muscles of the Human Body—Back View. The gastrocnemius and soleus muscles comprise the antigravity group known as the triceps surae. The biceps femoris, semitendinosus, and semimembranosus are called collectively the hamstrings. They flex the knee and extend the hip.

importance was explained in Chapter 2, pp. 21 and 22. The other muscles listed here for major emphasis in a conditioning program are large muscles that are not stressed to any great extent in daily activities, or even in many sports. Thus, they tend to be relatively weak in comparison with the other large muscles.

The fundamental principle of strength development is overload. Strength increase, although affected by the previously discussed factors of androgen levels and amount of

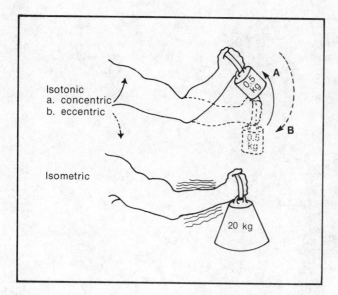

Isotonic
a. concentric
b. eccentric

Isometric

Figure 4-3. Types of Muscle Contraction. The top figure illustrates two isotonic contractions: *A,* a concentric contraction of the muscles in the anterior upper arm to move the weight upward; and *B,* an eccentric or antigravity contraction in the same muscles to slowly lower the weight. An isometric contraction in the bottom limb will not result in limb movement because the weight is too heavy for the muscle to lift. (Adapted from Ganong, W. F.: *The Nervous System.* Los Altos, CA, Lange Medical Publications, 1977, p. 37.)

existing development, appears to be a work-induced process. A strengthening exercise is one in which the agonist muscle is stimulated to contract against a load, and energy is expended for that contraction. In most cases, the muscle is attempting to shorten, and in a concentric isotonic exercise it does shorten. In an isometric exercise, the muscle still attempts to shorten, but the resistance is too great to overcome, or the muscle is simply held tense by volitional control. Therefore, no appreciable movement or muscle shortening occurs. The contractile unit remains the same length. In an eccentric isotonic contraction, the muscle is expending energy, but is gradually lengthening. Figure 4-3 illustrates isotonic and isometric contraction in elbow flexion. Each of these types of exercise has been used in strength training programs as a method of overloading the muscle, and each has resulted in significant gains in muscle strength and size. The decision about which type of contraction to use in a specific situation depends primarily on the objectives of the conditioning program. In general, isotonic contractions are favored by most strength training experts because they utilize a greater range of joint motion.

Another prolific area for research in strength development has been those studies concerned with the optimal combination of exercise variables to obtain maximal strength development. Examples of such experimental questions are as follows: (1) What percentage of maximal weight should be used for maximal strength development? (2) How many repetitions should be used? (3) How many sets is optimal? (4) How many days per week should the exercises be performed? Although tentative conclusions can be drawn from the review of research with these variables, a precise answer to each question is not yet available, especially when we consider that individuals may respond differently to various programs.

TYPES OF MUSCLE CONTRACTION AND TRAINING TECHNIQUES

Isometric Exercise

The development of strength by isometric methods has received widespread attention in recent years. This is largely due to the fact that strength is gained without bodily movement, and therefore the casual observer has assumed that no effort is required to perform such exercises. For many years, isometric exercise was popularized as the Charles Atlas "dynamic tension" program. It was not until 1953 that much serious scientific attention was given to this form of exercise. At that time, T. Hettinger and E. A. Müller of Germany reported several studies and observations on isometric exercise. Their method utilized static contractions applied at two-thirds maximal effort and held for 6 seconds. They reported that no further effort was required to yield gains of approximately 5 per cent per week above the beginning level. Subsequent investigations in the U.S. failed to verify such dramatic increases, and later studies by Müller and Rohmert showed weekly increases lower than those in the original studies. Furthermore, the later studies used maximal contractions with as much as 5 seconds' effort. More recent investigations have employed maximal efforts with varying amounts of time, and have demonstrated significant gains in strength. On the basis of these and similar studies, it appears that one maximal contraction held for 6 to 8 seconds is sufficient for maximal strength development in isometric training programs.

Although many research studies have demonstrated that strength can be increased by utilizing isometric contractions, the effect on sports performance is questionable. The strength gains appear to be limited primarily to the specific joint angle at which the isometric contraction occurs. Therefore, these gains do not transfer to increased strength throughout the range of motion, and they do not provide for improvement in the performance of isotonic skills. Also, there appears to be little increase in muscular endurance consequent to an isometric training program. Furthermore, there is little, if any, increase in cardiovascular function as a result of isometric training. The physiological training effect of isometric contractions thus appears to be limited solely to the strength aspect of fitness.

Unless there is a need to restrict joint movement, the use of isotonic contractions usually is preferred in conditioning programs. This preference is based on the fact that isometric exercises tend to develop strength at specific joint angles used for the exercise rather than throughout the full range of joint motion. Not exercising the full range of motion results in specific strength development for a particular joint angle and in less flexibility than with isotonic exercises, which utilize considerable movement at the joints. If, for some reason, one must omit or limit joint movement, isometric strength

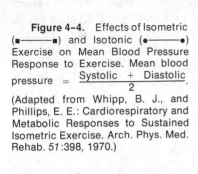

Figure 4–4. Effects of Isometric (■———■) and Isotonic (●———●) Exercise on Mean Blood Pressure Response to Exercise. Mean blood pressure $= \dfrac{Systolic + Diastolic}{2}$.
(Adapted from Whipp, B. J., and Phillips, E. E.: Cardiorespiratory and Metabolic Responses to Sustained Isometric Exercise. Arch. Phys. Med. Rehab. *51*:398, 1970.)

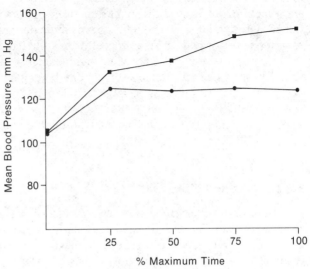

development can be invaluable. Otherwise, isotonic strength development is recommended.

Another reason is health-related. Most physical educators and physicians do not recommend isometric programs for persons over 30 years old unless they also are involved in a cardiovascular endurance program, and even then an isotonic strength program is preferred. It appears that the holding of maximal contractions tends to occlude blood flow through contracting muscles, significantly elevating blood pressure and hindering return of venous blood to the heart. This effect is particularly dangerous in persons with atherosclerosis, arteriosclerosis, high blood pressure, or other vascular problems. In contrast, the rhythmic contraction and relaxation of isotonic exercise is a valuable aid in venous return to the heart, and mean blood pressure elevations are less (Fig. 4–4). Although it is important to hold isometric contractions for the full 6 to 8 seconds for optimal strength development, holding for longer than 10 seconds does not result in additional strength gains and greatly increases the blood occlusion problem.

Isotonic Exercise

Concentric Isotonic Exercise

The type of exercise most widely applied and preferred for general use in the development of high levels of strength has been concentric isotonic exercise. Scientific investigations of weight-training procedures for the development of strength began with the work of Thomas DeLorme in the 1940s. At first, he proposed the use of 70 to 100 repetitions using weights, the repetitions being performed in sets of ten each. Originally terming this "heavy resistance exercise," he subsequently changed the name of the system to "progressive resistance exercise." Later, it was suggested that the original number of repetitions was too high and that 20 were sufficient for each exercise. The DeLorme method consists of determining by trial and error the most weight that can be lifted for ten repetitions. This is then called 10 RM, or ten repetitions maximum. The exercises are then performed in sets or bouts of ten repetitions each. The first bout is with one-half the 10 RM, the second with three-fourths 10 RM, and the last with the 10 RM. Most isotonic strength development programs currently in use employ this procedure or some modification of progressive resistance exercise. In general, modifications are in the total number of repetitions performed. Richard Berger, studying variations of resistance and repetitions, reported that 6 RM for three bouts yielded the greatest strength gains. Other investigations, when summarized, indicate that the use of one bout of five to 15 repetitions performed with maximal effort is sufficient for each exercise period. A greater number of repetitions does not yield significantly greater strength gains. In general, the use of progressive resistance exercise can be expected to result in significant strength gains over a wide range of resistance (60 to 100 per cent of the RM) and number of repetitions (2 RM for one set to 10 RM for three sets). The most widely accepted program appears to be Berger's three sets of 6 RM, but the number of RMs may vary from four to ten.

Eccentric Isotonic Exercise

Isotonic progressive resistance exercise normally contains two types of muscle contraction: (1) the uplift or power phase, in which the muscle shortens against a load; and (2) the lowering portion of the load, in which the same muscle is resisting gravity and gradually "letting the weight down," as illustrated in Figure 4–3. For example, if a person performs a bench press on the Universal Gym (Fig. 4–28*B*), moving the bar up is the concentric contraction. If one then drops the weights and lets the bar fall freely (certainly not a recommended procedure), the eccentric contraction would be omitted. If the weights are gradually returned to the starting position, an eccentric contraction is performed. The eccentric contraction explains why the same muscle group is controlling two opposite movements. For example, in arm curls (Figs. 4–3, 4–21), the biceps brachii is working concentrically as the elbow is flexed (upward movement) and eccentrically as the elbow is extended (downward movement). Thus, in this instance, the biceps brachii is contracting in both flexion and extension movements. These two types of contraction occur in almost all weight-training and calisthenic exercises.

Beside explaining a muscle's involvement in a particular exercise, exercise physiologists have been concerned with differentiating between concentric and eccentric contractions in their effect on strength development. Generally, it appears as if strength can be gained using either type of contraction. Strength improvements have been noted in both types of movement, but neither has been shown to be superior to the other. Since little is known about the training effect of eccentric programs, and most training apparatus is not designed to differentiate between the two movements in isotonic exercise, no *specific* eccentric program will be presented in this text.

Isokinetic Exercise (Accommodating Resistance Exercise)

A little over ten years ago, James J. Perrine, a bioengineering consultant, introduced a new concept of resistive exercise in which a special training device attached to the limb controls motion at a predetermined speed, and allows maximal resistance instead of increased acceleration throughout a range of joint motion. This form of contraction is referred to as "isokinetic exercise." No matter how much force the individual applies, the speed will not accelerate, thus allowing maximal resistance to be applied throughout the movement. In isotonic exercises, the speed is controlled by the individual, and the load remains constant throughout the range of motion. This limits the maximal stress of the exercise to the resistance that can be overcome at the weakest point in the range of motion. Because the resistance that can be overcome varies depending on the joint angle, there are resulting acceleration changes in the movement. In isokinetic exercise, the resistance offered by the machine matches the individual's capability throughout the range of motion. The resistance thus is said to accommodate. If maximal muscular force is applied throughout the movement, the lever arm remains at its preset, constant, motor-driven speed. Although there is not a great deal of experimental evidence, that available does support a superiority of isokinetic training and, more specifically, high-speed isokinetic training. It also has been reported that isokinetic training does not result in the initial muscle soreness commonly experienced early in more traditional programs. Obviously, isokinetic training involves special training devices that may not be available to the average student. For this reason, no specific isokinetic programs are presented in this text.

MUSCULAR STRENGTH/ENDURANCE RELATIONSHIPS

The major emphasis in optimal strength development is on the amount of resistance used to overload the muscle, but in muscular endurance work the emphasis shifts to the number of repetitions of a movement. Although the optimal programs for developing each are specific to the component, strength and muscular endurance are interrelated. How long a weight can be held, or how many repetitions of a movement can be made, surely depends on the percentage of maximal contractile force demanded by the exercise. For example, in absolute muscular endurance, a defined weight (e.g., 50 lbs) is moved. In this instance, muscular endurance is highly dependent on the strength of the individual, and improving strength will increase muscular endurance. Strength, however, is less related to relative endurance in which the number of repetitions or holding time is measured against a relative workload, e.g., 40 per cent of maximal strength. For example, if a 50-lb resistance must be overcome by two persons with different maximal strengths (e.g., 70 and 80 lbs for the exercise involved), the stronger person (80 lbs) will exhibit greater endurance. The reason is that, when the individual with 80 lbs max strength overcomes the 50-lb resistance, he is using only 62.5 per cent of his available strength, whereas the 70-lb strength individual is using 71 per cent. The weaker person has to recruit 10 to 15 per cent more motor units with each contraction. The motor units thus are working more and will fatigue at a faster rate. Therefore, improvements in strength will improve muscular endurance. This type of situation is termed "absolute endurance."

In situations of relative endurance in which each individual overcomes a resistance that is the same percentage of whatever the maximal strengths are, strength and endurance are not strongly related. In fact, it is even possible in that situation for high-strength individuals to exhibit less endurance than those of lower strength.

When the adaptations within the muscle as a result of training are considered, different training adaptations of muscle strength and muscle endurance are found. Increased blood flow during exercise as a result of muscle endurance training has been reported. In the muscle hypertrophy associated with increased strength, an increase in the contractile proteins of the muscle is evident. Myofibrils are also added to individual muscle cells. The changes associated with muscle endurance training primarily involve increases in the mechanisms within the muscle responsible for aerobic metabolism (more energy for repeated contractions) and additional functional capillary networks within the muscle (better blood flow in the muscle resulting in increased transport of nutrients and removal of waste from muscle cells). For example, it has been reported that endurance training increases the levels of over 20 enzymes that enhance capacity to use fatty acids as a fuel for muscle contraction. There is also an increase in mitochondrial mass per gram of trained muscle. (The mitochondria are the sites of oxidative metabolism in the muscle cell.) Changes in enzymes involved in anaerobic metabolism have not been demonstrated to any significant extent with either endurance or strength training.

Another example of this specificity of training is in the type of muscle fiber most heavily involved in the particular exercise. Human skeletal muscle has at least two types of muscle fiber, and possibly three: fast-twitch glycolytic (powerful, fast-fatiguing fibers), possibly fast-twitch oxidative (powerful, intermediate-fatiguing fibers), and slow-twitch oxidative (low-tension or -power, but slow-fatiguing fibers). These types of fiber differ in several ways: the size of the motoneuronal cell body controlling the muscle fibers; their enzymatic profiles; and their speed and strength of contraction. There is considerable evidence that the fiber types are selectively used in different types of movement. Heavy-strength involvement uses a greater proportion of fast-twitch, fast-fatiguing fibers, whereas endurance exercise involves more intermediate- and slow-fatiguing fibers.

Although it appears that the proportion of these fiber types varies within individuals, and especially among athletes in certain sports, the evidence as to whether training produces these differences or maximizes a predominant genetic endowment is still speculative. Current data favor the genetic explanation. However, significant training alterations in the oxidative capacity of fibers have been reported. Changes in the anaerobic (glycolytic) capacity do not appear to be significant.

It would seem that training adaptations, and thus optimal training procedures, are better if divided into more classifications than simply those of strength or muscle endurance. It is more likely that strength and endurance are really two points on a continuum of muscular contraction. Perrine described four categories of classification based on mechanical demands of common movements in muscular work: (1) a low-contraction speed, strength component; (2) a high-contraction speed, strength component; (3) a muscle endurance capacity for relatively high-rate, short-duration component; and (4) a muscle endurance capacity for relatively low-rate, extended-duration component. His approach is somewhat similar to one taken by Edington and Edgerton, who described the continuum very practically in terms of time duration of athletic events, as follows: 0 to 1 second—strength; 1 to 10 seconds—high power; 10 to 30 seconds—power; 30 seconds to 2 minutes—power endurance; 2 to 5 minutes—endurance; and longer— high endurance (Fig. 4–5). Using such classification systems as these, strength now takes on more meaning than slow maximal contraction, and endurance more than mere repetition of movement. If a person desires to maximize a particular combination of muscle strength and endurance, the training should involve most specifically that type of movement.

Behavioral studies involving muscle endurance training are complicated by a lack of any standardization in tests of endurance and training programs. Research on muscle endurance is less voluminous than strength research and very contradictory. The traditional programs for muscle endurance have involved an emphasis on the number of contractions—low resistance and high repetitions. Most programs have adjusted load and number of repetitions to subjectively fatigue the individual in a range of 20 to 100 repetitions. In light of the previous discussion, the load, speed of contractions, and number of repetitions should reflect the particular interests of the individual. Muscle hypertrophy is best accomplished at the strength end of the continuum, whereas the ability to make continued specific movements is gained at the endurance end of the continuum. Figure 4–6 presents an alternative way of viewing the exercise continuum of Figure 4–5 as it relates specifically to weight training.

Figure 4–5. Classification Scheme in Terms of Strength, Power, and Endurance for Physical Activities of Various Time Durations. Zero to 1 second (strength), 1 to 10 seconds (high power), 10 to 30 seconds (power), 30 seconds to 2 minutes (power-endurance), 2 to 5 minutes (endurance), over 5 minutes (high endurance). (From *The Biology of Physical Activity*. By Edington, D. W., and Edgerton, V. R. Copyright © 1976 by the Houghton Mifflin Company. Reprinted by permission of the publisher.)

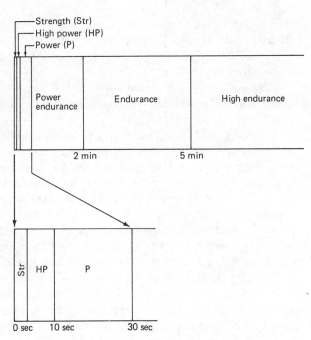

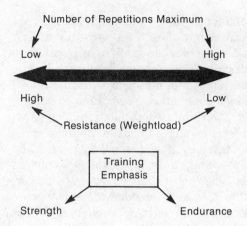

Figure 4-6. The Strength–Endurance Continuum. As the resistance increases, the number of repetitions maximum of necessity must be lower. Conversely, when resistance is low, repetitions maximum can be higher. A low number of repetitions maximum with high resistance emphasizes primarily strength. A high number of repetitions with a low resistance is primarily an endurance exercise. Both strength and endurance can be emphasized by an exercise in the 6 to 12 repetitions maximum range.

MUSCULAR STRENGTH AND ENDURANCE EXERCISES

Important Considerations

Warm-Up. Precede strengthening exercises with adequate warm-up and accompany with a flexibility program.

Number of Repetitions for Strength. Between six and 12 repetitions should be used; if the exercise cannot be performed at least six times, the weight should be decreased. If it can be performed more than 12 times, the resistance should be increased. At least two sets, preferably three, should be used each work-out period.

The Strength Plateau. When the tolerance for exercise has reached a very high level, only small gains can be expected. Often, no appreciable gains can be demonstrated; thus, a plateau is reached. In order to surpass the plateau, the regular work-out program can be supplemented with one of the following.

1. About once a week, attempt to lift a weight slightly heavier than would be used for one RM.

2. About once a week, "cheat" by moving through a comfortable range of motion with a slightly-heavier-than-maximal weight.

Regularity. Exercise at least three times per week, and usually not more than five, for strength.

Range of Motion. Normally perform the exercise throughout a comfortable range of motion. Do not "force" the movement. For safety, use flexibility procedures to increase the range of motion, *not weights*.

Breathing. There is a tendency to hold the breath during extreme efforts to overcome heavy resistances. This may be hazardous, as under these conditions the abdominal muscles contract and the glottis closes. Pressures in thoracic and abdominal areas are drastically increased by the breath being held. This pressure inhibits the venous return of blood to the heart, causing a fall in blood pressure. Arterial pressure decrease results in a reflex increase in the rate of the heart beat. After the effort of overcoming the heavy resistance, venous flow surges into the heart, causing an increase in blood pressure in the pulmonary pathways. At this time, the systolic blood pressure may rise to nearly twice its normal level. This effect is known as the Valsalva phenomenon.

Although this phenomenon may not be a hazard to someone with a normal, healthy circulatory apparatus, the possibility exists that medically undetected weaknesses in the system may be present. Therefore, in order to lessen the intensity of this potential hazard, it is recommended that the individual maintain an open glottis by breathing during the most difficult phase of the exercise. Also, by performing several repetitions with a lighter weight than could be lifted with one maximal effort, it is believed that the Valsalva phenomenon is less likely to result in injury.

It must be understood, however, that the way in which one breathes has nothing to do with the development of strength, but that maintenance of an open glottis is important only as a safety factor.

Maintenance of Strength. Once desired levels of strength are reached through a strength training program, the principle of progression need not apply. In order to maintain such levels, an increase in demand is not necessary; it is sufficient to work out about twice a week at the resistances used when the desired strength level was reached.

Use of Isometric Exercises. Although isotonic exercises normally are preferred, you may wish to perform isometric exercises.

1. Use a maximal contraction.

2. Hold each exercise the full 6 to 8 seconds, but no longer than 10 seconds. Holding for longer periods very significantly elevates blood pressure owing to occlusion of blood flow through the contracting muscles (see p. 67).

3. Perform each exercise two or three times per exercise session.

4. Isometric exercises are not recommended for persons over 30 years of age or with known vascular disease (see p. 67).

Number of Repetitions for Muscular Endurance. Perform each exercise a minimum of 20 times per set, two or three sets. A maximal number of repetitions should be set according to the specific desire of the individual. Adjust the resistance according to the number of repetitions.

Other Safety Precautions

1. Use chalk to avoid wet hands caused by perspiration. Chalk blocks in the form of carbonate of magnesium are available from gymnastic supply companies.

2. Use rubber soled shoes for safe footing and wear cotton clothing to absorb perspiration.

3. Be certain that detachable equipment is securely attached before lifting the weights. Metal plates should never be placed on the ends of bars without the use of collars. Many injuries result from insecurely attached equipment falling on the feet and legs.

4. The beginner especially should not attempt to overcome more resistance than can be safely handled. It is a wise procedure to begin with about 10 lbs less than one feels can be successfully overcome.

5. The use of spotters when performing such exercises as bench presses and squats is essential, particularly when heavy loads are lifted. Racks to hold the weight before the exercise help to eliminate some of the hazard. The development of the Universal Gym and similar machines has been a definite plus factor in this regard.

6. Protect the normal curvature of the back while performing any type of exercise, especially with weights. Severe damage can occur to the intervertebral discs of the spinal column. As the weight is lifted, uneven pressure (as illustrated in Fig. 4–7) is placed on the intervertebral discs, which forces the nucleus pulposus, the fluid-like center of the discs, to project posteriorly. If the discs have any weakness due to previous injury or other causes, they may herniate and exert pressure on the spinal cord. This pressure results in a number of complications that usually require medical attention.

One important protection for the back is to perform exercises with the knees slightly bent (approximately 15 degrees of flexion), never hyperextended (locked in a straight

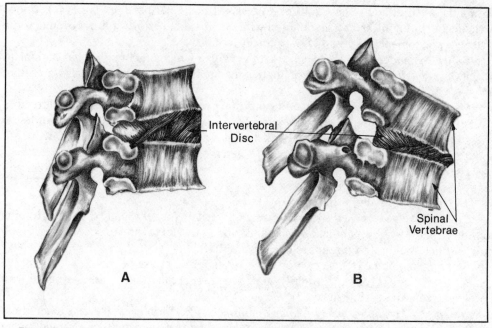

Figure 4–7. Pressure on the Intervertebral Discs During Movements. *A* shows the greater pressure toward the back of the spinal disc in hyperextension of the back. *B* illustrates the increased pressure toward the front of the disc in flexion movements. Because of these unequal pressures on the discs, the proper position of the low back is even more important when working with weights. The illustration shows thoracic (midback) vertebrae. Shifting of the intervertebral discs is even more of a problem with the lumbar vertebrae of the lower back. (Adapted from MacConaill, M. A., and Basmajian, J. V.: *Muscles and Movements: A Basis for Human Kinesiology.* Baltimore, Williams and Wilkins Co., 1969, p. 154.)

position). One common fault in performing weight-training exercises is to attempt to lift weights from the floor while standing with the knees locked in hyperextension and the hips bent to approximately 90 degrees' flexion. When lifting weights to move them from one place to another, the knees should be bent before the lift is made. This is sometimes called lifting from the number ''4'' rather than from the number ''7'' position (Fig. 4–8) (so-named because the body assumes positions similar to the numbers 4 and 7). When making such a lift, the *legs* and *not the back* should perform most of the action.

Another protection for the back is to develop strong abdominal muscles, and exercise with them in a shortened (slightly contracted) position. This position keeps the lower pelvis forward, the hips tucked, and the back flat—extremely important considerations in any exercise. In addition, overdevelopment of the hip flexor muscles (flexors of the leg on the anterior hip and upper thigh) should be avoided because these muscles (primarily the psoas major and minor) originate on the anterior surface of the lumbar vertebrae (see Fig. 4–9), and thus pull the back toward an exaggerated lumbar curvature (sway back). For this reason, straight leg sit-ups, double leg lifts, and other similar exercises are not recommended. Flexing the knees during the sit-up flexes the leg at the hip, thus reducing much of the action of the hip flexor muscles during the sit-up and placing more of the action on the abdominal muscles.

Specific Exercises for Muscular Strength and Endurance

For a well-rounded conditioning program, at least one exercise from each category should be chosen. Each category represents a body area and generally a muscle group for

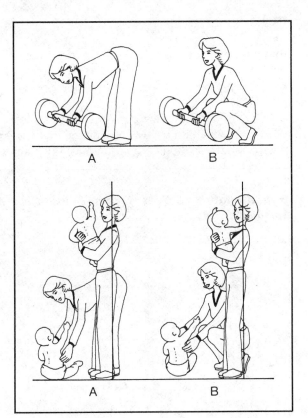

Figure 4–8. Lifting from the Number "4" *(B)* and Number "7" *(A)* Positions. *B* is the preferred position since most of the force is provided by the leg muscles, and the back is kept relatively straight.

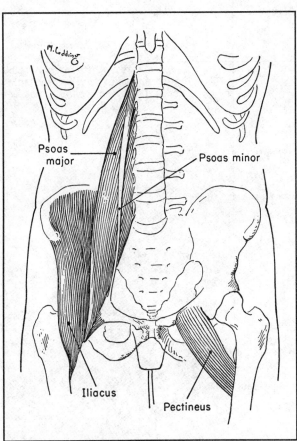

Figure 4–9. The Psoas Major and Minor Muscles. These two muscles are primarily involved in flexion of the upper thigh at the hip. Because they insert on the anterior surfaces of the verterbrae in the low back, over-development of these muscles from such exercises as straight leg sit-ups, double leg lifts, and flexion of the legs from a hanging position may cause an increased lordosis (swayback posture). These types of exercises generally are not recommended. (From Wells, K. F., and Luttgens, K.: *Kinesiology: Scientific Basis of Human Motion.* Philadelphia, W. B. Saunders Co., 1976, p. 151.)

some specific movement. Perform the exercise for either muscular strength and/or muscular endurance, as desired. The guidelines for strength and endurance were presented in previous sections of this chapter. Related concepts are discussed elsewhere in the chapter.

Each of the following sections begins with an illustration of dissected anatomy showing the major muscles conditioned by the exercises included in the section. Where possible, each section contains at least one each of weights, calisthenic, and isometric exercises.

Grip Strength and Wrist Flexors (Anterior Hand and Forearm Muscles)

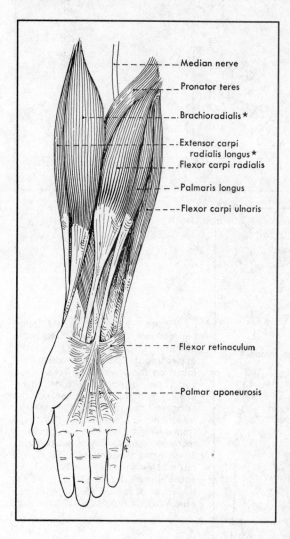

Median nerve

Pronator teres

Brachioradialis ★

Extensor carpi radialis longus ★

Flexor carpi radialis

Palmaris longus

Flexor carpi ulnaris

Flexor retinaculum

Palmar aponeurosis

Figure 4–10. The More Superficial Flexor Muscles of the Right Forearm. The starred muscles are extensor muscles visible from the anterior side. (From Hollinshead, W. H.: *Functional Anatomy of the Limbs and Back.* Philadelphia, W. B. Saunders Co., 1976, p. 151.)

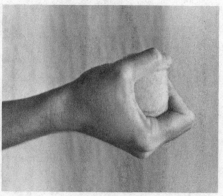

Figure 4–11. Ball Squeezing.

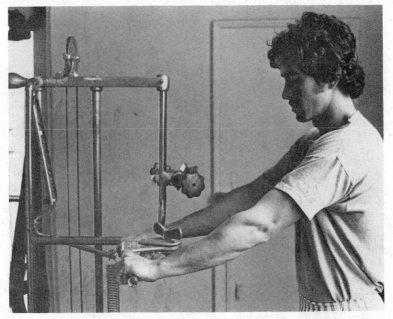

Figure 4–12.   Universal Gym—Hand Grip Stations.

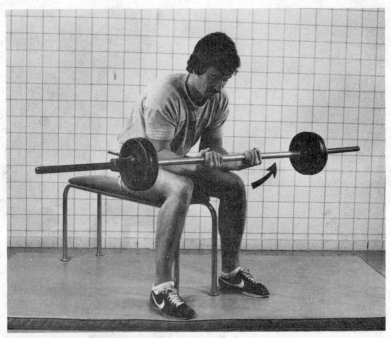

Figure 4–13.   Weights—Wrist Curls. With the forearms resting on the thighs, the wrists are flexed and extended through a full range of motion. With the weight held in the palms-up position, the wrist flexors are stressed. This exercise also may be performed on the curl station of the Universal Gym.

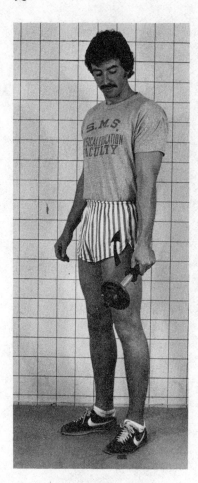

Figure 4–14. Weights. This exercise is used to strengthen the muscles on the thumb side of the wrist. The weight should be raised and lowered without movement of the elbow.

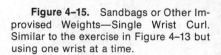

Figure 4–15. Sandbags or Other Improvised Weights—Single Wrist Curl. Similar to the exercise in Figure 4–13 but using one wrist at a time.

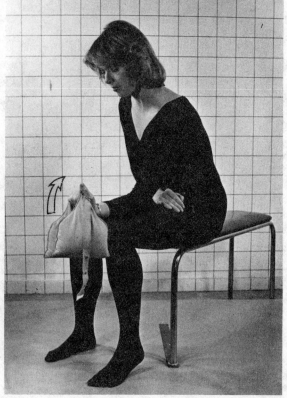

Grip Strength and Wrist Extensors (Posterior Hand and Forearm Muscles)

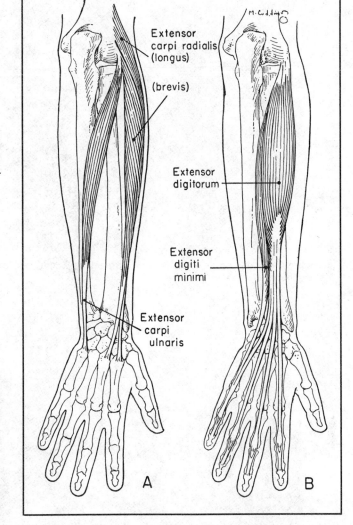

Figure 4–16. Muscles on Back of Right Forearm. (From Wells, K. F., and Luttgens, K.: *Kinesiology.* Philadelphia, W. B. Saunders Co., 1976, p. 123.)

Extensor carpi radialis (longus)

(brevis)

Extensor digitorum

Extensor digiti minimi

Extensor carpi ulnaris

A   B

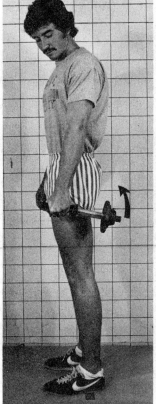

Figure 4–17. This exercise strengthens the muscles on the little finger side of the wrist. The weight should be raised and then lowered without movement of the elbow joint.

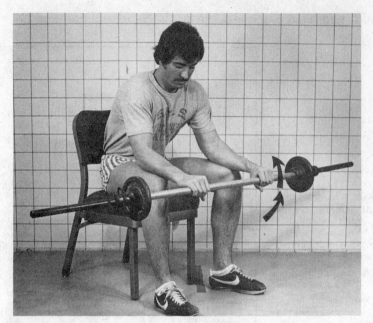

Figure 4–18. Weights—Reverse Wrist Curls. If the weight is held in the palms-down position, the wrist extensors are stressed.

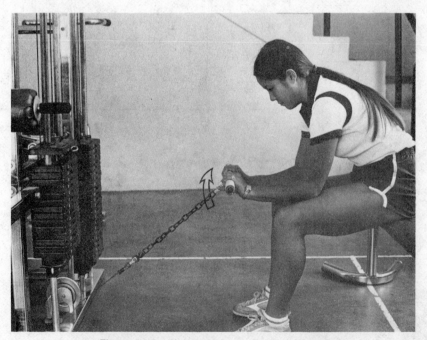

Figure 4–19. Universal Gym—Reverse Wrist Curl.

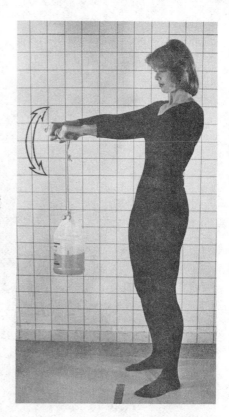

Figure 4–20. Weights—Wrist Roller. A cord connects a bar and a weight. The weight is moved up and down by rolling the cord around the bar. This exercise works both the flexor and extensor muscles of the wrist.

Elbow Flexion [*Anterior Upper Arm (Biceps Brachii and Brachialis Muscles)*]*

*For an illustration of these muscles, see Figure 2–2.

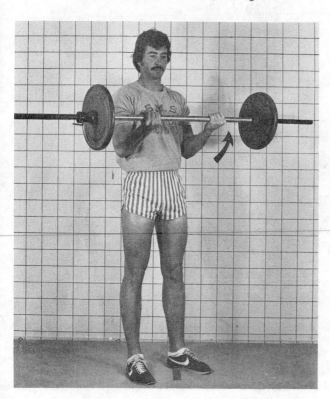

Figure 4–21. Weights—Arm (Biceps) Curls. This exercise strengthens the flexor muscles of the elbow and wrist. The palms-up position intensifies the action of the wrist flexors. If the weight is held with the palms down, greater stress is placed on the extensors of the wrist. As far as strengthening of the elbow flexors is concerned, there is little difference in the two hand positions.

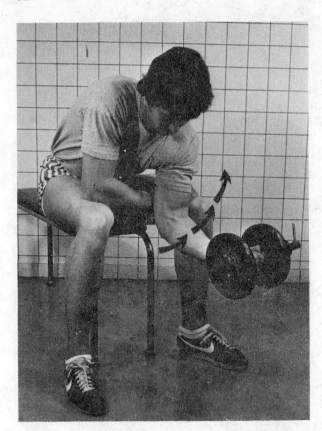

Figure 4–22. Weights—Single Arm (Biceps) Curl.

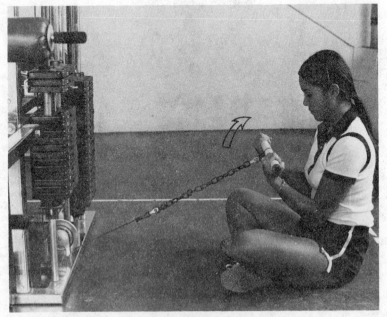

Figure 4–23. Universal Gym—Arm (Biceps) Curls.

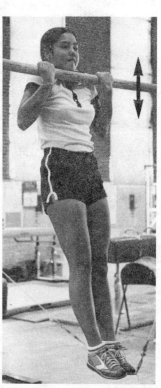

Figure 4–24. Pull-up—Reverse Grip (palms facing exerciser). Although this is an exercise for the back and shoulder muscles, the elbow flexors can be stressed by gripping the bar with the palms facing the exerciser. The body is raised and lowered as many times as possible.

Shoulder Pressing and Elbow Extension Exercises [*Upper Back and Chest Muscles; Superior Shoulder Muscles; Posterior Upper Arm (Triceps Brachii)*]

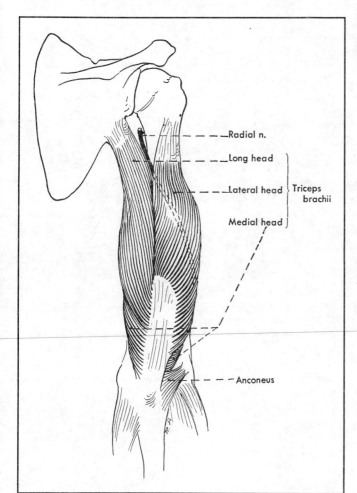

Figure 4–25. Posterior Muscles of the Right Arm. (From Hollinshead, W. H.: *Functional Anatomy of the Limbs and Back*. Philadelphia, W. B. Saunders Co., 1976, p. 131.)

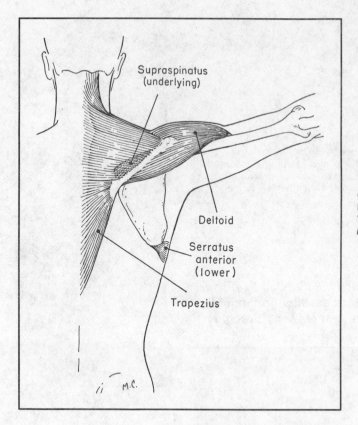

Figure 4–26. Muscles That Contract to Produce Sideward Elevation of the Arm. (From Wells, K. F., and Luttgens, K.: *Kinesiology.* Philadelphia, W. B. Saunders Co., 1976, p. 89.)

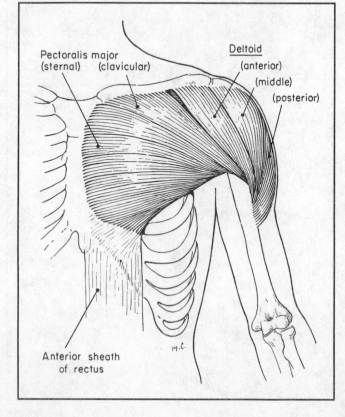

Figure 4–27. Anterior View of Muscles of the Shoulder Joint, Superficial Layer. (From Wells, K. F., and Luttgens, K.: *Kinesiology.* Philadelphia, W. B. Saunders Co., 1976, p. 79.)

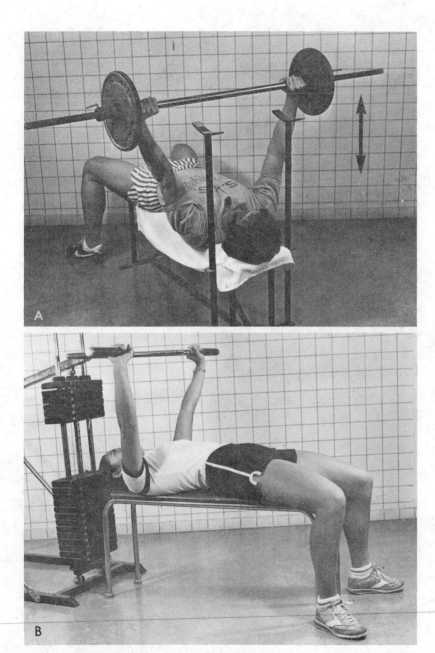

Figure 4–28. Bench Press—*A*, Free Weights; *B*, Bench Press Station on the Universal Gym. The bench press exercise is designed to strengthen the muscles of the chest and the posterior upper arm. In *A*, before one assumes the illustrated position, the barbell should be placed on the rack. Assistance may be required to place the weight in the exercise position as well as to remove it after several repetitions.

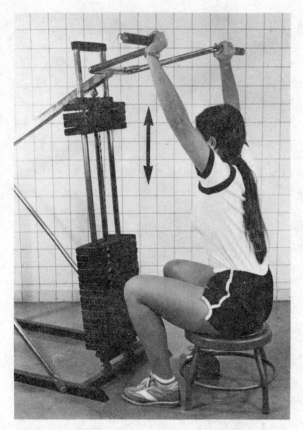

Figure 4–29. Shoulder Press—Press Station on Universal Gym or Free Weights. Although this exercise may be done standing, the sitting position is recommended in order to increase stability and avoid the possibility of excessive strain in the lower back. With the weight in front of the body, effort is concentrated on the anterior shoulder muscles.

Figure 4–30. Shoulder Press—Weights or Press Station on the Universal Gym. An alternate form of the shoulder press exercise, with the weight behind the head to increase emphasis on the elbow extensor muscles.

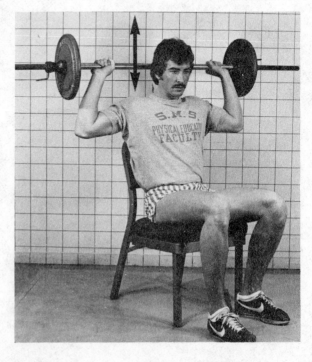

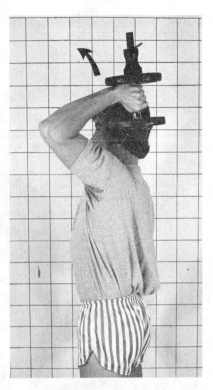

Figure 4-31. Weights. Emphasis is placed specifically on the elbow extensor muscles. The upper arm should remain in a nearly vertical position during the exercise.

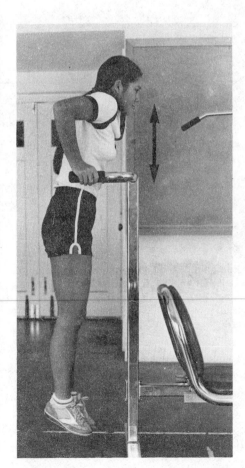

Figure 4-32. Dips—Parallel Bars or Dip Station on the Universal Gym. The body is moved up and down by flexing and extending the elbows. This exercise places a strong stress on the elbow extensors and chest muscles.

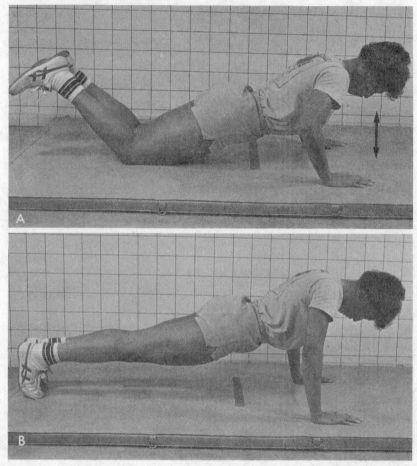

Figure 4–33. *A,* Modified Push-Up—Less difficult. Calisthenic. *B,* Extended Push-Up—More difficult. Calisthenic. *A* and *B,* The chest is lowered until it is about 6 inches from the mat. The body is then raised by extending the elbows.

Superior Shoulder [Deltoid and Upper Back (Trapezius)]*

Note: Most of the Shoulder Pressing and Elbow Extension Exercises place stress on the deltoid and upper back muscles. However, they differ from the Superior Shoulder Exercises below in that they are designed also to emphasize the chest and posterior arm muscles.

---

*For an illustration of these muscles, see Figure 4–26.

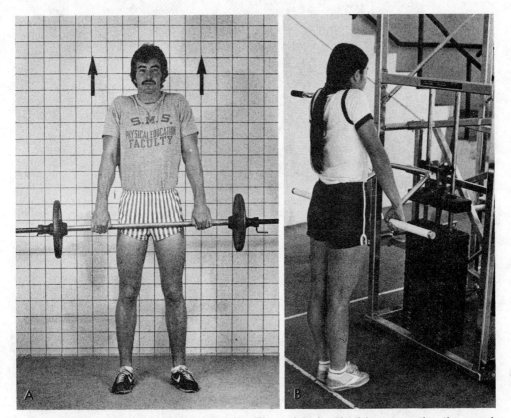

Figure 4–34. *A,* Shoulder Shrug—Weights. The weight is raised by contracting the superior shoulder and back muscles. The elbows should be kept extended throughout the exercise. *B,* Shoulder Shrug—Universal Gym.

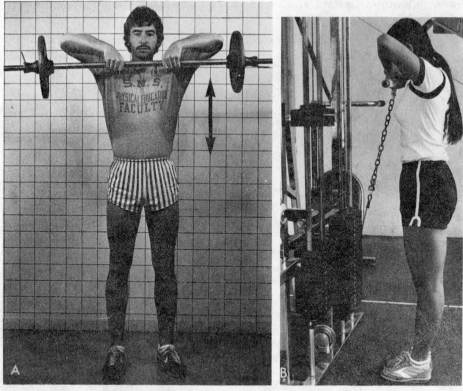

Figure 4–35. *A*, Upright Rowing—Weights. *B*, Upright Rowing—Universal Gym Curl Station. *A* and *B*, This exercise is designed to place strong emphasis on the deltoid muscles. The beginning position is with the weight held just below the waist.

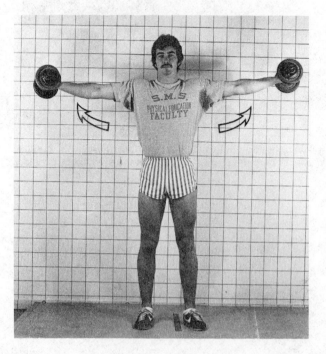

Figure 4–36. Shoulder Abduction—Weights. An alternate exercise for strengthening the deltoid. The starting position here is with the weights held at the sides.

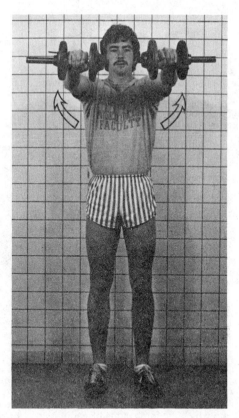

Figure 4–37. Shoulder Flexion—Weights. This exercise places most of the stress on the anterior portion of the deltoid. The starting position is with the weights at the sides.

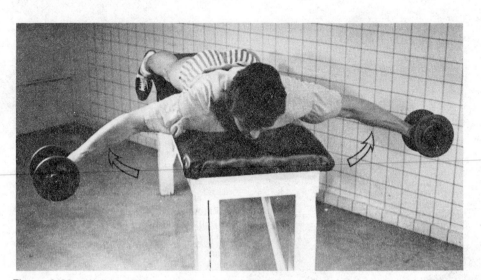

Figure 4–38. Weights. This exercise emphasizes the muscles of the upper back. The starting position is with the arms hanging downward at the sides of the table. The elbows should be kept extended throughout the exercise. Good tone in the muscles of the upper back is important in counteracting many of the postural problems associated with sedentary living.

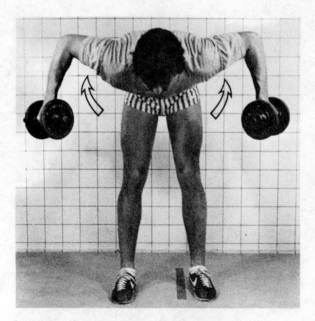

Figure 4–39. Weights. This is an alternate form of the exercise in Figure 4–38, but the latter is recommended because it gives greater stability to the lower back.

Figure 4–40. Bent-Over Rowing—Weights. The trunk must be kept horizontal so that the pull of gravity is in the proper direction. The use of the table on which the forehead is placed provides stability in the standing position.

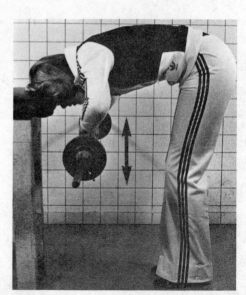

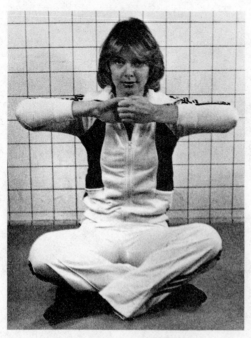

Figure 4–41. Isometric. Hook hands together and pull outward.

Anterior Shoulder and Chest Muscles (Anterior Deltoid and Pectoral Muscles)*

_____
*For an illustration of these muscles, see Figure 4–27. Exercises 4–28A and B, 4–32, and 4–33A and B may be repeated for these muscle groups.

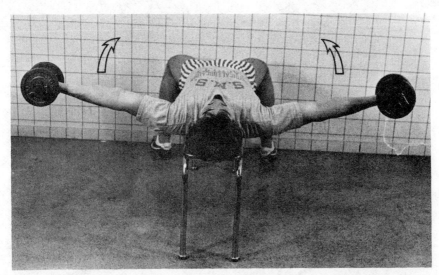

Figure 4–42. Weights. The weights should be raised and lowered through as great a range of motion as possible. It may be necessary to flex the elbows slightly to stabilize the elbow joint.

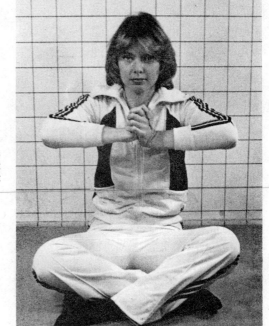

Figure 4–43. Isometric. Place hands together and push for tension development throughout the anterior shoulder and the chest muscles.

Cervical Spine Flexion (Anterior Neck Muscles)

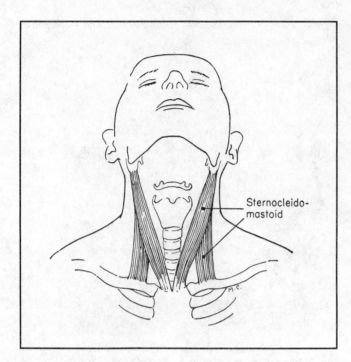

Figure 4–44. The Major Cervical Flexor Muscle. (From Wells, K. F., and Luttgens, K.: *Kinesiology.* Philadelphia, W. B. Saunders Co., 1976, p. 218.)

Sternocleido-mastoid

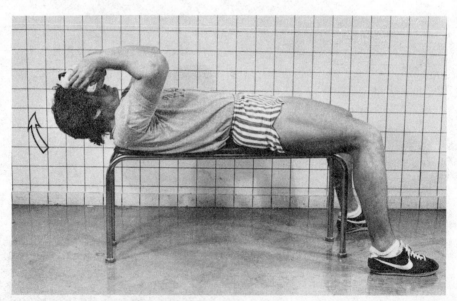

Figure 4–45. Weights. This exercise will strengthen the anterior neck muscles. The starting position is with the head hanging over the end of the bench. A folded towel on which the weight is placed is used for comfort.

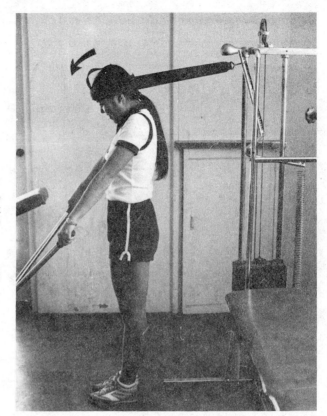

Figure 4-46. Universal Gym—Head Strap. The flexor muscles of the anterior neck are made to work against the resistance of the machine by bending the head forward.

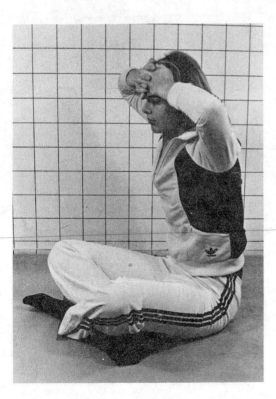

Figure 4-47. Isometric. Place hands against the forehead. Attempt to bend the head forward as the hands resist the movement. A folded towel may be placed under the hands for added comfort.

Cervical Spine Extension (Posterior Neck Muscles)

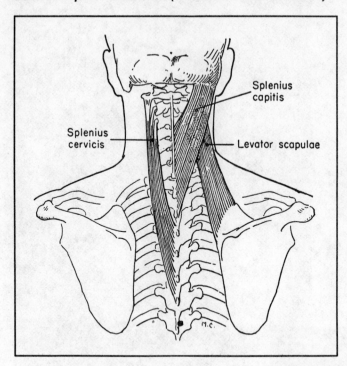

Figure 4–48. Posterior and Lateral Muscles of the Cervical Spine. (From Wells, K. F., and Luttgens, K.: *Kinesiology.* Philadelphia, W. B. Saunders Co., 1976, p. 213.)

Figure 4–49. Weights. The head should be moved upward and downward with a weight attached to a head harness.

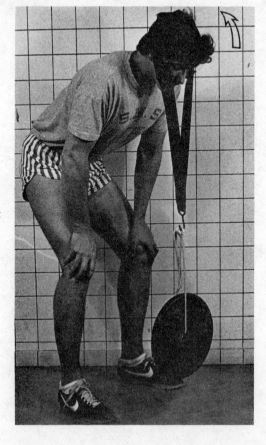

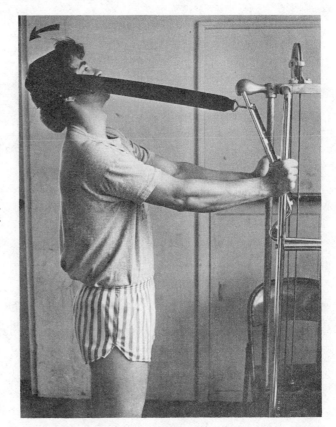

Figure 4–50. Universal Gym. The head should be moved backward against the resistance provided by the Universal Gym.

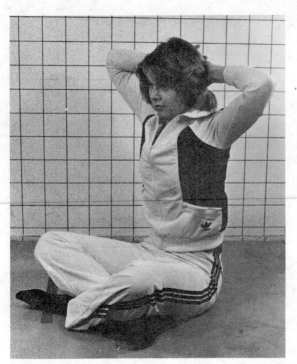

Figure 4–51. Isometric. The head should be pushed backward against the resistance provided by the clasped hands.

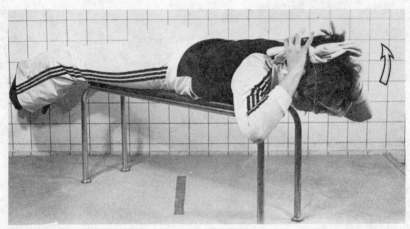

Figure 4–52. Weights. The starting position is with the head hanging over the end of the bench. The head should be moved upward against the resistance provided by the weight. A folded towel is placed under the weight for added comfort.

Trunk Flexion [*Anterior Trunk Muscles (Abdominals)*]

Anterior trunk muscle exercises are arranged in order of increasing difficulty. Most of these exercises begin from what is known as the "hook lying position" [supine (flat on back), knees and hips flexed, feet about 12 to 18 inches from the buttocks]. Preferably, the feet are not anchored or held down. This forces more action from the abdominal muscles and less from the hip flexors. Also, placing the feet higher than the hips, as in Figure 4–59, helps to eliminate some of the action of the hip flexors. *Note:* Double leg lifts and straight leg sit-ups are *not* recommended because they place undue strain on the lower spine owing to strong action of the hip flexor muscles (Fig. 4–9).

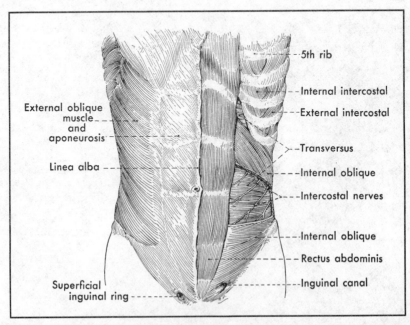

Figure 4–53. The Musculature of the Anterior and Lateral Abdominal Wall. (From Hollinshead, W. H.: *Functional Anatomy of the Limbs and Back*. Philadelphia, W. B. Saunders Co., 1976, p. 398.)

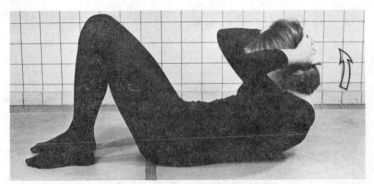

Figure 4–54. Trunk Curl—Calisthenic. Assume a hook lying position with the hands clasped behind the neck. Roll (curl) the head and shoulders forward and upward enough to feel tension in the abdominals. Keep the lower back on the floor or mat. Return to the starting position.

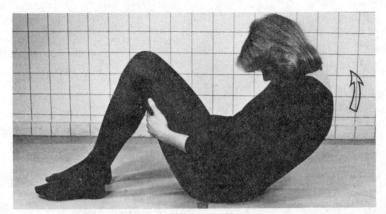

Figure 4–55. Assisted Flexed Knee Sit-Up—Calisthenic. Assume a hook lying position with the arms at the sides. Put hands under the thighs to help pull up. Use arms to help the sit-up only if the exercise cannot be done without using them.

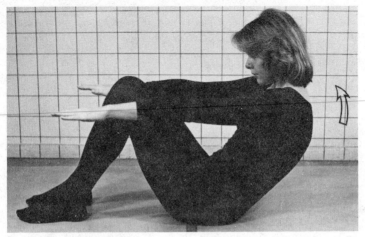

Figure 4–56. Flexed Knee Sit-Up; Arms at Sides—Calisthenic. A sit-up is done while the arms are held at the side.

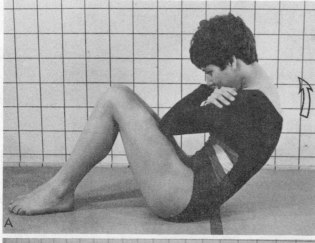

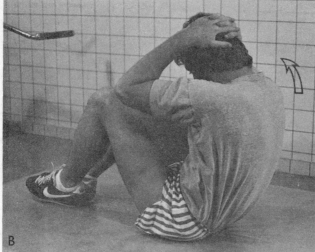

Figure 4–57. *A,* Flexed Knee Sit-Up, Arms on Chest—Calisthenic. In this version of the sit-up, the arms are kept folded across the chest throughout the exercise. *B,* Full Flexed Knee Sit-Up. Assume a hook lying position. Clasp hands behind the neck. Curl trunk forward and sit up until the elbows touch the knees. Keep head curled forward throughout. Do not arch the back.

Figure 4–58. Reverse Sit-Up—Calisthenic. Assume a hook lying position with feet flat on the floor and arms at the sides. Lift the knees to the chest, raising the hips off the floor. Return to the starting position. This exercise emphasizes the lower abdominal muscles.

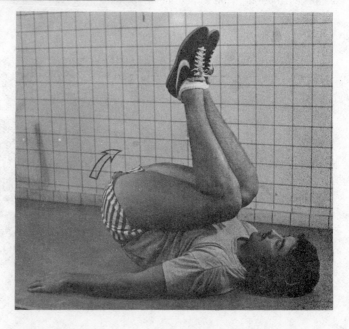

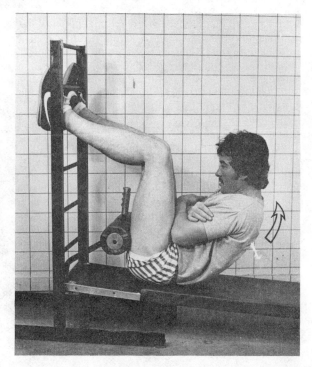

Figure 4–59. Feet High Sit-Up. By placing the feet up high during the sit-up, some of the assistance usually gained from the hip flexors is eliminated. This places a greater stress on the abdominals.

Trunk Curls or Sit-Ups with Resistance

To add resistance to the sit-up or trunk curl, it may be performed with a weight plate held behind the neck. An improvised form of resistance may be obtained with a plastic milk or bleach bottle with a lid. Fill the bottle with only enough water or sand to make it difficult to do three sets of six curls or sit-ups holding the bottle. Increase the repetitions until three sets of nine can be done. Then, increase the amount of water or sand until it is again hard to do three sets of six sit-ups or trunk curls. Resistance also can be added to the sit-up with an inclined board; these are commercially available or may be improvised.

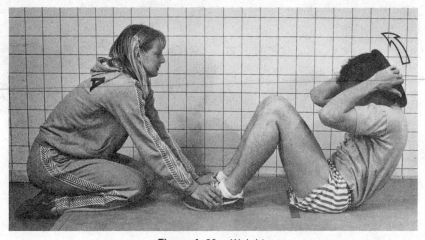

Figure 4–60. Weights.

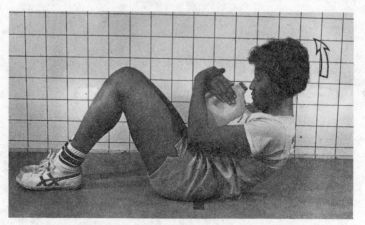

Figure 4-61. Improvised weights—Plastic Bottle.

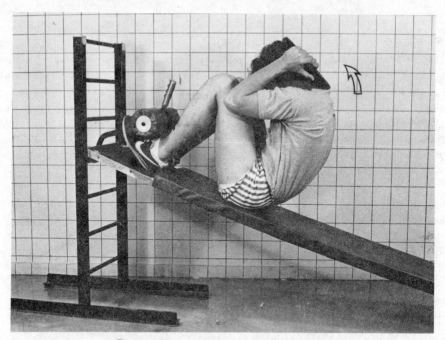

Figure 4-62. Weights Plus Inclined Board.

Lateral Flexion of Trunk (Lateral Trunk Muscles—External and Internal Obliques)*

In each exercise below, several repetitions to each side should be performed.

---

*For an illustration of the external and internal oblique muscles, see Figure 4–53.

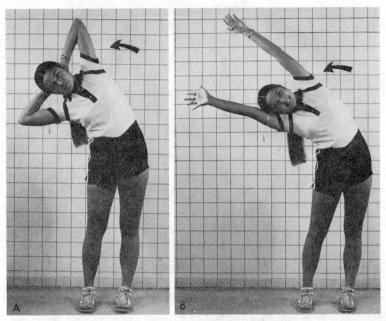

Figure 4–63. *A*, Side Bender—Calisthenic. Less difficult arm position. *B*, Side Bender. More difficult arm position.

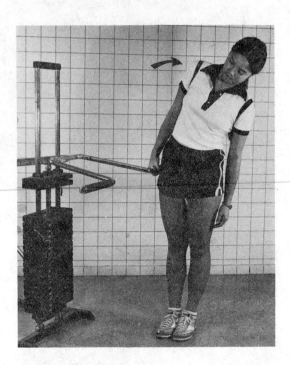

Figure 4–64. Lateral Flexion—Universal Gym or Hand-Held Weight. Weight should be lifted by contracting the lateral trunk muscles on the opposite side of the body. The elbow should be kept extended.

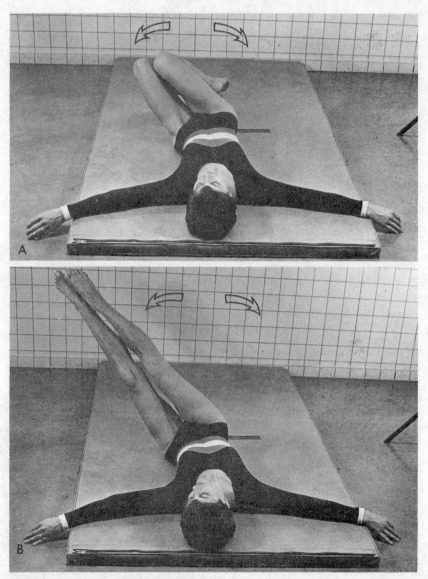

Figure 4–65. Calisthenic. Slowly move the legs and hips from one side to the other. The exercise is less difficult with the knees flexed, as in A. In B, weights may be added to the ankles to increase the resistance.

Shoulder Adduction and Extension (Latissimus Dorsi Muscle—Lower and Middle Back; Posterior Muscles of Shoulder)

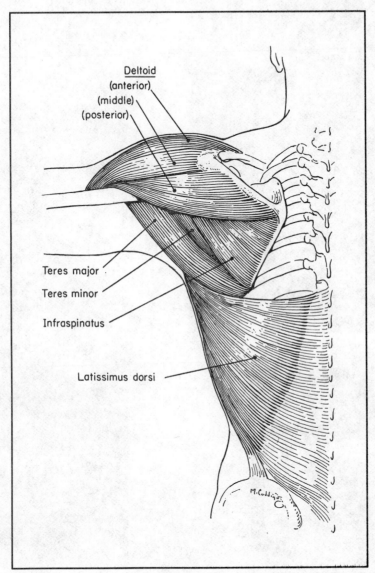

Figure 4-66. Posterior View of Muscles of the Shoulder Joint, Superficial Layer. (From Wells, K. F., and Luttgens, K.: *Kinesiology.* Philadelphia, W. B. Saunders Co., 1976, p. 77.)

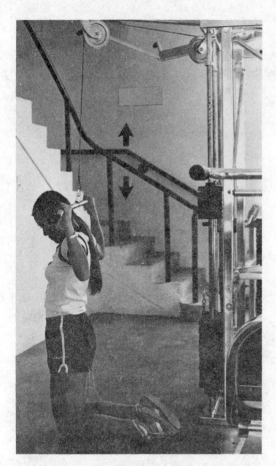

Figure 4–67. Latissimus Pulldown—Universal Gym or Similar Apparatus. This shows the use of a latissimus machine. Weights are attached by way of an overhead pulley. The exercise is begun with the elbows extended and completed, with the bar either in front or in back, depending on whether concentrated effort is desired in the upper chest or the upper back. In addition to the latissimus dorsi muscle, stress is placed on the elbow flexors.

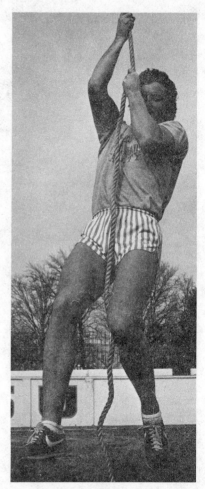

Figure 4–69. Rope Climbing.

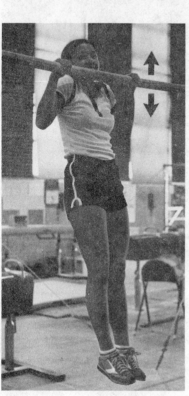

Figure 4–68. Pull-Up—Forward Hand Grip. When the pull-up is performed with the palms facing away from the exerciser, less assistance is provided by the elbow flexors, thereby concentrating more effort in the latissimus dorsi.

Extension of Spine [Posterior Trunk (Back) Muscles]

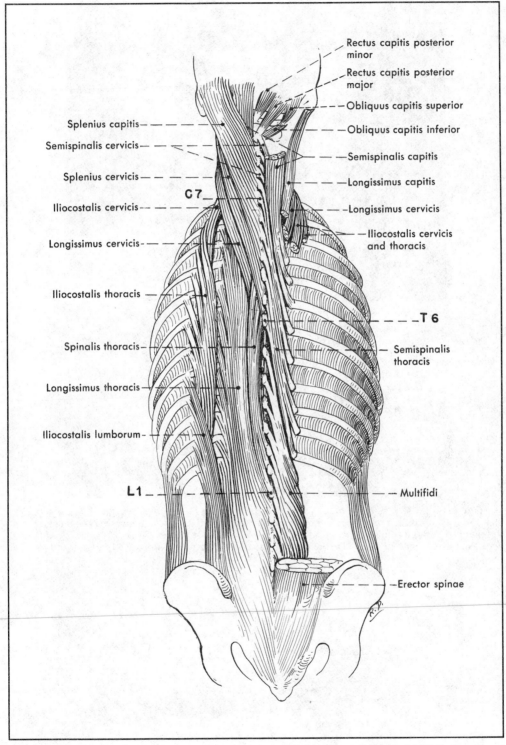

Rectus capitis posterior minor

Rectus capitis posterior major

Obliquus capitis superior

Splenius capitis

Obliquus capitis inferior

Semispinalis cervicis

Semispinalis capitis

Splenius cervicis

Longissimus capitis

C 7

Iliocostalis cervicis

Longissimus cervicis

Longissimus cervicis

Iliocostalis cervicis and thoracis

Iliocostalis thoracis

T 6

Spinalis thoracis

Semispinalis thoracis

Longissimus thoracis

Iliocostalis lumborum

L 1

Multifidi

Erector spinae

Figure 4–70. The Chief Muscles of the Back: Erector Spinae. (From Hollinshead, W. H.: *Functional Anatomy of the Limbs and Back*. Philadelphia, W. B. Saunders Co., 1976, p. 225.)

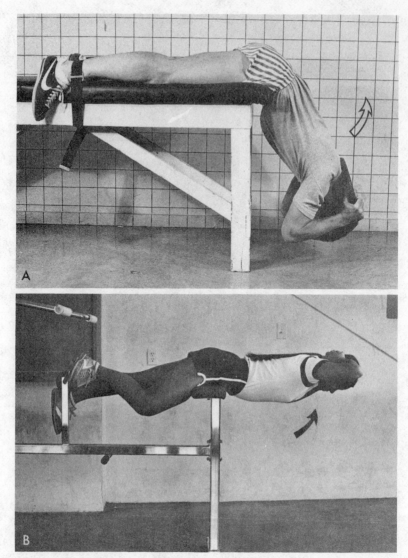

Figure 4–71. *A,* Weights—Upper Trunk Lift. *B,* Universal Gym—Upper Trunk Lift. *A* and *B,* This exercise may be performed with or without weights held behind the neck. A towel may be placed under the weight for added comfort. The feet may be held by a strap or a partner. *Note:* The upper body should *not* be moved higher than parallel to the table or apparatus, to prevent possible injury to the lower back.

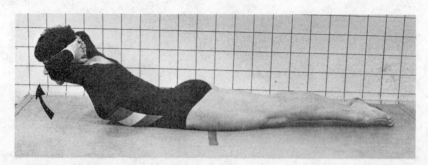

Figure 4–72. Trunk Raise—Calisthenic. The toes should be kept in contact with the mat or floor. The trunk should be raised to a moderate height only. Do *not* fully arch the back. Weights may be added behind the head for added resistance.

Knee and Hip Extension [*Posterior Hip (Gluteals) and Anterior Thigh (Quadriceps Femoris) Muscle Groups*]

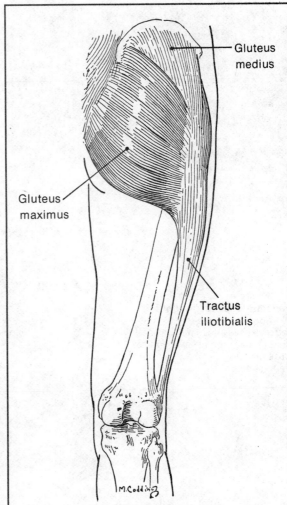

Figure 4–73. Posterior View of Gluteus Maximus, Gluteus Medius, and Iliotibial Tract. (Adapted from Wells, K. F., and Luttgens, K.: *Kinesiology*, Philadelphia, W. B. Saunders Co., 1976, p. 146.)

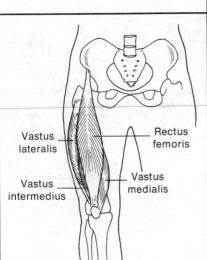

Figure 4–74. Muscles of the Anterior Thigh.

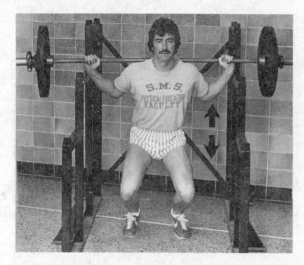

Figure 4-75. Half-Squat—Weights. A support should be placed under the heels for stability, and a towel may be rolled on the bar for protection of the neck. Before the exercise is begun, the barbell is placed on the supporting rack. The knees should *not* be flexed beyond the position illustrated because of possible injury to the joint. The starting position is standing straight with the knees fully extended. Lower to the half-squat position and return to the starting position.

Figure 4-76. Half-Squat—Weights. Raise the weight from the floor by completely extending the knees and hips. The back should be kept as straight as possible, and the elbows should be kept extended.

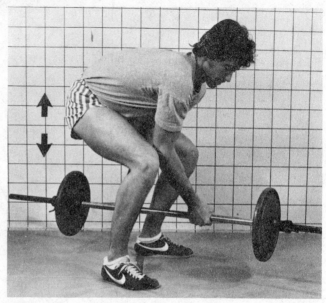

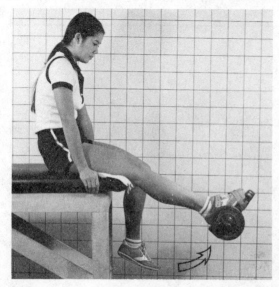

Figure 4-77. Knee Extension—Weights. This illustrates the use of an iron boot to which weights are attached. This exercise is used to concentrate the effort within the quadriceps femoris group of muscles. A folded towel is placed under the knee joint to promote comfort. Full extension of the knee should be attained on each repetition.

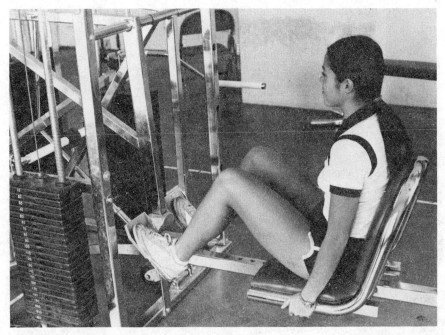

Figure 4–78. Universal Gym—Leg Press Station. On machines that have two positions for the feet, the upper position emphasizes the hip extensors. The lower foot position emphasizes the knee extensors.

Figure 4–79. Universal Gym—Knee Extension. An exercise similar to that in Figure 4–77. Full extension of the knee should be attained on each repetition. May be performed using one or both legs.

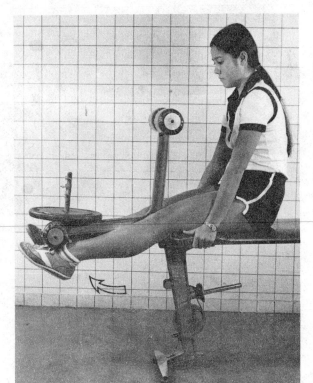

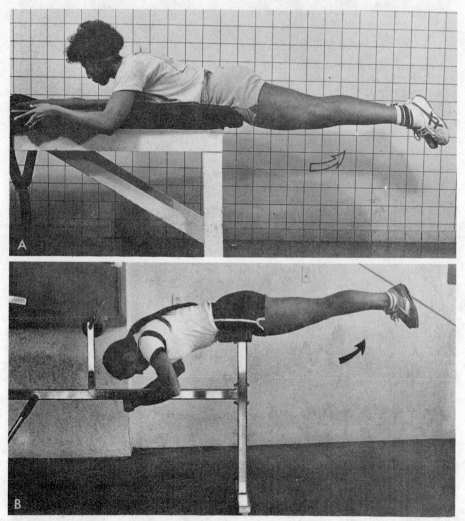

Figure 4–80. *A*, Lower Trunk Lift. Emphasizes the gluteal muscles. Weights may be added to the ankles for more resistance. *B*, Lower Trunk Lift—Universal Gym.

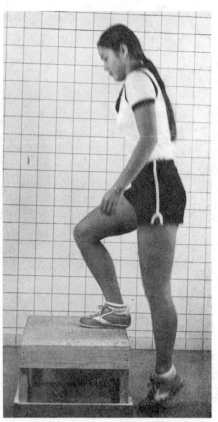

Figure 4–81. Bench Stepping. Step up and down on a 12- to 18-inch bench at a cadence of 15 to 25 steps per minute. When continued for several minutes, this exercise is an effective cardiovascular conditioner.

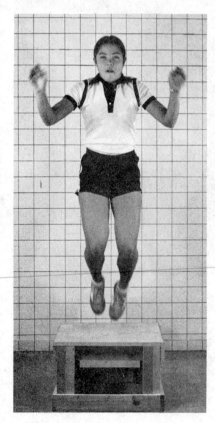

Figure 4–82. Jumping. Jump with both feet onto a high stair step, or onto or over a bench as shown.

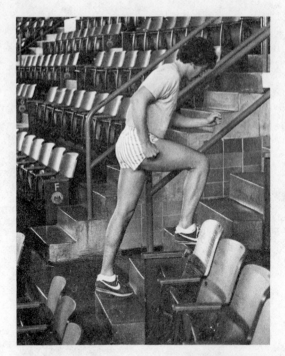

Figure 4–83. Stair Climbing. Walking or running up stairs, two steps at a time, will condition the hip and knee extensors. If continued for long enough (several minutes), it is also a good cardiovascular conditioning exercise.

Figure 4–84. Calisthenic. Extend knee and raise leg behind the body. Repeat several times with each leg. Emphasizes the gluteal muscles. Weight may be added to the ankle for increased resistance.

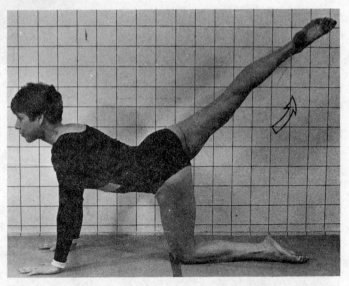

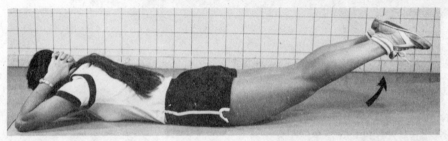

Figure 4–85. Back Leg Raise—Calisthenic. Hold the head and chest to the mat, extend the knees, and raise the legs a few inches from the mat. Weights may be added to the ankles for increased resistance.

Hip Abduction (Lateral Muscles of Hip and Upper Thigh)

The major muscles involved are the gluteus medius and tractus iliotibialis (Fig. 4–73).

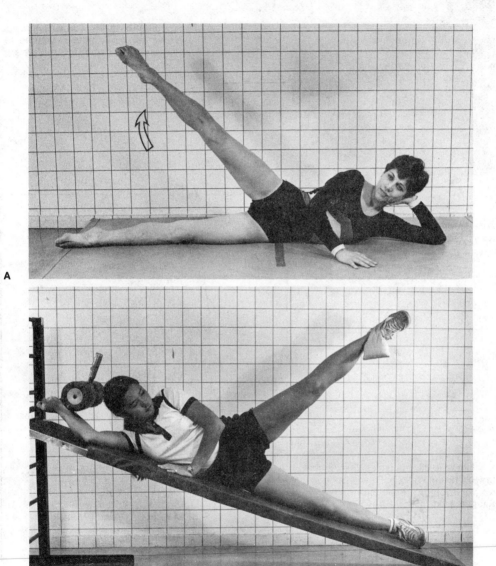

Figure 4–86. Calisthenics. *A*, The leg is alternately raised and lowered. Weight may be added to the ankle for increased resistance. *B*, same as *A*, but using an inclined board and sandbag to increase the resistance.

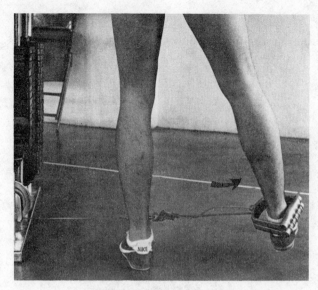

Figure 4–87. Universal Gym. Move leg outward to overcome resistance afforded by the machine.

Hip Adduction (Medial Muscles of Thigh and Hip)

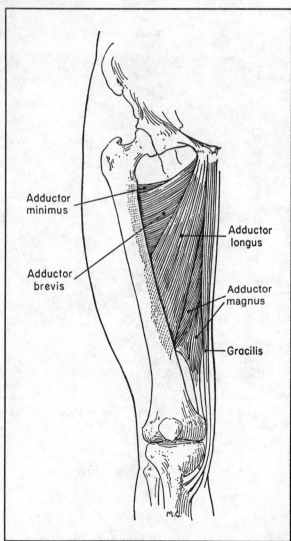

Figure 4–88. Muscles That Adduct the Hip. (From Wells, K. F., and Luttgens, K.: *Kinesiology*. Philadelphia, W. B. Saunders Co., 1976, p. 144.)

Adductor minimus

Adductor brevis

Adductor longus

Adductor magnus

Gracilis

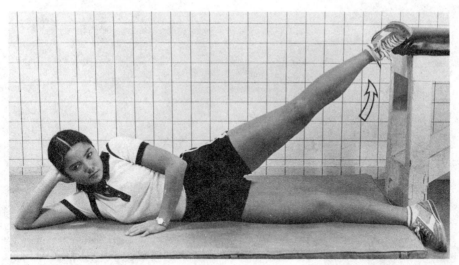

Figure 4–89. Calisthenic. Support upper leg on table edge. Move lower leg up to upper leg, then lower to starting position. Weights may be added to ankle for increased resistance.

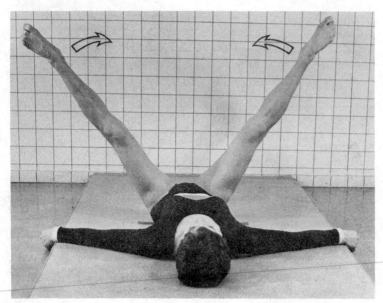

Figure 4–90. Calisthenic. Move legs together. Weights may be added to the ankles for increased resistance. If weights are secured to the ankles, this exercise may be performed effectively in the seated position with the legs extending out in front of the body. By opening and closing the legs in that position, *both* the lateral and medial thigh muscles can be exercised.

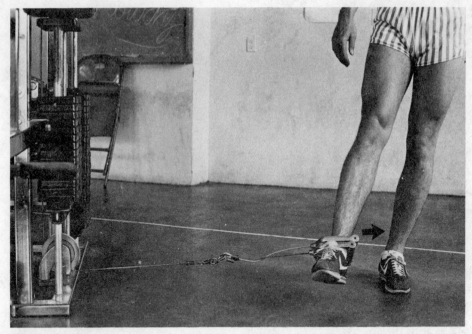

Figure 4–91. Calisthenic. Move the leg across the midline of the body to overcome the resistance afforded by the machine.

Flexion of Knee [*Posterior Thigh Muscles (Hamstrings)*]

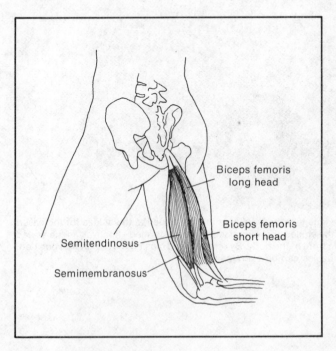

Biceps femoris long head

Biceps femoris short head

Semitendinosus

Semimembranosus

Figure 4–92. The Hamstring Muscles of the Posterior Thigh.

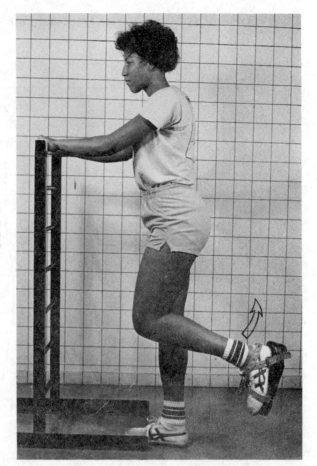

Figure 4–93. Weights. A support is used to assure body balance. The exercise may be done while standing on a low bench to allow the foot to move through a greater range of motion.

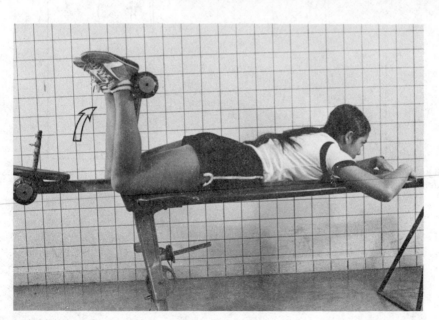

Figure 4–94. Knee Flexion—Universal Gym. The exercise may be performed with both legs or with one leg at a time.

Dorsi Flexion of Ankles (Anterior Lower Leg Muscles)

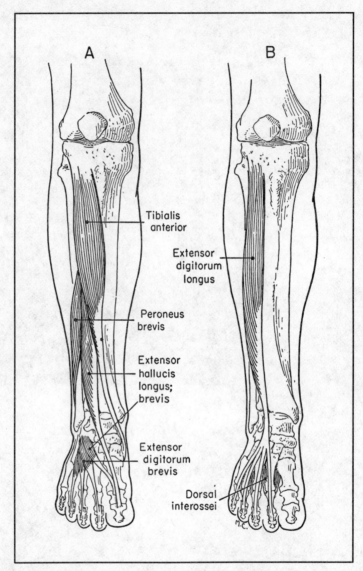

Figure 4–95. Anterior Muscles of the Leg. (From Wells, K. F., and Luttgens, K.: *Kinesiology.* Philadelphia, W. B. Saunders Co., 1976, p. 179.)

Figure 4–96. Improvised Weights. The weight is strapped over the front half of the foot, and the toes are moved up toward the anterior leg. Movement is at ankle only. This exercise may be performed with the leg hanging over the edge of a table, similar to Figure 4–77.

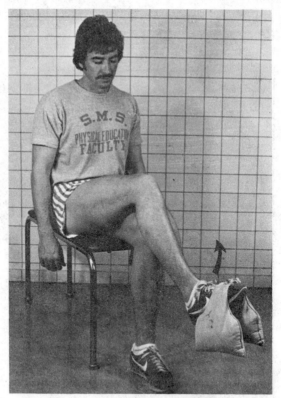

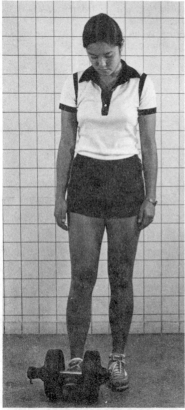

Figure 4–97. Isometric. The foot is hooked under weights, and an attempt is made to lift the weight off the floor by raising the toes. The exercise may be done by hooking the foot under any piece of low furniture or other suitable anchor.

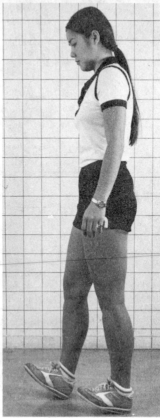

Figure 4–98. Isometric. Hold toes up toward anterior portion of lower leg while walking on the heels.

Plantar Flexion of Ankle [*Posterior Muscles of Lower Leg (Gastrocnemius and Soleus)*]

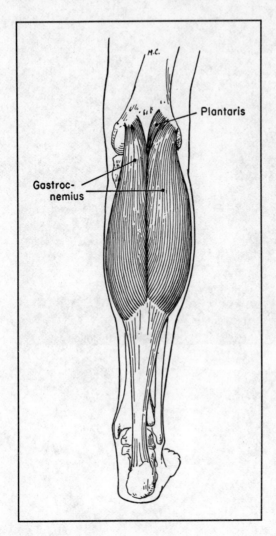

Figure 4–99. The Gastrocnemius Muscle. This large muscle is part of the triceps surae group. The other large muscle in this group lies directly underneath the gastrocnemius. It also inserts onto the heel by way of the Achilles tendon. (From Wells, K. F., and Luttgens, K.: *Kinesiology.* Philadelphia, W. B. Saunders Co., 1976, p. 181.)

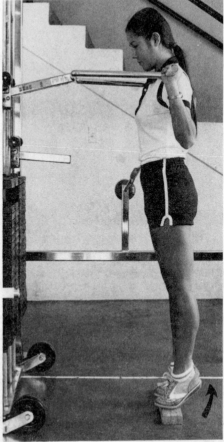

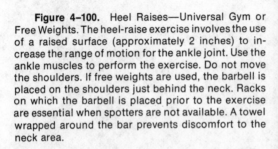

Figure 4–100. Heel Raises—Universal Gym or Free Weights. The heel-raise exercise involves the use of a raised surface (approximately 2 inches) to increase the range of motion for the ankle joint. Use the ankle muscles to perform the exercise. Do not move the shoulders. If free weights are used, the barbell is placed on the shoulders just behind the neck. Racks on which the barbell is placed prior to the exercise are essential when spotters are not available. A towel wrapped around the bar prevents discomfort to the neck area.

The Universal Gym leg press station (see Fig. 4–78) also may be used to condition the muscles in the posterior lower leg. To do this, the weight is pushed as far as possible with the toes at the end of the movement. If the machine has two foot placements, use the lower one.

Improvised Weights

Many of the exercises shown in the preceding sections have depicted the use of weights as the form of resistance. For the most part, traditional bars and weight plates have been pictured. These are usually found in schools, colleges, universities, health clubs, and the YMCA and YWCA. Similar sets suitable for home use may be purchased rather inexpensively at most sporting goods, department, and discount stores. Sandbag weights and weights with Velcro fasteners (Fig. 4–101) can be purchased commercially (one source is the J. A. Preston Corp., 71 Fifth Ave., New York, NY 10003). These may be improvised by a person with minimal sewing skills from strong cloth of various types. Another convenient method of improvising weights is to use plastic bottles containing sand or water (sand is heavier) (see Fig. 4–61). These bottles are obtainable in various sizes. Two bottles may be strapped together for hanging on various body segments. Old pantyhose or stockings make excellent straps.

LEARNING OBJECTIVES

After completing a study of Chapter 4, students should be able to
1. Indicate whether amount of resistance or number of repetitions is the most important element in strength development, and explain why.
2. Indicate whether amount of resistance or number of repetitions is the most important element in muscular endurance development, and explain why.
3. Explain why asking different individuals to perform 50 sit-ups may prove to be unequal workloads for them.
4. List some of the reasons why some people are stronger than others.
5. List the primary changes in the body which make individuals stronger as they train for strength.

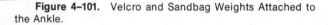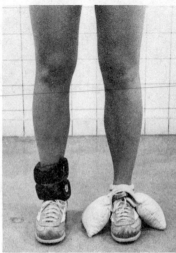

Figure 4–101. Velcro and Sandbag Weights Attached to the Ankle.

6. Indicate whether men and women are equal in strength, and explain.

7. Explain how strength gain is influenced by beginning level of strength.

8. List and explain which factors determine an individual's rate of progress in strength development.

9. Indicate how long it generally takes to experience significant gains after beginning a strength program.

10. Explain specificity of training as it relates to strength training.

11. List the areas of the body important to maintenance of posture.

12. List some areas of the body that are specifically neglected in everyday use.

13. List the fundamental principles of strength development.

14. Describe and/or demonstrate each of the following types of muscle contraction:
　　a. isotonic contraction.
　　　　(1) concentric.
　　　　(2) eccentric.
　　b. isometric contraction.

15. Indicate which of the above types of contraction is generally favored for strength development.

16. List some common criticisms of isometric exercises.

17. Indicate how long an isometric exercise should be held, and say why it should not be maintained any longer.

18. Explain the basic concept behind isokinetic training.

19. Evaluate isokinetic exercise in relation to other types of training.

20. Explain what is meant by absolute muscle endurance and by relative endurance.

21. List the primary changes in the body that accompany muscle endurance.

22. Explain what is meant by 1 RM, 6 RM, and 10 RM.

23. List how many times per week one should train for strength.

24. List the recommended number of repetitions and sets for weight training.

25. Explain how improper breathing during strengthening exercises can be a health hazard.

26. List some important safety precautions for strengthening exercises.

27. Explain why the position of the low back is so important in working with weights.

28. Name and/or demonstrate at least one exercise for each of the following body areas:
　　a. anterior hand and forearm (grip).
　　b. posterior hand and forearm.
　　c. anterior upper arm (biceps).
　　d. posterior upper arm (triceps).
　　e. anterior chest (pectoralis major).
　　f. posterior shoulders.
　　g. superior shoulder and back.
　　h. posterior trunk.
　　i. lateral trunk.
　　j. anterior trunk.
　　k. anterior neck.
　　l. posterior neck.
　　m. posterior hip and upper thigh (gluteus maximus).
　　n. lateral hip and upper thigh (gluteus medius).
　　o. posterior thigh (hamstrings).
　　p. anterior lower leg.
　　q. posterior lower leg (calf).

29. Explain how strengthening exercises differ from flexibility exercises; from muscular endurance exercises; from cardiovascular endurance exercises; and from weight control exercises.

30. Explain why warm up before strength training is or is not important.

REFERENCES

1. Ball, J. R., Rich, G. Q., and Wallis, E. L.: Effects of isometric training on vertical jumping. Res. Q. Am. Assoc. Health Phys. Educ. 35:231, 1964.
2. Berger, R. A.: Effect of varied weight training programs on strength. Res. Q. Am. Assoc. Health Phys. Educ. 33:168, 1962.
3. Booth, F. W., and Gould, E. W.: Effects of Training and Disuse on Connective Tissue. In J. H. Wilmore, and J. F. Keogh, (eds.) Exercise and Sport Sciences Reviews, Vol. 3. New York, Academic Press, 1975.
4. Brown, C. H., and Wilmore, J. H.: The effects of maximal resistance training on the strength and body composition of women athletes. Med. Sci. Sports 6:174, 1974.
5. Bruce, R. A.: Methods of Exercise Testing: Step Test, Bicycle, Treadmill, Isometrics. In E. A. Amsterdam, J. H. Wilmore, and A. N. DeMaria (eds.) Exercise in Cardiovascular Health and Disease. New York, Yorke Medical Books, 1977.
6. Burke, R. E., and Edgerton, V. R.: Motor Unit Properties and Selective Involvement in Movement. In J. H. Wilmore and J. F. Keogh (eds.) Exercise and Sport Sciences Reviews, Vol. 3. New York, Academic Press, 1975.
7. Burleigh, I. G.: On the cellular regulation of growth and development in skeletal muscle. Biol. Rev. 49:267, 1974.
8. Cheek, D. B., Hold, A. B., Hill, D. E., and Tabbert, J. L.: Skeletal muscle mass and growth: the concept of the deoxyribonucleic acid unit. Pediatr. Res. 5:312, 1971.
9. Clarke, D. H.: Adaptations in Strength and Muscular Endurance Resulting from Exercise. In J. H. Wilmore (ed.) Exercise and Sport Sciences Reviews, Vol. 1. New York, Academic Press, 1973.
10. Crakes, J. G.: An analysis of some aspects of an exercise and training program developed by Hettinger and Müller. Eugene, University of Oregon, MS Thesis, 1957.
11. DeLorme, T. L.: Restoration of muscle power by heavy resistance exercises. J. Bone Joint Surg. (Am.) 27A:645, 1945.
12. DeLorme, T. L., and Watkins, A. L.: Progressive Resistance Exercise. New York, Appleton, 1951.
13. Duncan, A.: Operation of the Size Principle in the Recruitment of Motoneurons. In D. M. Landers (ed.) Psychology of Sport and Motor Behavior II. University Park, PA, Pennsylvania State University HPER Series, No. 10, 1975.
14. Edington, D. W., and Edgerton, V. R.: The Biology of Physical Activity. Boston, Houghton Mifflin Co., 1976.
15. Fahey, T. D., Rolph, R., Moungmee, P., Nagel, J., and Mortara, S.: Serum testosterone, body composition and strength of young adults. Med. Sci. Sports 8:31, 1976.
16. Falls, H. B., Wallis, E. L., and Logan, G. A.: Foundations of Conditioning. New York, Academic Press, 1970.
17. Goldberg, A. L., Etlinger, J. D., Goldspink, D. F., and Jablecki, C.: Mechanism of work-induced hypertrophy of skeletal muscle. Med. Sci. Sports 7:185, 1975.
18. Goldspink, G.: The proliferation of myofibrils during muscle fibre growth. J. Cell Sci. 6:593, 1970.
19. Gollnick, P. D., and Hermansen, L.: Biochemical Adaptations to Exercise: Anaerobic Metabolism. In J. H. Wilmore (ed.) Exercise and Sport Sciences Reviews, Vol. 1. New York, Academic Press, 1973.
20. Gollnick, P. D., Ianuzzo, C. D., and King, D. W.: Ultrastructure and Enzyme Changes in Muscles with Exercise. In B. Pernow, and B. Saltin (eds.) Muscle Metabolism During Exercise. New York, Plenum Press, 1971.
21. Goss, R. J.: Hypertrophy versus hyperplasia. Science 153(3743):1615, 1966.
22. Heath, B. H., and Carter, J. E. L.: A modified somatotype method. Am. J. Phys. Anthropol. 27:57, 1967.
23. Hettinger, T., and Müller, E. A.: Muskelleistung and Muskeltraining. Eur. J. Appl. Physiol. 15:111, 1953.
24. Holloszy, J. O.: Biochemical Adaptations to Exercise. In J. H. Wilmore (ed.) Exercise and Sport Sciences Reviews, Vol. 1. New York, Academic Press, 1973.
25. Holloszy, J. O.: Adaptations of skeletal muscle to endurance exercise. Med. Sci. Sports 7:155, 1975.
26. Hudlicka, O., and Myrhage, R.: Growth of capillaries in adult skeletal muscle following chronic stimulation. J. Physiol. (Lond.) 258:25, 1976.
27. Johnson, B. L.: Eccentric vs concentric muscle training for strength development. Med. Sci. Sports 4:111, 1972.
28. Johnson, B. L., Adamczyk, J. W., Tennoe, K. O., and Stromme, S. B.: A comparison of concentric and eccentric muscle training. Med. Sci. Sports 8:35, 1976.
29. Johnson, M. A., Polgar, J., Weightman, D., and Appleton, D.: Data on the distribution of fibre types in thirty-six human muscles: an autopsy study. J Neurol. Sci. 18:111, 1973.

30. Jones, H. H.: The Valsalva procedure: its clinical importance to the physical therapist. Phys. Ther. *45*:570, 1965.
31. Keegan, J. J.: Alterations of the lumbar curve related to posture and seating. J. Bone Joint Surg. (Am.) *35A*:589, 1953.
32. Lamb, D. R.: Androgens and exercise. Med. Sci. Sports *7*:1, 1975.
33. Morehouse, L. E., and Rasch, P. J.: *Sports Medicine for Trainers*. Philadelphia, W. B. Saunders Co., 1966.
34. Paul, P., and Holmes, W. H.: Free fatty acid and glucose metabolism during increased energy expenditure and after training. Med. Sci. Sports *7*:176, 1975.
35. Perrine, J. J.: Isokinetic exercise and the mechanical energy potentials of muscle. J. Health Phys. Educ. Recr. *39(5)*:40, 1968.
36. Pipes, T. V., and Wilmore, J. H.: Isokinetic vs isotonic strength training in adult men. Med. Sci. Sports *7*:262, 1975.
37. Rasch, P. J., and Pierson, W. R.: Isometric exercise, isometric strength, and anthropometric measurements. Eur. J. Appl. Physiol. *20*:1, 1963.
38. Rich, G. Q., Ball, J. R., and Wallis, E. L.: Effects of isometric training on strength, and transfer of effect to untrained antagonists. J. Sports Med. Phys. Fitness *4*:217, 1964.
39. Royce, J.: Isometric fatigue curves in human muscle with normal and occluded circulation. Res. Q. Am. Assoc. Health Phys. Educ. *29*:204, 1958.
40. Royce, J.: Re–evaluation of isometric training methods and results, a must. Res. Q. Am. Assoc. Health Phys. Educ. *35*:215, 1964.
41. Sheldon, W. H., Stevens, S. S., and Tucker, W. B.: *The Varieties of Human Physique*. New York, Harper and Row, 1940.
42. Thistle, H. G., Hislop, H. J., Moffroid, M., and Lowman, E. W.: Isokinetic contraction: a new concept of resistive exercise. Arch. Phys. Med. Rehabil. *48*:279, 1967.
43. Tipton, C. M., Matthes, R. D., Maynard, J. A., and Carey, R. A.: The influence of physical activity on ligaments and tendons. Med. Sci. Sports *7*:165, 1975.
44. Vanderhood, E. R., Imig, C. J., and Hines, H. M.: Effect of muscle strength and endurance development on blood flow. J. Appl. Physiol. *16*:873, 1961.
45. Wells, K. F., and Luttgens, K.: *Kinesiology*. Philadelphia, W. B. Saunders Co., 1976.
46. Wilmore, J. H.: Alterations in strength, body composition and anthropometric measurements consequent to a 10-week weight training program. Med. Sci. Sports *6*:133, 1974.
47. Wisnes, A., and Kirkebo, A.: Regional distribution of blood flow in calf muscles of rat during passive stretch and sustained contraction. Acta Physiol. Scand. *96*:256, 1976.
48. Young, C. M.: Body composition and body weight: criteria of overnutrition. Can. Med. Assoc. J. *93*:900, 1965.
49. Zuckerman, J., and Stull, G. A.: Ligamentous separation force in rats as influenced by training, detraining, and cage restriction. Med. Sci. Sports *5*:44, 1973.

Chapter 5

Cardiovascular Fitness

INTRODUCTION

Chapters 1 and 3 of this text have emphasized the importance of physical activity in the possible prevention of cardiovascular diseases. The probability both of developing circulatory diseases and of mortality therefrom is reduced by regular vigorous exercise. In addition to the probable longevity benefits, optimal levels of cardiovascular fitness can make a significant contribution to the improvement of the quality of life. A moderate-to-high level of fitness provides a greater energy reserve for use in handling the day's mental and physical stresses. In terms of physical well-being, this means that a fit person can produce more work in a given time than one who is unfit when both are working at the same rate. Ergonomic studies have shown that, when workers set their own pace, they usually average an energy expenditure that is about 30 to 40 per cent of their aerobic power. Daily work at higher energy expenditure levels is likely to result in physical strain. A person with a higher fitness level is also more likely to have remaining at the end of a work day an energy reserve that can be invested in active recreational pursuits—a distinct advantage if one is to carry out a cardiovascular conditioning program.

It might be argued that cardiovascular fitness is likely to benefit only the person engaged in an occupation requiring physical labor, and therefore does not apply to salespeople, the professions, etc., but this is not true. Although the work of the latter is subjective and more difficult to quantify than physical work output, the added benefits of a sense of mental alertness, an enhanced feeling of well-being, and a generally elevated level of vitality do accrue to members of sedentary occupational groups who engage in physical activity on a regular basis. These latter factors may be more important to many persons than the more physical preventive medicine aspects of cardiovascular fitness.

THE CRITERION FOR CARDIOVASCULAR FITNESS

Simply stated, a high level of cardiovascular fitness implies a high level of functioning within the circulatory system and, more specifically, within the heart muscle itself. This functioning can best be assessed by two measures: (1) an electrocardiogram (ECG); and (2) a measurement of the heart's maximal capabilities for pumping blood into the body's systemic circulation.

The ECG is a measure of the transmission through the heart of the electrical impulses that cause contraction. Damage to the heart's muscle or valves, or other factors that interfere with the smooth flow of electrical activity, can be identified by persons trained in reading the ECG. A complete assessment of cardiovascular function would include a stress test ECG (one taken during exercise). The American College of Sports Medicine has recommended that all persons over age 35, and those younger than 35 with cardiovascular disease risk factors, should have an ECG before embarking on an exercise program (see p. 145).

Another measure, maximal cardiac output, is generally accepted as the ultimate criterion of dynamic circulatory function. The measure depends in large part on the quality of the contractile tissue within the heart's ventricles. The direct measurement of cardiac output is a complicated procedure accomplished only by highly trained personnel working in the best-equipped exercise physiology research laboratories. However, another, simpler measure, maximal oxygen consumption, is very highly related to maximal cardiac output. Figure 5–1 presents the relationship between cardiac output and oxygen consumption in athletes (Ath), sedentary normals (Sed), and patients with a form of valvular heart disease known as mitral stenosis (MS). It is clearly seen that a direct linear relationship exists between the two measures, and that the maximum achieved in one of the variables is highly related to the maximal value in the other. More specifically, the maximum that can be reached in oxygen consumption depends on the maximum that can be reached in cardiac output.

The relationship between the two variables is of such magnitude that maximal oxygen consumption is a valid substitute for maximal cardiac output when a measure of dynamic circulatory function is desired. In other words, cardiac output can be estimated easily from oxygen consumption measurements in a variety of different exercise situations. Furthermore, since the delivery of oxygen to the body also depends on respiratory function, the maximal oxygen consumption may be considered a combination measurement of both circulatory and respiratory capacity. For that reason it often is referred to as a circulorespiratory or cardiorespiratory test. It generally is considered to be the best single practical test of cardiovascular–respiratory function.

Although not as difficult as the measurement of cardiac output, the direct measurement of maximal oxygen consumption (max O_2 uptake) is also a laboratory procedure

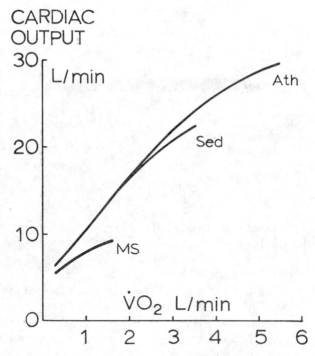

CARDIAC
OUTPUT

Figure 5–1. The Relationship Between Cardiac Output and Oxygen Consumption in Athletes, Sedentary Persons, and Heart Disease Patients (Mitral Stenosis). (From Rowell, L. B.: Human Cardiovascular Responses to Exercise. *In* Morse, R. L. (ed.) *Exercise and the Heart,* 1972. Courtesy of Charles C Thomas, publisher, Springfield, IL.)

that requires special equipment and knowledge (Fig. 5–2). Fortunately, some simple procedures for estimating maximal oxygen consumption are available, and are discussed on p. 147 and in Appendices A–7 and A–8. The measurement of max O_2 uptake is made in liters per minute. However, it is the oxygen consumption capacity per unit of body mass that is most important. Therefore, the measure usually is corrected for differences in

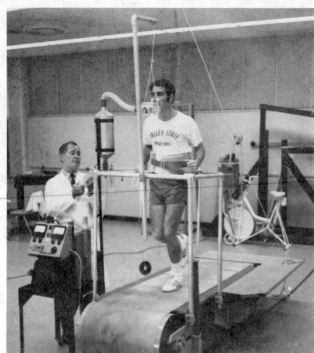

Figure 5–2. Laboratory Assessment of Physical Working Capacity (Maximum Oxygen Consumption). The subject runs to exhaustion on a treadmill while his expired air is collected and analyzed for its oxygen content. (Photo courtesy of Physical Education Research Laboratory, California State University, Northridge, CA.)

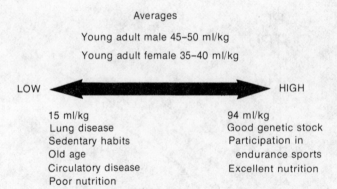

Averages

Young adult male 45–50 ml/kg

Young adult female 35–40 ml/kg

LOW   HIGH

15 ml/kg   94 ml/kg
Lung disease   Good genetic stock
Sedentary habits   Participation in
Old age   endurance sports
Circulatory disease   Excellent nutrition
Poor nutrition

Figure 5–3. The Continuum for Maximum Oxygen Consumption. Lowest known values are about 15 ml/kg/min. Highest known values (94 ml/kg/min) have been recorded in endurance athletes (cross-country skiers).

body size by dividing ml/min of oxygen consumption by the body weight in kilograms (1 kg = 2.2 lbs). The maximal oxygen consumption thus is finally expressed in ml/min per kg of body weight (ml/kg/min). This allows comparisons to be made among individuals of varying body size.

The maximal oxygen consumption expressed in the above manner exhibits a wide range within the population (Fig. 5–3). Lowest values are seen in old and/or sedentary individuals, and highest levels in young endurance athletes. There is also a sex relationship. Beyond the age of puberty, maximal oxygen consumption generally is higher in males than in females. Figure 5–4 shows max O_2 uptake values obtained from numerous research studies on males and females of various age and habitual level of physical activity. The data demonstrate quite clearly that max O_2 uptake values in the active person are consistently higher than those in the inactive. More importantly, it can be noted that the maximal oxygen uptake in the *active* person 50 to 60 years old is as high as that in the average person 20 to 30 years old. *This implies a heart function in the older active individual equal to or greater than that of the younger sedentary person.*

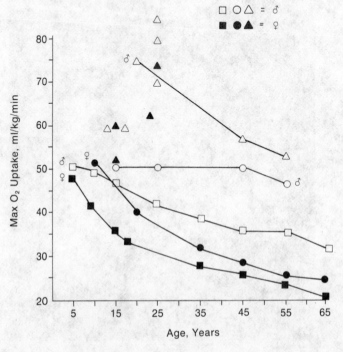

Figure 5–4. Maximum Oxygen Consumption in Relation to Age, Sex, and Habitual Level of Physical Activity. Curves have been constructed using values presented in numerous studies. Most values shown are for North Americans. Average values in the nonactive are somewhat higher in Scandinavian populations. △ ▲ athletes; ○ ● active nonathletes; □ ■ inactive (sedentary). Filled symbols are female, and open symbols male, values respectively.

There are several explanations for the decline in maximal oxygen consumption with age. For one thing, it is related to the general decline in various physiological functions that occurs during the aging process. Aging curves for such functions as basal metabolic rate, work rate, cardiac output, vital capacity of the lungs, maximal voluntary breathing capacity, nerve conduction velocity, body water content, filtration rate of the kidney, kidney plasma flow, maximal heart rate, and maximal muscle strength are similar in nature to those for maximal oxygen consumption in Figure 5–4. However, much of the decline must be due to lack of exercise and to other sedentary living habits. This is implicit in the fact that active individuals of all ages, and both sexes, generally have a higher maximal oxygen consumption than that of nonactive persons. Major factors contributing to the lower values in the sedentary are excess body fat accumulation, decrease in skeletal muscle function, and a decrease in blood pumping capacity of the heart.

Since oxygen consumption in liters is divided by body weight in kilograms to derive the measure, ml of oxygen/kg body weight/minute, it follows that any increase in body weight by the addition of "excess baggage" in the form of fat deposits will reduce the size of the max O_2 uptake expressed per unit of body weight. Skeletal muscle, on the other hand, is an active tissue. In the trained state, it is more capable of extracting oxygen from the blood passing through its capillary beds than when it is in the untrained state.

Sex differences in maximal oxygen consumption are accounted for primarily by: (1) differences in body fat percentage (females have approximately twice as much body fat as males for all ages beyond the early teens); (2) a smaller heart size per unit of body weight in the female; (3) a lower hemoglobin concentration in the blood of the female, thus reducing its oxygen-carrying capacity; and (4) a smaller active muscle mass in the female.

ACUTE AND CHRONIC EFFECTS OF EXERCISE ON CARDIOVASCULAR FUNCTION

When one engages in exercise, several changes in the body's physiology are immediately noticeable. The frequency and depth of breathing are increased. The heart pounds at a faster rate, and the pounding sensation is an indirect indication of an elevated blood pressure. Also, after the exercise has continued for a short period, the sweat glands begin to secrete sweat that collects on the surface of the body.

All the above are acute (rapidly occurring) physiological changes which are associated with *each* bout of physical activity. If the body is stimulated to respond acutely in this manner on a regular basis, certain chronic (more or less long-lasting) physiological changes will take place. It is these chronic changes that are beneficial to the over-all functioning of the cardiovascular system, and are the ones that a conditioning program should seek to stimulate. They are discussed in some detail in the following sections of this chapter.

Over-all Effect of Chronic (Regular) Vigorous Exercise on Maximal Oxygen Consumption

Figure 5–5 dramatically illustrates the differential effects of regular physical activity and sedentary pursuits on maximal oxygen consumption. In the study from which this

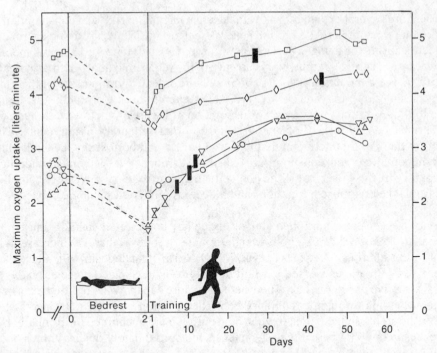

Figure 5–5. Changes in Maximum Oxygen Consumption, Before and After Bed Rest and at Various Intervals During Training. Individual data on five subjects. Heavy bars mark the point during the training period at which the maximum oxygen uptake had returned to the control value before bed rest. (From Saltin, B., Blomquist, G., Mitchell, J. H., Johnson, R. L., Jr., Wildenthal, K., and Chapman, C. B.: Response to Submaximal and Maximal Exercise After Bed Rest and Training. Circulation *38*: Suppl. 7, 1968. By permission of the American Heart Association, Inc.)

illustration was taken, the researchers investigated the effect of a 20-day period of bed rest followed by a 50-day period of physical training in five male subjects aged 19 to 21. The initial difference in max O_2 uptake is explained by the fact that three of the subjects previously had been sedentary, and two of them had been physically active. The max oxygen uptake fell from an average of 3.3 liters/min at the beginning of the study to 2.4 liters/min after bed rest (a 27 per cent drop). After training, it had risen to 3.9 liters/min, or an average 18 per cent higher than at the beginning.

If values for the sedentary individuals are considered alone (three lowest curves), an even more dramatic improvement in max oxygen uptake is seen. The average for these subjects after bed rest was 1.74 liters/min. It increased to 3.41 liters/min after training—a 100 per cent improvement!

The max oxygen uptake of the sedentary subjects before bed rest was 2.52 liters/min. Other analyses on the data indicated that the decrease to 1.74 liters/min with bed rest was due to a decline in cardiac output, and that most of the subsequent increase with training to 3.41 liters/min was due to further large improvements in cardiac output, with a small contribution from maximal A—V O_2 difference (Fig. 5–6).*

---

*Maximal A–V O_2 difference is the difference between arterial and venous blood concentrations of oxygen at maximal exercise. It is a measure of the degree to which the working muscle is extracting oxygen from the blood passing through the capillary bed. A large A–V O_2 difference indicates that the muscles are taking up more of the oxygen made available to them by the blood circulation. The measurement is related to functional capacity within the muscle and *not* to cardiovascular function.

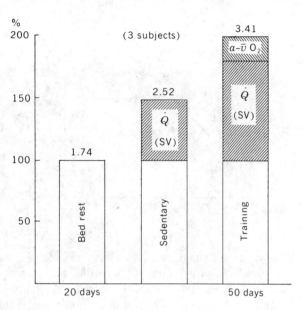

Figure 5–6. Maximum Oxygen Consumption (1) After Bed Rest (= 100%), (2) When Subjects are Habitually Sedentary, and (3) After Intensive Training, Respectively. The higher oxygen uptake under sedentary conditions compared with bed rest is due to an increased maximal cardiac output (Q̇). The further increase after training is possible owing to a further increase in maximal cardiac output and A—V O₂ difference. The maximal heart rate was the same throughout the experiment. Therefore, the increased cardiac output was due to a larger stroke volume (SV). (From Astrand, P. -O., and Rodahl, K.: *Textbook of Work Physiology.* New York, McGraw-Hill Book Co., 1977. Based on data from reference 39.)

Cardiac Output and Stroke Volume

Cardiac output (Q̇) is a function of the number of times the heart beats per minute (HR) and the volume of blood pumped per beat [stroke volume (SV)].

(Eq. 5–1) $$\dot{Q} = HR \times SV$$

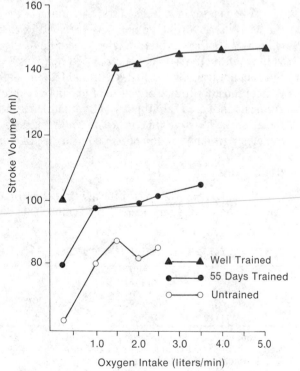

Figure 5–7. Stroke Volume of the Heart at Various Exercise Intensities in Subjects Untrained and After 55 Days of Intensive Training, and Compared with Subjects who had Trained for Several Years. (Adapted from Saltin, B.: Physiological Effects of Physical Conditioning. Med. Sci. Sports *1*: 50, 1969.)

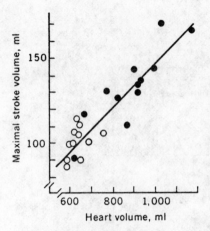

Figure 5-8. Relationship Between Heart Volume and Maximal Stroke Volume. (From Astrand, P. -O, Cuddy, T. E., Saltin, B., and Stenberg, J.: Cardiac Output During Submaximal and Maximal Work. J. Appl. Physiol. *19*:268, 1964.)

Since the maximal heart rate was unchanged throughout the study represented by Figures 5–5 and 5–6, changes in cardiac output undoubtedly were due solely to changes in stroke volume. In other words, bed rest decreased the heart's capability to pump blood with each beat, and physical conditioning increased this capability.

Similar large increases in the stroke volume of the heart have been demonstrated by many other investigations into the effect of physical conditioning on cardiac function. The data shown in the lower two curves of Figure 5–7 were obtained pre- and post-training from three subjects who trained for 55 days. The values for well-trained subjects are averages from a cross-sectional study on six subjects who had trained for several years. These data indicate the tremendous differences that may exist in heart function when the effects of regular, vigorous exercise are considered.

Heart Volume

A key factor in increased stroke volume of the heart is apparently the over-all size of the heart itself. Stroke volume has been shown to be highly related to total heart volume (Fig. 5–8). In the study from which the data of Figure 5–5 were taken, the average heart volume of the five subjects before bed rest was 867 ml. Bed rest decreased it to 778 ml. Subsequent training for 50 days brought about an increase to 900 ml. Further corroboration for the importance of heart volume in over-all cardiac function comes from extensive studies conducted on athletes and nonathletes in the Soviet Union. In both males and females, the heart volume is greater in the athlete (Table 5–1). This is especially true of athletes participating in sports requiring a large amount of endurance training.

Heart Rate

Physical conditioning, or the absence thereof, does not have any significant effect on the volume of oxygen needed by a muscle as it performs a given amount of work.

Table 5-1.   HEART VOLUMES OF ATHLETES AND NONATHLETES*

	Males	Females
Athletes	860†	725
Nonathletes	670	580

*Adapted from data presented by Abramyan, K. A., and Dzhuganyan, R. A.: Athlete heart measurements. Theory and Practice of Physical Culture *12*:27, 1969.
†Measurement in milliliters.

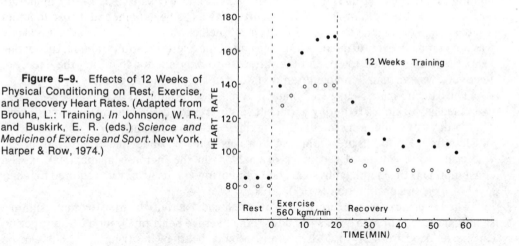

Figure 5–9. Effects of 12 Weeks of Physical Conditioning on Rest, Exercise, and Recovery Heart Rates. (Adapted from Brouha, L.: Training. *In* Johnson, W. R., and Buskirk, E. R. (eds.) *Science and Medicine of Exercise and Sport.* New York, Harper & Row, 1974.)

Therefore, the blood flow required by a muscle performing a given amount of work is unchanged following physical conditioning. In other words, the cardiac output associated with running 2 miles in 16 minutes is the same after a training program as before it. However, an adequate training program will increase the stroke volume of the heart. Therefore, since $\dot{Q}$ in Equation (5–1) remains unchanged, a reduction in heart rate will occur. The run will have been accomplished with fewer heart beats after training than before.

The effect of training on heart rate response to a standardized amount of exercise is illustrated in Figures 5–9 and 5–10. The data in Figure 5–9 were obtained from a middle-aged male who rode a stationary bicycle at a workload of 560 kilogram-meters/

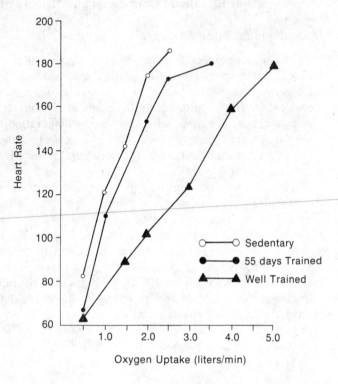

Figure 5–10. Heart Rate at Various Oxygen Consumptions in Subjects Untrained and After 55 Days of Intensive Training, and Compared with Subjects who had Trained for Several Years. (Adapted from Saltin, B.: Physiological Effects of Physical Conditioning. Med. Sci. Sports *1*: 50, 1969.)

minute, 20 minutes per day, four days per week for 12 weeks (this is a very moderate workload). Before training, the resting heart rate was 85 beats/min, and it rose to about 170 beats/min during the exercise. Recovery of the heart rate to the normal resting level was not complete even 40 minutes after the end of the exercise. After training, the resting heart rate was reduced to 80, and the rate rose to only about 140 during the exercise. Recovery was virtually complete ten minutes after the exercise ended.

The data in Figure 5–10 were obtained from the same subjects as in Figure 5–7. They exercised at workloads requiring various levels of oxygen consumption up to maximum. The 55 days of training increased the maximal oxygen consumption of the sedentary subjects from 2.5 to 3.5 liters/min, but that was still well under the 5 liters/min of the well-trained individuals. Even more dramatic than the increase in maximal oxygen consumption is the fact that physical conditioning lowers the heart rate required for *each* level of oxygen consumption (workload).

The lowering of rest, exercise, and other physical activity heart rates can result in a significant saving of heart beats per day. If the average heart rate over a 24-hour period can be reduced from 90 to 70 beats/min, a daily heart beat saving of 28,800 can be accomplished. Some medical authorities have estimated that this saving can be as great as 43,000 beats/day in a well-trained athlete compared with a sedentary person. At this rate, over 15,000,000 heart beats could be saved in a year. Over a lifetime that kind of efficiency undoubtedly results in a great deal less "wear and tear" on this most vital organ. The heart can be considered analogous to an automobile engine in this regard. As mileage on the engine increases, the likelihood of breakdowns and necessary repairs increases and the same can be said of the heart. Physical conditioning reduces its total mileage. This improved efficiency of cardiac output is perhaps the major explanation for a reduced incidence of circulatory diseases and a subsequently greater longevity among active, compared with inactive, persons.

Other Beneficial Cardiovascular Effects of Chronic Exercise

Reductions in Blood Pressure

As blood is pumped from the heart, there is an alternating rise and fall in pressure as it flows into the arterial tree. At rest the pressure rises to about 110 to 120 mm of mercury (Hg) per square centimeter of arterial wall surface in the arteries nearest the heart. Between beats the pressure drops to about 70 to 80 mm Hg. Typical measurements of this pressure change are made with special instrumentation from the brachial artery in the upper arm through an inflatable cuff placed around the arm. Blood pressure curves measured in this way resemble the configuration in Figure 5–11. It is called the *pulse wave*.

The baseline, or point at which the first heart sound (closing of A–V valves) is detected, is the minimal pressure during the rest phase (diastole) of the cardiac cycle. The pressure at the baseline is called the *diastolic* blood pressure. During the work phase (systole) of the heart cycle, the pressure rises to a peak. This peak pressure is called the *systolic* blood pressure. After the peak is reached, pressure declines again to the diastolic level. A person's blood pressure is expressed as systolic pressure over diastolic pressure. At rest, the average is about 120/75 in young adults. During exercise, the systolic pressure increases greatly, sometimes reaching levels above 200 mm Hg, while the diastolic pressure ordinarily remains relatively constant. The large increase in systolic pressure helps to overcome the peripheral resistance to blood flow imposed by the contracting muscles, and speeds the blood to the areas of the body where it is most needed.

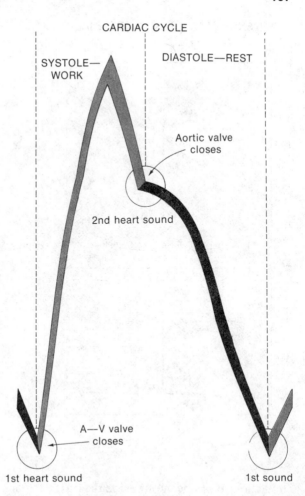

CARDIAC CYCLE

SYSTOLE— WORK

DIASTOLE—REST

Aortic valve closes

2nd heart sound

A—V valve closes

1st heart sound

1st sound

Figure 5–11. The Cardiac Cycle as Represented by the Brachial Pulse Wave. With each heart stroke, the pressure in the arteries increases during systole and decreases during diastole.

Although 120/75 is about the average normal resting blood pressure for a young adult, there is a considerable range of normal for both systolic and diastolic pressures (Fig. 5–12). As aging takes place, the blood pressure normally increases somewhat, owing primarily to some loss of elasticity in the major arteries (arteriosclerosis). Despite the fact that arteriosclerosis and higher blood pressure levels normally occur with aging, they definitely are not desirable consequences! One of our major health problems is abnormal elevation of blood pressure (hypertension). Long-standing elevations in blood pressure are likely to lead eventually to heart disease, atherosclerosis, kidney disease, and/or brain disease. The mortality rate at all ages in the adult population is significantly higher in those with hypertension than it is among those with normal blood pressure levels.

Whether or not a given individual's blood pressure is within the normal range is a matter best determined by a physician. However, in general, the *upper* limits of normal blood pressure for young adults are approximately 140 mm Hg for systolic and 90 mm Hg for diastolic pressure. In older individuals (50+ years of age), somewhat higher systolic pressures (up to 160 mm Hg) are accepted as normal.

High blood pressure can arise from several different disorders that either increase blood flow, the resistance to blood flow, or both. Consistent elevations of systolic and diastolic blood pressures over long periods of time, however, almost always are primarily due to an abnormally high resistance to blood flow in the small arteries of the systemic

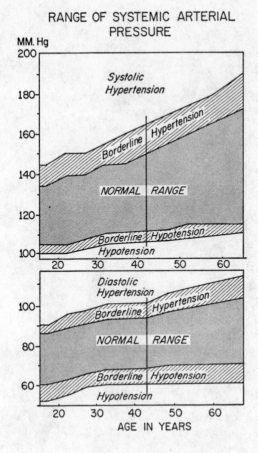

RANGE OF SYSTEMIC ARTERIAL PRESSURE

Figure 5–12. Blood Pressure as a Function of Age. Normal and abnormal ranges are shown. (From Rushmer, R. F.: *Cardiovascular Dynamics.* Philadelphia, W. B. Saunders Co., 1976.)

circulation. It has been estimated that up to 15 per cent of the general population has an abnormally elevated blood pressure. In the large majority of these individuals, no specific cause for the high pressure can be found. In these cases a medical diagnosis of *essential hypertension* is made. If a specific disease process can be identified, a diagnosis of *secondary hypertension* is established.

There are several possible complications of persistent blood pressure elevation. One focus for damage is found in the small arteries of the body. There may be abnormal thickening of the muscular walls of these arteries. Later, there may be a decrease in the size of the channel within the vessels. These changes may occur in any part of the circulation, but they are most damaging in the coronary arteries of the heart, and the vessels of the eye, kidney, and brain. Small areas of tissue damage may occur in these organs as a result of inadequate blood supply. In addition, a consistently high blood pressure may affect larger arteries through a tendency to stimulate atherosclerosis, the formation of yellowish plaques containing cholesterol and fats on the inner walls of the arteries. By accelerating this process, persistent hypertension can further adversely affect the blood supply to the heart, kidneys, and brain.

High blood pressure may also affect other vital tissues by causing hypertrophy (thickening) of the ventricular wall of the heart; enlargement and thickening, or destruction, of the muscle in the wall of the aorta; and/or stroke (damage to brain tissue by inadequate blood supply). In many hypertensive individuals the high blood pressure can be treated very effectively with drug therapy and/or dietary restriction of sodium. However, since many of the drugs used have undesirable side-effects, it is better if hypertension can be prevented or relieved in some other way. Several recent studies have shown that regular exercise may provide such a medium. In several groups of individuals with essential hypertension, and also in persons with normal blood pressure, both systolic and diastolic pressures were significantly reduced after a period of regular physical activity. Figures 5–13 and 5–14 present the results from one of these studies. Both diastolic and systolic pressures were reduced at rest as well as during exercise. It should be noted that the pressures were reduced not only in the hypertensives, but also in the subjects with normal tension. This is an especially important finding in view of the fact that mortality experience of life insurance companies has revealed that individuals with blood pressures nearer the *low end* of the normal ranges have a lower risk of circulatory disease compared with all those who have blood pressures *within* the normal ranges.

The exact mechanism whereby regular exercise helps to reduce hypertension and maintain normotension has not been clearly established by the research thus far conducted. One major factor is very likely—a restoration and/or maintenance of the elastic properties of the muscle within the arterial walls. As stated previously, one of the deleterious effects of high blood pressure is the progressive deterioration of the muscles that control the arterial diameters. The term *arteriosclerosis* (hardening of the arteries) refers to a loss of elastic properties within the muscular walls of the arteries. Regular exercise may help to counteract this adverse condition in at least two ways. In the first place, vigorous exercise produces constantly changing demands for shifts in blood flow at various points within the body. These shifts are controlled by contractions and/or relaxations of the smooth muscles within the arterial walls. In essence, when we exercise we work not only our skeletal muscles, but also the muscles of the arterial walls as they constantly control the shifts of blood flow within the body.

The relative elasticity in blood vessels may be gauged by measuring the velocity of the pulse wave as it travels down the vessels and away from the heart. The distensibility

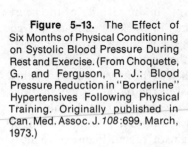

Figure 5–13. The Effect of Six Months of Physical Conditioning on Systolic Blood Pressure During Rest and Exercise. (From Choquette, G., and Ferguson, R. J.: Blood Pressure Reduction in "Borderline" Hypertensives Following Physical Training. Originally published in Can. Med. Assoc. J. *108*:699, March, 1973.)

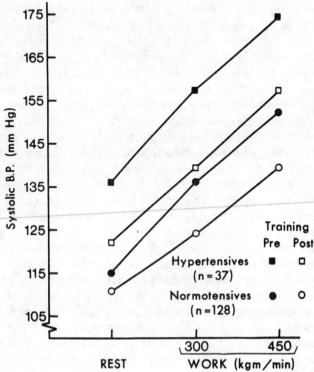

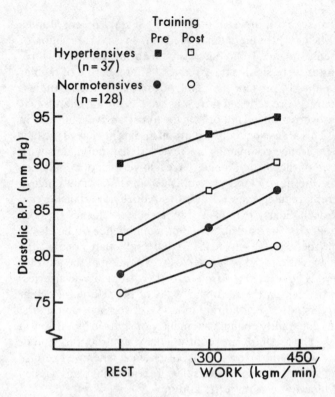

Figure 5–14. The Effect of Six Months of Physical Conditioning on Diastolic Blood Pressure During Rest and Exercise. (From Choquette, G., and Ferguson, R. J.: Blood Pressure Reduction in "Borderline" Hypertensives Following Physical Training. Originally published in Can. Med. Assoc. J. *108*:699, March, 1973.)

of the arteries can be determined based on a classic calculation in physics for the velocity of propagation of transverse elastic waves. The faster the pulse wave travels, the less elastic, and hence, the less distensible is the artery. Pulse wave velocity is also a measure of aging within the artery. "Young" arteries demonstrate greater elasticity than "old" arteries. Aging in arteries is characterized by their elastic fibers' undergoing a form of thickening of the fiber, a fragmentation of the ends, and sometimes aggregation of the fibers to form great irregular masses. It has been shown that elastin removed from old aortas is a heavy type that sinks in water, whereas elastin from young aortas floats.

Normal "young" arteries have an elastic recoil function that helps to transform the pulsatile flow of blood from the heart into a uniform flow at the periphery of the body. This facilitates a uniform circulation in the capillaries, and in the vicinity of the heart itself. It also helps the heart muscle to achieve an economy of work by allowing a large fraction of the stroke volume to be stored in the aorta after it is pumped from the heart. This volume can then be forwarded during diastole by the aorta's elastic recoil. If the elasticity of the vascular wall is reduced, as much as one-half of the heart's stroke volume can no longer be stored in the aorta during systole. Most of the blood thrown into the aorta with each ventricular contraction must then be forwarded *during* systole. This greatly increases the work of the heart, because it now has to take over a function of moving the blood formerly accomplished by the aorta's elastic recoil. Figure 5–15 illustrates the increase in cardiac workload brought on by aortic arteriosclerosis.

It seems apparent from studies comparing blood vessel elasticity in active and inactive people that exercise is a potent factor affecting elasticity and tone within the muscular walls of the arteries. In one large study from the Soviet Union, 70 per cent of middle-aged and older persons who participated in a physical conditioning program exhibited a decrease in arterial pulse wave velocity, along with significant decreases in systolic and diastolic blood pressures. Similar results have been obtained from several

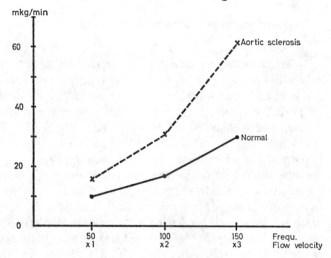

Heart work with increasing strain

Figure 5–15. Effect of Arteriosclerosis on Work of the Heart. (From Anschutz, F.: Aortic Sclerosis and Cardiac Strain in Elderly People. *In* Brunner, D., and Jokl, E. (eds.) *Physical Activity and Aging.* Basel, S. Karger, 1970.)

other investigations. Figure 5–16 is an excellent illustration of the effect that a lifetime of participation in physical activity can have on maintaining blood pressure during aging at levels well within the normal range for young adults. The mean systolic pressure for a group of 107 athletes at age 70 was only slightly above the average systolic pressure for the general population at age 25, and very significantly below the level for the general population at age 70.

A second plausible factor in blood pressure reduction involves the effect of exercise on the development of atherosclerotic plaques within the small arteries of the body. These plaques, as they develop, tend to cause progressive deterioration of the vessel wall, with subsequent loss of vessel elasticity and eventual narrowing of the vessel diameter. Both these situations can lead to an increase in the resistance to blood flow, and thus a rise in blood pressure. Moderate exercise increases the use of circulating blood fats as an energy source. Therefore, there are less of these fats available for distribution along the arterial walls.

Experimental evidence suggests that regular exercise is effective in reducing the resistance to blood flow in at least two other ways. One of these is through an increase in the size of the coronary tree; this type of adaptation consists of the development of new coronary branches or collaterals (collateral circulation). Second, exercise has been shown to increase the lumen area of the coronary arteries. Similar adaptations also occur within other vascular beds in the body.

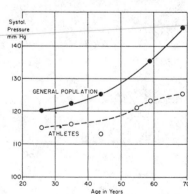

Figure 5–16. Systolic Blood Pressure in Relation to Age in Athletes and Untrained Subjects. (From Jokl, E.: *Heart and Sport.* Springfield, Ill., Charles C Thomas, 1964.)

Increased Myocardial Oxygen Supply

Development of Collateral Circulation

When vigorous exercise is taken on a systematic basis, it stimulates the development of additional capillary networks within the muscles being exercised. This occurs in both skeletal and heart muscle tissue. The magnitude of the increase is illustrated in Figure 5–17. In the experiment represented by the graph, guinea pigs were trained by being made to run on a special animal treadmill. The volume of training was thus quantified by the total distance run. At various intervals throughout the training program, members of the experimental group were sacrificed, and the capillary density per square millimeter of muscle was determined in the gastrocnemius (calf), heart, and masseter (jaw) muscles. One can readily see from the illustration that capillary density increased in both the heart and gastrocnemius muscles, but not in the masseter. It increased in the gastrocnemius because that muscle is used in the running, and in the heart because the heart increased its activity to pump more blood to the leg muscles. There should have been no increase in the work of the masseter associated with the running, and this is verified by the fact that its capillary density did not increase with the training. Similar experimental results have been reported more recently by other investigators.

Increased collateral circulation greatly aids the blood supply to any muscle in which it occurs. It thus helps prevent hypoxia within the muscle. This is especially important in the case of the heart, since hypoxic conditions, often caused by atherosclerotic fat deposits in the coronary vessels, account for about 50 per cent of all forms of heart disease. Figure 5–18*A* illustrates the normal coronary arterial blood supply without collateral circulation. In 5–18*B*, the effect of a coronary occlusion is shown, with the corresponding shaded area indicating the area of infarct. Figure 5–18*C* illustrates how

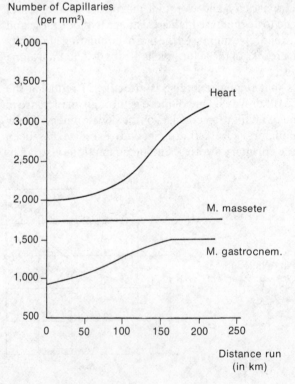

Figure 5–17. Capillary Density in Heart, Masseter, and Gastrocnemius Muscles of Trained and Untrained Guinea Pigs. (From Jokl, E.: *Heart and Sport.* Springfield, Ill., Charles C Thomas, 1964.)

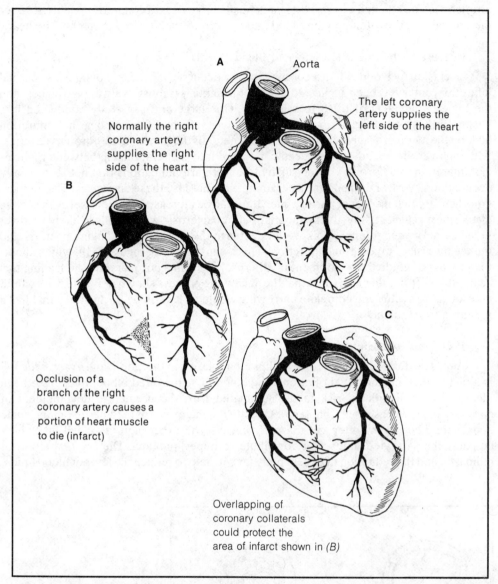

A

Aorta

The left coronary
artery supplies the
left side of the heart

Normally the right
coronary artery
supplies the right
side of the heart

B

Occlusion of a
branch of the right
coronary artery causes a
portion of heart muscle
to die (infarct)

C

Overlapping of
coronary collaterals
could protect the
area of infarct shown in (B)

Figure 5-18. Possible Protective Effect of Coronary Collateral Development in Myocardial Infarction. (Adapted from Miller, B. F., and Burt, J. J.: *Good Health: Personal and Community.* Philadelphia, W. B. Saunders Co., 1972.)

overlapping of collateral vessels developed through exercise might protect the area of infarct shown in 5–18*B*.

This could well be one of the most important cardiovascular benefits of exercise. Atherosclerosis is a very prevalent disease that begins early in life, and autopsy studies on young air force personnel and men killed in Korea (average age 22 years) revealed that 75 to 80 per cent had lipid deposits in their arteries. The authors of this book believe that atherosclerosis can be prevented, or at least kept to a minimal level, by a combination of prudent dietary practices and regular exercise. However, even if it could not be prevented, collateral networks of extra blood vessels within the heart musculature would provide an enormous protective mechanism if one of the branches of the coronary arteries became blocked as a result of fat deposits. These extra collaterals could take over the critical function of supplying blood and oxygen to the affected area(s) of the heart.

Increase in the Intrinsic Caliber of Blood Vessels

Occlusion by blood clot in a coronary artery occurs in most cases of fatal myocardial infarction, and it has been suggested that the thrombosis is most likely to take place when the lumen (diameter) of the artery is small. One large autopsy study conducted in a hospital in Oxford, England, revealed that those suffering fatal myocardial infarction had, on the average a significantly smaller diameter of the lumen in the coronary arteries. Although very few studies have been conducted into the relationship between myocardial infarction and coronary artery diameter, there are indications that active-to-heavy occupational work and/or endurance training may increase these diameters. The implications here are that if coronary artery diameters can be increased by exercise, as the above cited reports suggest, any given amount of atherosclerosis would be less likely to lower myocardial oxygen supply. This would decrease the likelihood of angina pectoris and reduce the risk of myocardial infarction. This is illustrated by Figure 5–19, which shows the process of gradual development of atherosclerosis in a coronary artery, leading to a heart attack. It should be obvious that the narrowing process shown in Figure 5–19 would take longer to occur, and complete narrowing would be less likely, in an artery that had a greater normal diameter,

Decreased Hyperlipidemia

Lipids are fats. *Lipidemia* refers to lipids circulating in the blood, and *hyperlipidemia* is a higher-than-normal level of circulating blood fats. Elevated blood lipids have been identified as a significant risk factor associated with the premature development of coronary heart disease (see Chapter 3). Obesity is a major factor in hyperlipidemia, since obese individuals very often get that way because of a diet high in animal fat, which contains the saturated lipids that contribute to hyperlipidemia. Dietary restriction of animal fat and the reduction of excess body fat will help to reduce the level of blood lipids.

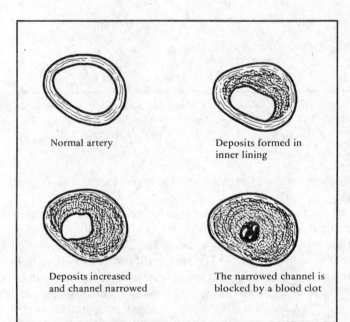

Normal artery

Deposits formed in inner lining

Deposits increased and channel narrowed

The narrowed channel is blocked by a blood clot

Figure 5–19. Schematic of the Gradual Development of Atherosclerosis in a Coronary Artery, Eventually Leading to a Heart Attack. (From Briney, K. L.: *Cardiovascular Disease: A Matter of Prevention.* © 1970 by Wadsworth Publishing Co, Inc., Belmont, CA 94002. Reprinted by permission of the publisher.)

Exercise also can be very effective. Triglycerides (a form of blood fats) are an important energy source during most forms of light-to-moderately heavy exercise, and the blood levels of these fats can be reduced with vigorous activity. However, these reductions are temporary, and the triglycerides return to previous levels within 72 to 96 hours after exercise. Therefore, the chronic exercise program should consist of at least three sessions per week, more or less evenly spaced, so that the triglycerides can be kept at a consistently lower level. Although it has been shown recently that other cardiovascular benefits of exercise may be derived from a program consisting of less than three sessions per week, the positive effect that lowered triglyceride levels may have in counteracting the development of atherosclerosis is a most important consideration. Therefore, at least three sessions per week are recommended as optimal in this regard.

DEVELOPING AND MAINTAINING CARDIOVASCULAR FITNESS

Many of the cardiovascular benefits to be derived from regular physical activity have been described in previous sections of this chapter. These include improved efficiency of respiratory and cardiovascular function and increased work capacity. As a result of training, one is less likely to suffer from chronic debilitating problems such as cardiovascular disease and obesity.

In order to obtain optimal or maximal benefit from exercise, one must regularly engage in a systematic, planned program of physical activity of an endurance nature. This section presents some suggestions for such a regular program.

Prerequisites

The Medical Examination

Exercise may be one of the most severe stresses that can be placed on the human organism. Although the healthy person cannot be harmed by rational physical activity, an already existing heart or kidney disease, joint injury, or similar condition might be aggravated. However, this does not mean that the person with such problems cannot exercise. Modified exercise has proved to be a very effective therapeutic or rehabilitative adjunct in many acute and chronic disease or injury conditions. If disease or injury does exist, the physician is in a position to assess the degree of severity within a given individual, and then recommend the type of activities that are appropriate and indicate those to be avoided.

The medical examination should include a comprehensive medical history including information about personal health history and current health-related habits, such as cigarette smoking, medications, habitual level of alcohol use (if any), and the amount of physical activity in which one currently is engaged. The American College of Sports Medicine has recently established guidelines stressing that a comprehensive medical examination is a "must" for anyone over the age of 35 years before they embark on an exercise program. It also is recommended for persons younger than 35 with symptoms of heart disease, or having a significant number of coronary heart disease risk factors. The examination should include: a standard 12–lead electrocardiogram (ECG); resting systolic and diastolic blood pressure; fasting blood sugar, cholesterol, and triglyceride determinations; evaluation of any orthopedic problems; urinalysis; and a graded, ECG-monitored exercise test. Similar recommendations have been made previously by the American Medical Association's Committee on Exercise and Physical Fitness.

For those under 35 years of age who are free of heart disease symptoms, have no previous history of cardiovascular disease, and are not *known* to have any primary coronary heart disease risk factors, the risks associated with an increase in habitual physical activity usually are sufficiently low for them to proceed without any medical clearance. However, if they smoke, develop heart disease symptoms, have not had a medical examination in the last two years, or have any doubts, they should consult with their personal physician.

The importance of the exercise ECG in the medical screening profile should not be overlooked. In persons over age 35, abnormal ECGs are seen with increasing frequency, reaching as high as 10 per cent in certain age-groups of otherwise normal individuals without symptoms of heart disease. By placing a controlled stress on the heart during the graded exercise test, the physician is able to evaluate how the heart will react to the later, somewhat uncontrolled stresses of the exercise program.

Adequate Rest and Nutrition

If nutrition and rest are inadequate, the body may suffer from chronic fatigue. The purpose of proper dietary practices is to supply the body with its essential nutrients in optimal amounts. These are discussed in specific detail in Chapter 8. Let it suffice here to say that optimal results will not be achieved from a cardiovascular training program if nutrition is poor.

Rest and relaxation are important restorative mechanisms. During sleep the body should have sufficient time to recover from the day's ravages. It is impossible to prescribe exactly the proper amount of sleep that an individual needs since these requirements vary quite widely. Some can get by on four to five hours of sleep, whereas others may need eight to ten. Also, any one individual's sleep needs will vary depending on the degree of stress that person is being subjected to at the time. Through experience one should be able to determine one's sleep needs. A basic principle is the establishment of a regular pattern. Often, less sleep is needed than might be expected. If nutrition is adequate, emotional tension is light, and there is no reason to suspect organic disease, but one feels tired after arising in the morning, it is likely that sleep has been inadequate. If this is the case, sleep should be increased.

Proper relaxation during the waking hours can augment sleep as a restorative mechanism and help to relieve emotional tension that may interfere with adequate sleep. Although exercise itself can be a form of relaxant, the individual can engage in certain other beneficial relaxation techniques. Some are suggested in Chapter 7 and Appendix A–14.

Prevention and Care of Injuries

Musculoskeletal injuries are often painful. They can also interfere with a training program, if they are severe enough, by making it necessary to stop exercising for varying periods of time. During the early stages of a conditioning program, the possibility of injury to muscles, tendons, and ligaments is high because the body has not yet adapted to the added stress being placed on these structures. Therefore, one should take it easy during these early stages and progress slowly into the conditioning program.

A proper warm-up is essential. Exercise participants should engage in a few minutes of slow jogging or similar exercise to increase the temperature of the muscles and their connective tissues. Then, they should slowly stretch the major muscle groups (see Chapter 6). Soreness in some muscles is to be expected during the early stages of an exercise program. This can be prevented to a certain extent by slowly stretching the muscles used during a work-out *after* the work-out has ended. It is important to stretch the muscles in the thigh (front and back), lower back, upper back, and calf both before and after exercise.

If, and when, an injury does occur, the best form of self-treatment is rest for the affected body part. This may mean discontinuing exercise for a time or altering its form. If the injury is such that it prevents jogging or running, swimming or bicycling still may be possible. If the lower limbs cannot be used at all, an effective means of cardiovascular exercise consists of turning the crank on an inverted bicycle with the arms.

Many injuries are caused by improper mechanics in the execution of the bodily movements involved. This is especially true in jogging. Do *not* run on the toes. The proper technique is to run almost flat-footed, with the heel striking the running surface just a split second ahead of the main portion of the foot. The push-off for the next stride is from the ball of the foot. The toes should be pointing as straight ahead as possible.

One common problem is pronation at the ankle. This is a condition where the toes turn out and the weight rolls over the inside border of the foot. You can help avoid it by keeping the feet pointing straight ahead and emphasizing transferrence of the weight along the outside border of the foot. If you have difficulty running in this manner, any time spent on developing the technique will pay big dividends in the future.

A point to remember is that, if injuries persist in spite of rest and other efforts to rehabilitate them, it is advisable to seek medical treatment.

Clothing

In almost every activity except aquatics, the most important consideration is the shoe. The training type of shoe used by most long-distance runners is recommended for jogging. These have a leather or nylon upper; a good, cushioned, multilayered, sponge-like sole; and a strong heel counter. Quality is the key here. Exercise participants should buy the best shoe they can afford. Anyone unsure about what shoes to purchase would be wise to consult with a track coach or someone who does a lot of long-distance running. Several popular periodicals on running, such as *Runner's World* and *Running Times,* regularly feature articles rating the models of shoes distributed by various manufacturers.

In general, clothing should be light and loose-fitting. Cotton clothing is better than synthetic fabrics, especially in warmer weather, because it has a looser weave and will allow heat and water vapor to pass through more readily. Avoid the rubberized weight reduction outfits and heavy warm-up suits; these are not necessary, even in the coldest weather. They trap in body heat and produce sweat on the surface of the body, thus hindering sweat evaporation. They are very dangerous in hot and/or humid weather because they raise body temperature. They will *not* help you to lose weight. Any weight loss associated with an exercise bout in these is simply the dehydration effect of sweat loss, and will be replaced within a few days. Light cotton or wool socks are recommended. If you are participating in a sport requiring sudden stopping and shifting movements of the feet, i.e., basketball, handball, or tennis, two pairs of socks are recommended to prevent blisters. (See also p. 155 on environmental aspects of cardiovascular fitness training programs.)

Evaluation of Cardiovascular Fitness

Before a cardiovascular training program is begun, an assessment should be made of one's condition in comparison to established standards for fitness. This will satisfy

Table 5–2. CLASSIFICATION OF CARDIOVASCULAR FITNESS BASED ON MAXIMAL OXYGEN UPTAKE VALUES (ML/KG BODY WT/MIN)*

Sex and Age	Poor	Low	Average	Good	High
Males					
15–30	<39	39–43	44–51	52–56	>56
31–40	<34	35–39	39–46	47–51	>51
41–50	<30	31–35	36–41	42–46	>46
51–60	<25	26–31	32–38	39–42	>42
61–70	<23	23–26	27–33	34–38	>38
Females					
15–30	<28	29–34	35–43	44–48	>48
31–40	<25	26–31	32–39	40–44	>44
41–50	<24	25–30	31–37	38–41	>41
51–60	<21	22–26	27–34	34–40	>40
61–70	<19	20–23	24–30	31–37	>37

The symbols < and > are mathematical terms meaning "less than" and "more than," respectively.
*Adapted from data presented in Astrand, I.: Aerobic capacity in men and women, with special reference to age. Acta Physiol. Scand. *49* (Suppl. 169): 1960, *and* Hodgson, J. L.: Age and Aerobic Capacity of Urban Midwestern Males. Ph.D. Dissertation, Minneapolis, University of Minnesota, 1971.

natural curiosity and also enable participants to plan better the type of program they need. The assessment can also be repeated at periodic intervals to chart progress.

In a previous section of this chapter it was established that the maximal oxygen consumption is the best relatively pratical over-all measure of cardiovascular fitness. The measure is expressed in ml/kg body wt/min, and standards are available for evaluating the measure once it has been obtained (Table 5–2).

The accurate measurement of maximal oxygen consumption requires time-consuming laboratory procedures and is not something that would be done by average individuals in determining their fitness levels. Fortunately, several reasonably valid short-cut procedures are available that provide rapid and inexpensive methods for evaluating cardiovascular fitness level.

The 12-Minute Run Test

One of the best procedures for estimating maximal oxygen consumption is the 12-minute run test (aerobics test) devised by Dr. Kenneth Cooper, based on the earlier work of Dr. Bruno Balke. The test is very simple. All one need do is determine how far one can go by running and walking in a 12-minute period, the object of the test being to cover as much distance as possible. A running track is a convenient place to conduct the test, but any flat, accurately measured area where one can run conveniently is suitable.

The test has a sound scientific basis. Both Dr. Cooper and Dr. Balke validated it by correlating the distance covered in 12 minutes with laboratory measurements of maximal oxygen consumption in a large group of U. S. Air Force personnel ranging in age between 17 and 52 years. An excellent relationship has been established (Fig. 5–20). Subsequent to this work, many other investigators have studied the relationship between maximal oxygen consumption and runs of various distances. Most of these studies have supported the use of the 12-minute run, or some similar test, in the estimation of maximal oxygen consumption.

The test is based on the way the body uses anaerobic and aerobic sources of energy. As pointed out in Chapter 2, the anaerobic sources of energy are very powerful, but useful only in short bursts of activity. In activities lasting more than a few minutes, most of

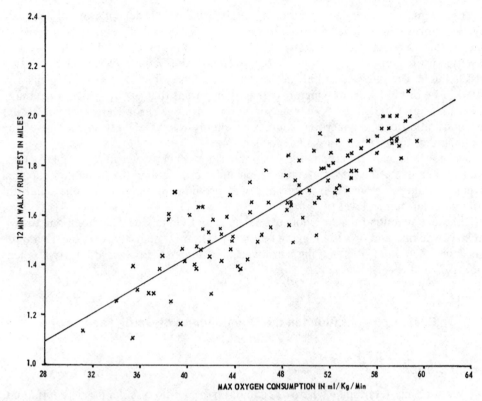

Figure 5–20. Relationship Between Maximal Oxygen Consumption and a 12-Minute Run-Walk Performance in Normal Males Age 17–52. (From Cooper, K. H.: A Means of Assessing Maximal Oxygen Intake. J.A.M.A. *203*:201–204, 1968. Copyright 1968 by American Medical Association.)

Table 5–3. PREDICTED MAXIMAL OXYGEN CONSUMPTION ON THE BASIS OF 12-MINUTE RUN PERFORMANCE*

Distance (Miles)	Laps (¼ Mile Track)	Predicted Maximal O₂ Uptake (ml/kg/min)
1.000	4	28.2
1.065	4¼	30.0
1.125	4½	31.9
1.187	4¾	33.8
1.250	5	35.7
1.317	5¼	37.5
1.375	5½	39.2
1.437	5¾	41.0
1.500	6	42.7
1.565	6¼	44.6
1.625	6½	46.4
1.687	6¾	48.2
1.750	7	50.0
1.817	7¼	51.8
1.875	7½	53.5
1.937	7¾	55.3
2.000	8	57.0

*Based on data from Balke, B.: A Simple Field Test for the Assessment of Physical Fitness. Oklahoma City, Publication 63-6, Civil Aeromedical Research Institute, 1963; Cooper, K. H.: A means of assessing maximal oxygen intake. J.A.M.A. *203*:201, 1968; *and* Margaria, R. P., et al.: Energy cost of running. J. Appl. Physiol. *18*:367, 1963.

the energy must be supplied by aerobic metabolism, which depends on an adequate oxygen supply to the muscles. In order to supply a large volume of oxygen, such as would be necessary to cover a great distance in 12 minutes of running, the circulatory system must function to pump a large volume of blood. Hence, the maximal oxygen consumption must be high. The interaction between aerobic and anaerobic oxygen supply was presented in Figure 2–18, from which it is readily apparent that, as the length of running increases, a larger and larger percentage of the work is done aerobically; this cancels out the contribution of the anaerobic sources of energy and gives a truer picture of the functioning of the oxygen transport mechanism.

Once the distance covered in the 12-minute run has been determined, Table 5–3 can be used to estimate the maximal oxygen consumption. Finding the estimated maximal oxygen consumption value in Table 5–2 will provide an estimate of one's current cardiovascular fitness level.

It is recommended that previously sedentary individuals participate in one to two weeks of walking and/or slow jogging before self–testing themselves on the 12-minute run. Other methods for estimating cardiovascular fitness are presented in Appendices A–6, A–7, and A–8.

Basic Considerations in the Development of Cardiovascular Fitness

Getting Started

Once one has determined where one stands on the cardiovascular fitness continuum, one needs to decide on the most appropriate type of fitness program. If the estimated maximal oxygen consumption from Table 5–2 is in the good or high category, one may wish merely to maintain the present condition. However, one may want to improve it, and there is no reason why one cannot. Examination of Figures 5–4 and 5–5 indicates that those who participate in regular vigorous physical activity easily achieve the high category or above on oxygen consumption. If the maximal oxygen consumption is estimated to be average or below, there is considerable room for improvement up to a more desirable fitness level.

All persons who previously have been sedentary, or nearly so, should start slowly, and gradually approach the desired level of physical activity. It is recommended that such persons should begin the program with walking as the exercise mode. The walking should be at a comfortable pace so that it is always kept well within the individual's capacity. The intensity of exercise should always be kept low enough so that the associated fatigue can be relieved with a few minutes' rest. Initially, walking should be at a speed to cover 1 mile in 15 minutes. Later, the distance can be extended till 3 miles can be completed in 45 minutes. After that pace and distance have been achieved, almost everyone can progress to jogging or other activities.

The above may seem a very light amount of exercise, especially for a young person, but the relative stress of any given exercise is dependent on the individual's relative state of fitness. The poorer-conditioned one is, the less strenuous will be the exercise needed to raise the pulse rate. It might require a 1-mile run in less than 5 minutes to raise the pulse rate of a champion miler to 150, whereas someone who is sedentary in habits might need only to walk at a brisk pace to reach the same pulse rate. Therefore, it is possible for the sedentary, poorly-conditioned person to start out with relatively light exercise and still receive a training benefit. This individual might take several weeks to work up to more strenuous activities.

Intensity, Frequency, Duration, and Type of Exercise

A large volume of research has been conducted on intensity, frequency, and duration of exercise as they affect the cardiovascular conditioning aspects of various modes of exercise. There is a definite interaction among these factors, but it is impossible to prescribe the specific best combinations of them for males and females at all ages. However, certain generalities are apparent from the research, and recommendations are possible that will provide reasonable improvements in cardiovascular function for most persons. In general, these studies have shown that there is a threshold of exercise intensity below which a cardiovascular training effect will not occur. This threshold appears to be at approximately 75 per cent of the individual's maximal heart rate capacity. Therefore, it is very easy to monitor exercise intensity by simply counting the heart rate. This is best done by palpating either the temporal artery just in front of the ear, or the radial artery on the thumb side of the wrist, with slight finger pressure (Fig. 5–21A and B). The pulse should *not* be counted at the carotid artery in the throat (5–21C), since pressure on this artery apparently invokes a circulatory reflex in most persons that slows the heart rate abnormally and causes changes in the ECG.

In order to assess the intensity of an exercise, it is recommended that the individual participate in the exercise for 3 to 4 minutes at a steady pace. Then, *immediately* upon terminating the exercise, the pulse is counted for 10 seconds. The number of heart beats

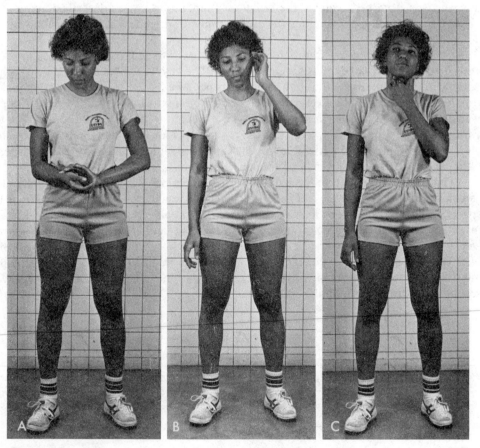

Figure 5–21. Suggested Arterial Locations for Counting Pulse Rate, A, B. Pulse should *not* be counted at carotid artery, C, as pressure on this artery causes a reflex change in the rate.

counted in the 10-second period is multiplied by six to change the count to a minute rate. If the minute rate thus determined is at least 75 per cent of the individual's age-adjusted maximal heart rate, a cardiovascular training effect is to be expected if duration and frequency of exercise are optimal. The age-adjusted maximal heart rate is used in this calculation because the maximal heart rate decreases with age: it is about 195 beats/min at age 20, but decreases at the rate of about 1 beat/year thereafter. The rates to be expected at various ages are shown in Table 5–4. There is no apparent sex difference in the level of maximal heart rate at a given age, nor in its rate of decline with aging.

The age decline in maximal heart rate is an important consideration in the choice of exercise intensities for a training effect, especially in older persons. Seventy-five per cent of maximal heart rate for a 20-year-old is 146 beats/min, but for a person 50 years of age it is 125 beats/min. The 146 figure would be almost 90 per cent of the older person's maximal heart rate. Training heart rate must be established on an individual basis. It is a questionable practice to use a standard heart rate such as 150/min for all ages; this rate may place a greater than optimal stress on some older persons.

The technique described above for estimating training intensity is applicable for all those who have resting heart rates between about 55 and 75 beats/min. If the resting heart is *above* 75 beats/min, the individual can expect a training effect at 65 to 70 per cent of age-adjusted maximal heart rate. If the resting heart rate is normally *below 55,* exercise intensity should be at 80 to 85 per cent of age-adjusted maximal heart rate.

Resting heart rate is best determined in the morning after one is fully awake but has not yet risen from bed. Palpate the radial or temporal artery, as described above, for about 5 to 6 minutes, and average the counts taken during the last three minutes of the counting period.

Optimal frequency and duration of exercise appear to be three to four days a week, with 20 to 40 minutes of exercise at each session. The key word here is *optimal,* for other combinations of intensity, duration, and frequency of exercise may produce significant training effects. Certainly, exercise at 90 per cent of maximal heart rate, seven days per week, and for one hour each session may be expected to provide a large stimulus for cardiovascular training. However, for the average person the additional time invested above the recommended optimal level will yield less return relative to the time spent. Also, injuries and other stress and trauma will increase.

The reader will note that three to four exercise periods per week are recommended as being an optimal frequency. It generally is recommended, also, that these periods be spaced more or less at even intervals throughout the week, i.e., every other day. Recent investigations have compared this approach to exercise frequency with fewer periods per week, and with exercise periods bunched together with a three-or four-day break between them. In one study, college age male subjects trained for ten weeks with high-intensity interval-type running on Monday, Tuesday, and Wednesday of each week. A second group trained in a similar manner but on Monday, Wednesday, and Friday. At the

Table 5–4.   MAXIMAL HEART RATE AT VARIOUS AGES

Age	Maximal Heart Rate
20	195
30	185
40	175
50	165
60	155
70	145

end of the ten weeks, both groups had made significant improvements in maximal oxygen consumption, and there was no noticeable difference in the rate at which they had improved. In another study, training for two days per week was compared with training for four days over periods of seven and 13 weeks. There was no difference in the improvement of maximal oxygen consumption with four days vs. two days per week of training. However, *heart rate at a standard submaximal work load decreased more in the four days/week group.*

The results of the above studies make it obvious that significant improvements in maximal oxygen consumption can be elicited from training frequencies fewer than three per week and from sessions not spaced evenly throughout the training week. However, there are other important considerations. In the latter study cited above, it was shown that the submaximal exercise heart rate decreased more with greater frequency of training. This is an important factor in circulatory economy. Second, there is research evidence suggesting that the exercise development of cardiac hypertrophy is related to the frequency of the exercise. The same is true for the enlargement of the main coronary arteries, and there is a linear relationship between coronary artery diameter and heart weight. Furthermore, it was pointed out earlier in this chapter that circulating blood levels of triglycerides, even though reduced by exercise, return to higher levels within 72 to 96 hours unless the exercise is repeated. These factors argue in favor of more frequent exercise bouts, interspersed with nonexercise intervals of no more than 48 to 72 hours.

Let us reiterate the consensus in regard to intensity, frequency, and duration of training for a cardiovascular training effect. The first consideration is intensity. The exercise intensity must be such that it achieves a level equal to, or greater than, the training threshold. For most persons, this is 75 per cent of the individual's age-adjusted maximal heart rate. This is not to say that the heart rate must be above this level throughout the entire exercise period. However, it should at least average 75 per cent of maximum. Intermittent-type exercise in which the heart rate alternately rises above and falls below 75 per cent of maximum can be very effective as a training stimulus (i.e., interval training: see Appendix A–10).

An optimal cardiovascular function training program is one in which the exercise is at an average intensity of 75 per cent of maximal heart rate for a period of 20 to 40 minutes per session, with the sessions repeated at least three to four times per week within 48- to 72-hour intervals.

The type of exercise used within these training sessions is relatively unimportant as long as the above criteria are met. It is preferable that the activity be one that emphasizes an endurance component. Walking, jogging in place or while moving, running, cycling, swimming, rope skipping, Nordic (cross-country) and Alpine (downhill) skiing, ice and roller skating, rowing, and stair climbing are all excellent in this regard. Various sport activities that require an element of running also can be good (e.g., basketball, handball, tennis, badminton). In order to assure continuation it is best to provide variety in the program; repeated participation in the same exercise causes many people to lose their motivation. Jogging, swimming, cycling, and Nordic skiing are prehaps the best all-round activities for cardiovascular conditioning because they require a high percentage of aerobic energy output. Participation in a sport such as badminton may not yield as great a cardiovascular training effect as jogging, swimming, or cycling, but if the participant dislikes these latter activities and enjoys badminton, it should be the activity of choice, even though it may take longer to gain the same cardiovascular training effects.

Table 5–5 can be used in selecting sport activities for participation. Emphasis should be placed on sports yielding at least a score of 20 from column C. Activities with more than 70 showing in column A are primarily speed and strength activities, with very little emphasis on the cardiovascular component of fitness.

Table 5–5. VARIOUS SPORTS AND THEIR PREDOMINANT ENERGY SYSTEM(S)*

| | % Emphasis According to Energy Systems | | |
| | A | B | C |
Sports or Sport Activity	ATP-PC and LA	LA-O₂	O₂
1. Baseball	80	20	—
2. Basketball	85	15	—
3. Fencing	90	10	—
4. Field Hockey	60	20	20
5. Football	90	10	—
6. Golf	95	5	—
7. Gymnastics	90	10	—
8. Ice Hockey			
a. forwards, defense	80	20	—
b. goalie	95	5	—
9. Lacrosse			
a. goalie, defense, attack men	80	20	—
b. midfielders, man-down	60	20	20
10. Rowing	20	30	50
11. Skiing			
a. slalom, jumping, downhill	80	20	—
b. cross-country	—	5	95
c. pleasure skiing	34	33	33
12. Soccer			
a. goalie, wings, strikers	80	20	—
b. halfbacks, or link men	60	20	20
13. Swimming and Diving			
a. 50 yds, diving	98	2	—
b. 100 yds	80	15	5
c. 200 yds	30	65	5
d. 400, 500 yds	20	40	40
e. 1500, 1650 yds	10	20	70
14. Tennis	70	20	10
15. Track and Field			
a. 100, 220 yds	98	2	—
b. field events	90	10	—
c. 440 yds	80	15	5
d. 880 yds	30	65	5
e. 1 mile	20	55	25
f. 2 miles	20	40	40
g. 3 miles	10	20	70
h. 6 miles (cross-country)	5	15	80
i. marathon	—	5	95
16. Volleyball	90	10	—
17. Wrestling	90	10	—

*From Fox, E. L., and Mathews, D. K.: *Interval Training: Conditioning for Sports and General Fitness.* Philadelphia, W. B. Saunders Co., 1974.

At this point, a comment is appropriate in regard to sports competition among persons differing significantly in ability. In competitive games, persons not closely matched in ability may expend quite different amounts of energy from those expended when they are matched more closely. This is illustrated in Figure 5–22, which shows energy expenditures of handball players under different competitive situations. Players evenly matched, or an inexperienced player matched against an experienced player, expended energy at a rate 45 to 63 per cent greater than did an experienced player against one who was inexperienced. The same type of situation would be expected to hold true for other competitive sport situations. Even in noncompetitive participation in jogging-running or swimming, the less skilled and less experienced participant will expend more energy at a given speed of progression than the more skilled and experienced.

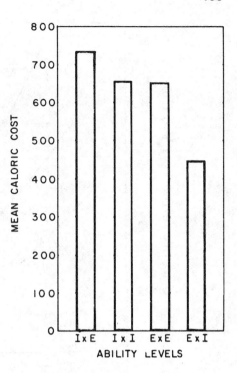

Figure 5-22. Total Mean Caloric Cost Per Hour of Experienced Handball Players *(E)* and Inexperienced Players *(I)* Playing Against a Player of Their Own Ability and Also One of Either Superior or Inferior Ability. (From Banister, E. W., and Brown, S. R.: The Relative Energy Requirements of Physical Activity. *In* Falls, H. B. (ed.) *Exercise Physiology.* New York, Academic Press, 1968.)

Initial Level of Fitness and Age in Determining the Cardiovascular Training Effect

The age of participants and their initial level of fitness are important factors in determining the degree of improvement that can be expected from a cardiovascular conditioning program. In general, the older person is less "trainable" than one who is younger. The same holds true for a person who already possesses a relatively high level of cardiovascular fitness. Figure 5–23 illustrates these interactions: it can be noted that those who are younger and less fit at the beginning of a conditioning program can be expected to show the greatest percentage improvement for any given combination of intensity, duration, and frequency of exercise.

Other Special Considerations in Training for Cardiovascular Function

Environmental Factors

HEAT STRESS

Exercise when the environmental temperature and/or humidity is high can lead to heat stress wherein the circulation and other physiological mechanisms are taxed because the body encounters difficulty in removing the heat generated by the increased metabolism of exercise. Heat stress may even occur at lower temperatures and humidity, in sports such as skiing, if the clothing is too heavy and interferes with the evaporation of sweat from the surface of the body.

During heat stress, as much as 25 per cent of the blood that ordinarily would be flowing through the capillary beds in the muscles is diverted to the skin in order to carry heat from the core of the body to the surface. That means that the oxygen it carries,

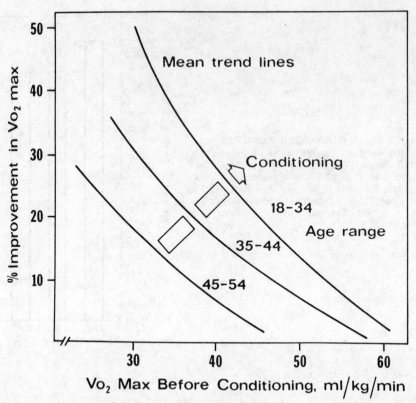

Figure 5–23. Percentage Improvement that can be Expected from an Optimum Cardiovascular Conditioning Program, Relations to Age and Initial State of Fitness. (From Buskirk, E. R.: Cardiovascular Adaptation to Physical Effort in Healthy Men. *In* Naughton, J. P., and Hellerstein, H. K. (eds.) *Exercise Testing and Exercise Training in Coronary Heart Disease.* New York, Academic Press, 1973.)

ordinarily used for metabolism in the muscle, returns to the heart without diffusing into the muscle cells. In addition, the water content of sweat comes from the blood plasma: in a literal sense we "sweat blood." These problems have several implications.

1. The work capacity will be reduced. The blood being shunted away from the muscles to the skin will make it such that any given amount of work will impose a greater stress on the circulatory system. The individual cannot then work as long or as hard at any given task. This may lead to excessive levels of fatigue. Even prolonged and excessive sweating alone (without heat stress) can cause extreme fatigue.

2. Loss of water in sweating can lead to dehydration. Significant dehydration triggers the body's reflex regulatory mechanisms that make it tend to conserve the remaining water. Sweating is the chief means of dissipating heat, and if sweating is reduced, body heat tends to accumulate abnormally, driving body temperature upward. This can lead to a failure of the body's temperature regulating mechanism and can result in heat stroke, which has a fatality rate of approximately 50 per cent.

Certain procedures can be followed by the exercise participant to reduce the adverse effects of heat stress. Dehydration can be prevented by replacing the body fluid that is lost in sweating. The thirst mechanism is not an adequate criterion of body water replacement, however. Research studies have shown that, when people drink to satisfy their thirst after exercising in a heat stress situation, they almost always end up with a water deficit. A better procedure is to use body weight. By measuring body weight before and after exercise, one can determine how much was lost as a result of the exercise. Nearly 100 per cent of such weight loss is sweat loss. Therefore, the basic principle is to drink enough water to bring the body weight back to its normal level.

It is also good to have the water as cold as tolerable. Water that is less than body temperature will take up some of the heat stored in the body as it is warmed to the body temperature. For instance, if the body temperature is 100°F, and one drinks only a pint of water at 60°F, the water will take up about 12 kilocalories of the heat stored in the body. Water at colder temperatures will take up even greater quantities of heat. There is no physiological reason why an individual should not drink even very cold water, as long as it does not cause headache and nausea.

Some of the fatiguing effects of excessive sweating can be counteracted by taking a little extra salt in hot weather. This can be accomplished by adding a few extra sprinkles to food at mealtime, or by salt dissolved in fluids that are drunk. Only a small amount is needed—about 1 tablespoon per gallon of water. Salt tablets are relatively ineffective as they do not readily dissolve in the gastrointestinal tract, and often pass completely through virtually in their original form.

Drinking one of the special electrolyte solutions such as Gatorade, Body punch, or Sportade, etc., is effective since they contain salt in approximately the same quantity as that needed for replacement in the body. However, they are expensive and unnecessary. A great deal of research has been conducted, and there is no conclusive evidence that they are any more effective at relieving heat stress than plain salt and water.

A word of caution is warranted in regard to the taking of salt and other electrolytes (sugar). One can get too much. Too high an electrolyte concentration in the gastrointestinal tract will interfere with water absorption by the body and actually may cause reabsorption of fluid back into the tract. This is due to the osmotic effect of the electrolyte concentration.

Because of the reduction in muscle blood flow that occurs with exercise in heat stress, it is recommended that the intensity and/or duration of exercise be reduced by 25 per cent in these situations. This will tend to compensate for the larger reduction in blood flow to the muscle, and still give approximately the same cardiovascular training effect without inducing either excessive stress during the exercise or undue postexercise fatigue.

Environmental conditions may be considered to be conducive to heat stress any time when the relative humidity is above 60 per cent and/or the temperature is above 83°F. The body temperature usually is effectively regulated below these levels as long as the clothing is light and loose and there is no external barrier, such as a sweatsuit, that interferes with the vaporization of sweat from the body surface. Rubber and plastic suits should not be worn during exercise, even in cold weather. The body must vaporize sweat in order effectively to control its temperature, and these suits impose a severe impediment to that mechanism.

EXERCISE IN COLD WEATHER

Although problems are not as likely to occur during cold weather exercise as in hot weather, they do arise for some individuals. Exercising in very cold temperatures (less than 30°F) increases the mean systemic blood pressure by up to 20 mm Hg. This increases the work of the heart and causes a concomitant increase in the oxygen required by the heart muscle. This should pose no difficulty, other than a reduction in work capacity, for those with a completely healthy circulatory system. However, in persons with diseases of the coronary circulation (diagnosed or unsuspected), it can cause angina pectoris, severe reduction in work capacity, and perhaps other adverse consequences. Those with known heart disease and/or low working capacity (low max O_2 consumption) would be particularly susceptible to the above-mentioned problems, and should be especially cautious when exercising outdoors in cold weather. They should reduce their exercise intensity well below the levels normally applied during moderate weather.

The effects of wind are an important consideration in cold weather exercise. A strong wind can cause the effective environmental temperature to be much less than the actual air temperature reading. This effect is referred to as "wind chill," and often is given as part of the weather report on radio and television. Running into the wind raises the wind chill factor. For example, if the wind speed is 10 mph, and one runs against the wind at a speed of 10 mph (6-minute mile pace), the effective wind speed is increased to 20 mph. Running with the wind has the opposite effect—wind chill is decreased. If one is jogging against the wind as part of a work-out, it is always preferable to do this in the early part of the work-out, and then do the running with the wind in the latter stages. If one runs against the wind after sweating has increased, and the sweat has collected on the surface of the body and in the clothing, the chilling effects of the wind will be accentuated. Running with the wind after one has worked up a sweat will decrease the chilling effect. Table 5–6 shows the wind chill effect by presenting various environmental temperature and wind speed combinations, and the associated effective temperatures. The exercise participant may use it in planning the type of clothing and other precautions for exercise sessions. One important thing to remember is that exposed flesh can suffer frostbite damage within a very short period whenever the effective temperature is below −20°F.

There is a tendency for persons inexperienced at exercising in the cold to dress too warmly. The objective is to dress so that one feels comfortably warm during the exercise period but not so that profuse sweating is caused. Usually, one or two layers of light clothing, a knit cap for the head and ears, and knit jersey gloves for the hands are sufficient. In very cold weather, a ski mask can be worn to protect the face. It is recommended that clothing which traps heat and sweat vapor should not be worn as this usually makes the exercise participant uncomfortably warm. The authors have found from their own experience that a suit of cotton or cotton and polyester blend thermal underwear makes an excellent cold weather exercise outfit. It can be worn underneath the usual shorts and tee shirt or blouse. A heavyweight suit will usually protect the arms and legs sufficiently, even in very cold weather, and a lighter-weight suit can be worn, if preferred, when the temperature is not quite so cold. Some of the irritating effects of inhaled cold air can be eliminated by breathing through a ski mask or muffler wrapped across the nose and mouth.

Table 5–6. WIND CHILL INDEX

Wind Speed mph	Actual Temperature, °F					
	50	40	30	20	10	0
	Effective Temperature, °F					
Calm	50	40	30	20	10	0
5	48	37	27	16	6	−5
10	40	28	16	4	−9	−21
15	36	22	9	−5	−18	−36
20	32	18	4	−10	−25	−39
25	30	16	0	−15	−29	−44
30	28	13	−2	−18	−33	−48
35	27	11	−4	−20	−35	−49
40*	26	10	−6	−21	−37	−53

*Wind speeds greater than 40 mph have little additional effect.

Smoking and Cardiovascular Conditioning

Smoking tobacco is a practice that nearly everyone knows to be detrimental to general health in many ways. Well-publicized effects are the increased risk of coronary heart disease and lung cancer. Tobacco smoking also contributes to a less-than-optimal improvement in cardiovascular fitness during a training program. Cigarette smoking deposits tars and other impurities on the surface of the lung membranes, thereby reducing their diffusing capacity for oxygen. It also causes changes in the respiratory airway and increases the resistance to breathing. This results in a greater proportion of the maximal oxygen consumption being used for the work of the respiratory muscles. In addition, the nicotine in the smoke causes constriction of peripheral blood vessels, which elevates the heart rate and blood pressure above normal nonsmoking levels, both at rest and during exercise. Furthermore, the carbon monoxide in tobacco smoke reduces the oxygen-carrying capacity of the blood by displacing some of the oxygen that ordinarily would be combined with the hemoglobin in the red blood cell.

All the above factors combine to reduce working capacity, as shown in Figure 5–24. In the study on which the illustration is based, 60 college-age males trained with interval training techniques three times a week for a period of eight weeks. As can be seen, both smokers and nonsmokers increased in estimated maximal oxygen consumption, but the nonsmokers started out in better condition and maintained their advantage throughout the training program. In a similar study on several hundred U.S. Air Force recruits, it was noted that at the beginning of basic training nonsmokers could cover more distance on the 12-minute run test of cardiovascular fitness than could smokers. Both smokers and nonsmokers steadily increased the distances they could cover in 12 minutes throughout the six-week basic training period, but the nonsmokers maintained a higher level of performance, just as in the study shown in Figure 5–24. It was also noted that the level of cardiovascular fitness was inversely related to the number of cigarettes habitually smoked, i.e., the heavier smokers exhibited lowest cardiovascular fitness. In addition,

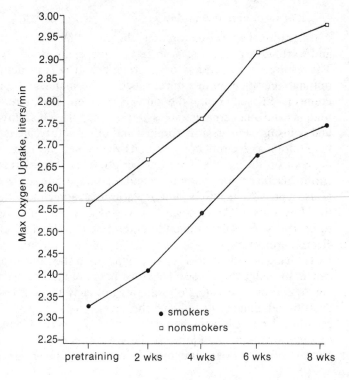

Figure 5–24. Effect of Interval Training on Maximum Oxygen Consumption in Smokers and Nonsmokers. (From data presented by Peterson, F. J., and Kelley, D. L.: The Effect of Cigarette Smoking Upon the Acquisition of Physical Fitness During Training as Measured by Aerobic Capacity. J. Am. Coll. Health Assoc. *17*:250, 1969.)

Max Oxygen Uptake, liters/min

• smokers
□ nonsmokers

pretraining   2 wks   4 wks   6 wks   8 wks

the smokers had higher heart rates at all levels of submaximal exercise when compared with the nonsmokers, an indication that their hearts had to work harder to help the body to accomplish any given amount of work.

These studies suggest that, even though smokers can improve their cardiovascular function through training, they always will have a lower level of fitness than would be the case if they did not smoke. Thus, the circulatory and respiratory systems are always operating under an additional burden imposed by the effects of the cigarette smoke.

Alcohol Consumption and Cardiovascular Conditioning

Chronic consumption of ethanol (alcohol) in moderate amounts is not known to have any deleterious effects on the level of cardiovascular function or on the ease with which that function may be improved through physical training. However, if alcohol consumption has progressed to the point at which it has caused liver deterioration or other adverse physiological and/or anatomical changes, work capacity and training potential may be reduced. Perhaps the major concern in regard to alcohol consumption is the possible effect it may have if it is closely followed by exercise. Alcohol consumption causes vasodilation in peripheral blood vessels, sending more blood to the skin. This is similar to the effect of heat stress. The potential muscle blood flow and maximal work capacity thus are reduced. Alcohol also has a diuretic effect that may cause dehydration. This can be a special problem when exercising in hot weather, even one or two days after the alcohol consumption. In industries in which heat stress is a significant problem, medical personnel have always noted a higher incidence of heat illness on Mondays than on other days of the week. This has been attributed to increased consumption of alcohol over the weekend.

In view of the above problems, the exercise participant is advised to use caution when exercising shortly after anything but very moderate alcohol consumption. On the two or three days immediately following moderately heavy-to-heavy bouts of drinking, the exercise intensity should be reduced accordingly.

Warm-up and Warm-down

In rational exercise programs, the three "W"'s are important—warm-up, work-out, and warm-down. The warm-up serves to prepare the body for the stresses of exercise. The respiratory and circulatory systems are stirred into action, muscles are warmed to an optimal operating temperature, much in the manner of an automobile engine, and the connective tissue around the joints is warmed. Slow stretching exercises make muscle tendons and other connective tissue more supple. This allows a greater ease of movement and helps prevent strains, sprains, and other soft tissue injury. The mobilization of the respiratory and circulatory systems decreases the body's need to rely on anaerobic metabolism during the work-out period. This insures that the exercise is primarily a cardiovascular training stimulus, and reduces undue stress on the body's systems. There is also a possible health benefit of warm-up in some individuals. At the medical school of the University of California at Los Angeles, men 21 to 52 years of age and asymptomatic to heart disease were studied to determine the effect of sudden, strenuous exertion on electrocardiographic responses. When sudden exertion was not preceded by warm-up, ECG changes indicating a relative hypoxia in the myocardium were observed in 60 per cent of the subjects. These changes were not related to age or state of physical conditioning. Warm-up, consisting of 2 minutes of easy jogging-in-place just before the sudden exertion, eliminated or reduced the severity of the ECG changes in most cases. Blood pressure also was lower when the exertion was preceded by warm-up. It was noted, too, that the warm-up could precede the strenuous exercise by as much as 10 to 15 minutes and still provide a benefit in terms of modifying the ECG responses. It thus appears that warm-up may be important in reducing the possibility of hypoxia in the heart muscle at the beginning of strenuous exercise. This could be especially crucial in any person with a degree of underlying coronary artery disease.

Warming down (sometimes referred to as *cool-down*) is a term describing the continuation of exercise at low intensity for a few minutes following a normal work-out. The purpose is to allow the body slowly to readjust to the resting state. Walking is the most commonly used activity for gradually decreasing the intensity level. When exercise ends abruptly, the heart is still sending blood to the muscles at an increased rate. Since the muscles are no longer contracting and helping to move the blood back toward the heart, the blood has a tendency to pool in the muscles. This may result in insufficient blood for other organs of the body. Fainting may even occur if blood flow to the brain is decreased. Also, continuation of exercise at a low intensity helps to speed recovery by removing accumulated lactic acid at a faster rate.

Insuring Continued Improvement Through the Conditioning Program

If the recommendations earlier in this chapter in regard to intensity, duration, and frequency of exercise are followed for a period of several weeks, a definite improvement in cardiovascular function should occur. This should be noticeable in a subjective sense by the way the individual feels. A given intensity of exercise should cause less circulatory and respiratory distress; there should be less chronic fatigue; sleep may be improved; and there should be a greater over-all sense of well-being. In addition, it is suggested that participants make an objective check on progress by retesting themselves periodically on the 12-minute run or by other procedures.

In all conditioning programs, a leveling-off point, or plateau, is eventually reached. This occurs because the cardiovascular capacity will have improved to the point at which the intensity of exercise is no longer providing a stimulus for further development (e.g., the level of heart rate during the exercise may be below 75 per cent of age-adjusted maximum). When this point is reached, the individual may be able to maintain the achieved level of function, but no further improvement will be noted until the combined stimulus of intensity, duration, and frequency is increased. Therefore, exercise participants periodically should retest their fitness level and also check the heart rate being reached during the exercise period, to assure that improvement is occurring and that the intensity of exercise is still sufficient. An exercise intensity that raises the heart rate to 150 beats/min in a sedentary person will not cause the rate to go as high when that person becomes physically fit (see Fig. 5–9). The intensity of exercise will need to be adjusted accordingly.

Six week-intervals are sufficiently short periods for making the above checks on progress. The procedure is known as the principle of progressive resistance. It originated with, and is still widely used in, weight-training programs. When a plateau of strength improvement occurs, more weight (resistance) is added to the exercise. The concept is applicable to all forms of conditioning. In training programs for cardiovascular function, the "resistance" is intensity and/or duration of the exercise being used.

Loss of Training Effects with Decreased Levels of Exercise

A point of special interest in regard to cardiovascular conditioning programs is the rate at which training effects are dissipated if exercise is terminated or reduced in frequency. The effects of training do not suddenly disappear if training stops! They are gradually dissipated. This is illustrated in Figure 5–25. Two groups of young adults were given one half-hour of training daily for four weeks. At the end of that period, they showed an increase of 20 per cent in work capacity. Group I subsequently continued to

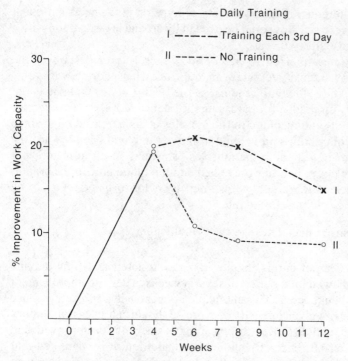

Figure 5–25. Effect of Decreased Training on Retention of Cardiovascular Fitness. (Adapted from Roskamm, H.: Optimal Patterns of Exercise for Healthy Adults. Originally published in Canadian Medical Association Journal *96*:895, March 1967.)

train every third day (about twice per week). Although there was some drop-off, they were able to sustain the increased working capacity at near the level it had reached through the four weeks of intensive training. Group II stopped all training after the four weeks. The working capacity decreased rapidly during the first two weeks of no training, but tended to plateau during the next six weeks. Even after eight weeks without training, the improved work capacity was still approximately midway between the initial level and the level reached with training.

Similar results have been obtained from other research. It seems apparent that cardiovascular condition, once attained, can be maintained with only a moderate effort on the part of the individual. Some fitness experts have speculated, on the basis of available research data, that two periods per week of training only on the weekend might be sufficient to improve and/or maintain cardiovascular function. However, before readers are encouraged to follow such an exercise regimen, they should reread the earlier comments in this chapter in regard to the relationships between exercise frequency and cardiac hypertrophy, coronary artery enlargement, and the reduction of serum triglycerides. These are important in the total circulatory health picture. It could well be that, even though training twice per week improves or maintains maximal oxygen consumption, such a pattern of training may have no beneficial effect on other desirable qualities related to the circulation. Following that type of program, therefore, would be a less desirable health-related fitness practice.

LEARNING OBJECTIVES

After completing a study of Chapter 5 on cardiovascular fitness, students should be able to

1. Demonstrate a knowledge of average values for maximal oxygen consumption for both sexes in young adulthood in ml/kg body weight/min.

2. Define maximal oxygen consumption.

3. Estimate maximal oxygen consumption from 12-minute run performance.

4. Explain the effect of aging on maximal oxygen consumption.

5. Define endurance and explain why maximal oxygen consumption is a significant factor in endurance.

6. Explain the effects of tobacco smoking on the respiration and circulation, and say what effect it has in a conditioning program.

7. Identify the best method(s) for measuring cardiovascular function.

8. Explain, in general, the purpose of an electrocardiographic measurement.

9. Define what is meant by cardiac output.

10. Explain the effect that physical conditioning has on resting, exercise, and recovery heart rates.

11. Define stroke volume of the heart.

12. Explain why heart rate decreases when there is an increase in stroke volume as a result of physical conditioning.

13. Define blood pressure and explain how it is commonly measured.

14. Indicate the approximate normal ranges for blood pressure at various ages.

15. Define essential and secondary hypertension.

16. Describe how blood pressure changes during exercise as compared to rest.

17. Write a general definition of interval training.

18. Explain the inter-relationships between intensity, duration, and frequency of exercise as they relate to improvement in cardiovascular function.

19. Explain the meaning of the terms *systole* (systolic) and *diastole* (diastolic) as they relate to the heart function and blood pressure.

20. Demonstrate a knowledge of what collateral circulation means in regard to heart function, and indicate how it might affect the health of the circulatory system.

21. Explain the coronary circulation.

22. Define coronary heart disease (CHD).

23. Define the terms *atherosclerosis* and *arteriosclerosis*, and indicate in what way(s) they may be related.

24. Define heart volume; indicate sex differences.

25. Explain in what way(s) chronic exercise would be expected to affect heart volume.

26. Explain the relationship between heart volume and stroke volume of the heart.

27. List and explain the primary factors responsible for sex differences in circulatory function.

28. List and explain the primary factors that account for individual variations in maximal oxygen consumption, i.e. say what makes one person have a max O_2 uptake of 60 ml/kg/min whereas another has only 40.

29. List and explain the major benefits of an optimal level of cardiovascular fitness.

30. Explain how atherosclerosis and arteriosclerosis may be implicated in hypertension.

31. Define cholesterol and triglycerides of the blood; explain how these may affect cardiovascular health.

32. Explain what effect decrease in elasticity of the arteries of the body has on cardiovascular health.

33. Demonstrate a knowledge of how to evaluate an individual's cardiovascular health.

34. Explain the procedures involved in Cooper's 12-minute run test, and the scientific basis for it.

35. Explain how to estimate exercise heart rate from a rate taken postexercise.

36. Explain the SAID principle as it relates to cardiovascular conditioning.

37. Demonstrate a knowledge of average, above average, and below average performance on Cooper's 12-minute run test for both sexes at various ages.

38. Explain how reduction of excess body fat possibly may affect an individual's cardiovascular health.

39. Demonstrate a knowledge of average resting and maximal exercise heart rates in young adult males and females.

40. Explain why the 12-minute run test is called the "aerobics" test.

41. Convert a maximal oxygen consumption measurement to ml/kg wt/min when given the measure in liters/min.

42. Explain what medical screening procedures should be followed as a prerequisite for participation in a cardiovascular conditioning program.

43. Demonstrate a knowledge of the possible significance of "warming-up."

44. Explain the concept of progressive resistance exercise as it relates to cardiovascular conditioning.

45. Explain in what way(s) the antigravity musculature is important in cardiovascular conditioning.

46. Explain in what way(s) the initial level of fitness affects the degree of improvement that can be expected from a cardiovascular conditioning program.

47. Define hyperlipidemia and explain how exercise, or the lack thereof, may affect it.

48. Explain why wearing rubber or plastic suits while exercising is not an effective way to lose weight; indicate possible dangers of this practice.

49. Explain why it is not appropriate to count pulse rate by palpating the carotid artery in the throat.

50. Determine threshold intensity of exercise for a cardiovascular training effect from age-adjusted maximal heart rate.

51. Explain why the recommended frequency of training for cardiovascular fitness is at least three times per week.

52. List and explain the precautions that should be taken when performing endurance exercise under heat stress conditions.

53. Define "wind chill" and explain how it may affect exercise performance.

54. Explain what factors must be considered when one exercises within 24 to 48 hours after alcohol consumption.

REFERENCES

1. American College of Sports Medicine: *Guidelines for Graded Exercise Testing and Exercise Prescription.* Philadelphia, Lea and Febiger, 1975.
2. American College of Sports Medicine: The recommended quantity and quality of exercise for developing and maintaining fitness in healthy adults. Med. Sci. Sports *10*:vii, 1978.
3. American Medical Association: Evaluation for exercise participation: the apparently healthy individual. J.A.M.A. *219*:900, 1972.
4. Anschutz, F.: Aortic Sclerosis and Cardiac Strain in Elderly People. *In* D. Brunner, and E. Jokl (eds.), *Physical Activity and Aging.* Baltimore, University Park Press, 1970.
5. Astrand, I.: Aerobic capacity in men and women, with special reference to age. Acta Physiol. Scand. *49*(Suppl. 169):1960.
6. Astrand, P.-O., and Rodahl, K.: *Textbook of Work Physiology.* New York, McGraw-Hill Book Co., 1977.
7. Balke, B.: A Simple Field Test for the Assessment of Physical Fitness. Oklahoma City, Publication 63–6, Civil Aeromedical Research Institute, 1963.
8. Barnard, R. J.: Long-term Effects of Exercise on Cardiac Function. *In* J. H. Wilmore, and J. F. Keogh (eds.), *Exercise and Sport Sciences Reviews,* Vol. 3. New York, Academic Press, 1975.
9. Barnard, R. J., et al.: Cardiovascular responses to sudden strenuous exercise—heart rate, blood pressure, and ECG. J. Appl. Physiol. *34*:833, 1973.
10. Bonanno, J. A.: Effects of physical training on coronary risk factors. Am. J. Cardiol. *33*:760, 1974.
11. Bourne, G. H.: Structural Changes in Aging. *In* N. W. Shock (ed.), *Aging: Some Social and Biological Aspects.* Freeport, New York, Books for Libraries Press, 1972.

12. Boyer, J. L., and Kasch, F. W.: Exercise therapy in hypertensive men. J.A.M.A. *211*:1668, 1970.
13. Bransford, D. R., and Howley, E. T.: Oxygen cost of running in trained and untrained men and women. Med. Sci. Sports *9*:41, 1977.
14. Choquette, G., and Ferguson, R. J.: Blood pressure reduction in "borderline" hypertensives following physical training. Can. Med. Assoc. J. *108*:699, 1973.
15. Cooper, K. H.: A means of assessing maximal oxygen intake. J.A.M.A. *203*:201, 1968.
16. Cooper, K. H., Gey, G. O., and Bottenberg. R. A.: Effects of cigarette smoking on endurance performance. J.A.M.A. *203*:189, 1968.
17. Davies, C. T. M.: Limitations to the prediction of maximum oxygen intake from cardiac frequency measurements. J. Appl. Physiol. *24*:700, 1968.
18. Disch, J., Frankiewicz, R., and Jackson, A.: Construct validity of distance run tests. Res. Q. Am. Assoc. Health Phys. Educ. *46*:169, 1975.
19. Epstein, S. E., et al.: Effects of a reduction in environmental temperature on the circulatory response to exercise in man. N. Engl. J. Med. *280*:7, 1969.
20. Faulkner, J. A.: Physiology of Swimming and Diving. *In* H. B. Falls, (ed.), *Exercise Physiology*. New York, Academic Press, 1968.
21. Faulkner, J. A., Heigenhauser, G. F., and Schork, M. A.: The cardiac output–oxygen uptake relationship of men during graded bicycle ergometry. Med. Sci. Sports *9*:148, 1977.
22. Fox, E. L., et al.: Frequency and duration of interval training programs and changes in aerobic power. J. Appl. Physiol. *38*:481, 1975.
23. Gilliam, T. B., Katch, V. L., Tharland, W., and Weltman, A.: Prevalence of coronary heart disease risk factors in active children, 7 to 12 years of age. Med. Sci. Sports *9*:21, 1977.
24. Hanson, J. S., and Nedde, W. H.: Preliminary observations on physical training for hypertensive males. Circ. Res. *26, 27* (Suppl. 1): 49, 1970.
25. Hattenhauer, M., and Neill, W. A.: The effects of cold air inhalation on angina pectoris and myocardial oxygen supply. Circulation *51*:1053, 1975.
26. Hodgson, J. L.: Age and Aerobic Capacity of Urban Midwestern Males. Ph.D. Dissertation, Minneapolis, University of Minnesota, 1971.
27. Leithead, C. S., and Lind, A. R.: *Heat Stress and Heat Disorders*. Philadelphia, F. A. Davis Co., 1964.
28. Leon, A. S., and Bloor, C. M.: Effects of exercise and its cessation on the heart and its blood supply. J. Appl. Physiol. *24*:485, 1968.
29. Leon, D. F., Morteza, A., and Leonard, J. J.: Left heart work and temperature responses to cold exposure in man. Am. J. Cardiol. *26*:38, 1970.
30. Letounov, S.: The importance of physical education and sport as preventive measures for healthy and sick persons. J. Sports Med. Phys. Fitness *9*:142, 1969.
31. Margaria, R. P., Cerretelli, P., Aghemo, R., and Sassi, G.: Energy cost of running. J. Appl. Physiol. *18*:367, 1963.
32. Meerson, F. A.: Mechanism of hypertrophy of the heart and experimental prevention of acute cardiac insufficiency. Br. Heart. J. *33* (Suppl.):100, 1971.
33. Miller, B. F., and Burt, J. J.: *Good Health: Personal and Community*. Philadelphia, W. B. Saunders Co., 1972.
34. Moffatt, R. J., Stamford, B. A., and Neill, R. D.: Placement of tri-weekly training sessions: importance regarding enhancement of aerobic capacity. Res. Q. Am. Assoc. Health Phys. Educ. *48*:583, 1977.
35. Neill, W. A.: Coronary and Systemic Circulatory Adaptations to Exercise. *In* E. A. Amsterdam, J. H. Wilmore, and A. N. DeMaria (eds.) *Exercise in Cardiovascular Health and Disease*. New York, Yorke Medical Books, 1977.
36. Rode, A., and Shephard, R. J.: The influence of cigarette smoking upon the oxygen cost of breathing in near-maximal exercise." Med. Sci. Sports *3*:51, 1971.
37. Rose, G., Prineas, R. J., and Mitchell, J. R. A.: Myocardial infarction and the intrinsic calibre of coronary arteries. Br. Heart J. *29*:548, 1967.
38. Ross, J., Jr., and O'Rourke, R. A.: *Understanding the Heart and its Diseases*. New York, McGraw-Hill Book Co., 1976.
39. Saltin, B., Blomquist, G., Mitchell, J. H., Johnson, R. D., Jr., Wildenthal, K., and Chapman, C. B.: Response to submaximal and maximal exercise after bed rest and training. Circulation *38*(Suppl. 7): 1968.
40. Scheuer, J., Penparqkul, S., and Bhan, A. K.: Experimental Observations on the Effects of Physical Training upon Intrinsic Cardiac Physiology and Biochemistry. *In* E. A. Amsterdam, J. H. Wilmore, and A. N. DeMaria (eds.). *Exercise in Cardiovascular Health and Disease*. New York, Yorke Medical Books, 1977.
41. Shock, N. W.: The physiology of aging. Sci. Am. *206*:100, 1962.
42. Skinner, J. S.: Age and Performance. *In* J. Keul (ed.) *Limiting Factors of Physical Performance*. Stuttgart, Germany, Georg Thieme, 1973.
43. White, J. R.: EKG changes using carotid artery for heart rate monitoring. Med. Sci. Sports *9*:88, 1977.
44. Wilmore, J. H.: Individualized Exercise Prescription. *In* E. A., Amsterdam, J. H. Wilmore, and A. N. DeMaria, (eds.) *Exercise in Cardiovascular Health and Disease*. New York, Yorke Medical Books, 1977.
45. Wilmore, J. H., and McNamara, J. J.: Prevalence of coronary heart disease risk factors in boys, 8 to 12 years of age. J. Pediatr. *84*:527, 1974.

Chapter 6

Flexibility

INTRODUCTION

Imagine a football punter who does not have the range of motion necessary to punt the football and allow the leg to follow through. If he is not flexible enough, the movement will not be executed as planned (inferior performance), or if the movement is forced under these conditions the possibility of injury is very great. A dancer who does not have adequate flexibility cannot move with ease through movements requiring extreme ranges of motion at the joints. Inadequate flexibility in the dancer either greatly reduces the movement repertoire and/or increases the chances for injury in movements requiring increased range of movement. For the agonist muscles to contract and cause joint movement, the antagonist muscles must be capable of lengthening to the extent necessary for that range of motion. Otherwise, movement is impaired and injury possibilities are greater.

Although the need for flexibility varies with the movement requirements of an individual, a degree of flexibility is important to general physical fitness. In addition, adequate flexibility in certain areas of the body (e.g., the low back, posterior thigh, and hip) has been identified as an important component of health-related fitness (see also Chapter 1, p. 7). Beside increasing movement capabilities and reducing the possibility of "low back syndrome," maintenance of an adequate range of motion about the joints through a flexibility program is believed to prevent or help relieve some of the aches, pains, and other problems associated with aging.

Flexibility commonly is defined as the range of motion about a joint. Flexibility differences are seen from one person to the next, and great differences occur within a single individual. One very obvious cause of these differences within an individual is the type of joint structure. Of the freely movable joints, the hinge joints and ball-and-socket-type joints present the greatest problems for flexibility—especially the latter (hip and shoulder). Another potential limiting factor is the amount of muscle and fatty tissue around the joint. Body type does not appear to be highly related to flexibility.

A flexibility program, no matter how good, cannot change the basic joint structure. It is designed instead to increase the extensibility of muscles and connective tissue. In joints that can receive the most benefit from flexibility exercise, the limitation of the range of motion is imposed by the muscle and its fascial sheaths, connective tissue (tendons, ligaments, and joint capsules), and the skin.

It is quite easy to conceive of a muscle sheath that is seldom stretched beyond its normal resting length becoming so shortened that range of motion is limited. In a flexibility program an individual must devise a safe means of periodically stretching the muscle and connective tissue. Because flexibility is very specific to the joint involved, no one general exercise can be used. A person must select flexibility exercises that will adequately cover the areas of the body needing the exercise. These areas may differ, depending on the activity requirements of the individual, but the following areas are usually important in most persons: the muscles around the ball and socket joints (hip and shoulder); the posterior lower leg (especially in those who often wear high-heeled shoes and in joggers or runners); the muscles of the middle and low back (also the lumbosacral fascia); the anterior chest muscles; and the muscles of the posterior thigh (hamstrings).

Until recently, flexibility exercises and programs have appeared to be more popular with females than with males. Men, who appear to have the biological edge in muscular strength and cardiovascular endurance, have not experienced the same advantage in flexibility programs. In fact, their greater emphasis on strength development programs in the absence of flexibility programs probably has contributed to their lower flexibility by building larger muscle bulk and stronger, more developed muscle fascia and tendons. Because of muscle bulk development, men probably have experienced more difficulty with flexibility exercises than have women. This does not mean that a person cannot be both strong and flexible. It does mean that those who develop the muscle and its connective tissue should work concurrently to develop and retain flexibility. Individuals who have developed muscles and connective tissues in a strength program without concomitant flexibility development have a stronger system limiting their range of motion than those who have not experienced as much strength development.

In recent years, it appears that men have become more involved with flexibility programs. The myth that stretching tears away muscle tissue has finally been dispelled. Much of the increased interest may be attributable to the importance many athletic coaches are now placing on development of flexibility for improved performance. In addition, people in general seem to be more knowledgeable about the importance of development of the various components of health-related fitness.

STATIC VS. BALLISTIC STRETCHING

The trend in safe flexibility programs has been away from *ballistic* or bouncing-type stretches, where the movement is suddenly and forcefully ended by an abrupt pull on muscle and connective tissue. These types of stretch have been replaced in preference by slow *static stretches,* where the resistance of the stretch is gradually developed to a point slightly beyond comfort and held for a short time before it is released. Both programs appear to be about equal in the development of flexibility, but the static approach is preferred for several reasons.

1. There is less danger of exceeding the extensibility limits of the tissues because the force is gradually applied and held. Therefore, injuries resulting from the stretching program can be reduced or eliminated.

2. The gradual application of force in the static program has also resulted in much less muscle soreness than the ballistic stretch. In fact, the static stretch has been advocated as a method to relieve muscular soreness and as a form of warm-up.

3. The static stretch is less energy-consuming than the ballistic method.

In addition to the above, the static method has another major advantage over the ballistic method. A slow static stretch tends to counteract what is known as the *stretch reflex* of the muscle, which was explained in Chapter 2. A common example of the stretch reflex is tapping someone just below the kneecap on the patellar tendon [tendon from the quadriceps femoris (anterior thigh) muscles]. This places a sudden stretch on the muscle and causes it to contract reflexly. The knee is extended in a sort of kicking action. This often is referred to as the "knee-jerk" reflex. The primary endings of muscle spindles (stretch receptors in muscle) respond to the sudden stretch by reflexly exciting some of the motor neurons controlling the stretched muscle. The end result of this reflex is a contraction of the muscle which is not injurious to the muscle, but does negate the purpose of the exercise. An exercise designed to lengthen the muscle and connective tissue is suddenly reversed by a reflex contraction of the muscle and thus the benefit is lost.

Another common procedure for enhancing stretch in a muscle is to use *reciprocal innervation,* which also was discussed in Chapter 2. Muscles are interconnected with the nervous system in such a way that, when muscles on one side of the limb contract, the opposing or antagonistic muscles reflexively relax. At the same time that a contraction message is sent from the brain to the agonist muscle, an anticontraction or inhibition message is sent to the motor neurons responsible for the antagonistic muscle's activity. Thus, many people contract the muscle which is antagonistic to the muscle they are stretching—a sound approach to flexibility exercise.

Still another reflexive influence involves a special tendon receptor, the *Golgi tendon organ* (discussed in Chapter 2), which is also sensitive to muscle stretch, especially when the muscle is actively contracting. The Golgi tendon organ has an opposite function from the stretch reflex. When the tendon is stretched, this receptor sends an inhibition message back to the motor neurons of the muscle, thereby lessening the contraction causing the stretch. Owing to inhibitory neurons in this neural circuit, the effects of this receptor slightly outlast the contraction. Flexibility enthusiasts and therapists have used this tendon receptor to their benefit by preceding the stretch with a strong isometric contraction in the muscle to be stretched. They immediately follow this with a static stretch of that muscle. A very interesting Canadian program has used this concept, described in *Scientific Stretching for Sport*[5].

It should be emphasized, however, that the concept underlying these techniques is to attain and maintain relaxation in the muscles being stretched. If the primary resistance to flexibility is not in the contractile elements of the muscle, as is likely the case, programs using reciprocal innervation and tendon reflexes probably are adding little to the effect of the static stretching exercise. In special rehabilitation cases where the contractile elements may be more of a problem, therapists may find significant gains associated with these techniques.

FLEXIBILITY EXERCISE PRINCIPLES

1. Choose at least one flexibility exercise from each of the exercise categories below.

2. Gradually increase the force of the stretch until the position is slightly beyond comfort ("moderately miserable") or slightly past the point at which pain is initiated.

AT LEAST 10 SEC

3. Hold the static stretch for 20 to 30 seconds. *Do not bounce or stretch rapidly*.

4. Repeat the exercise. *3 X*

5. In performing stretches for the legs, keep the toes pulled back toward the body (not pointed). This position stretches the muscles of the posterior lower leg (calf muscles). If you point the toes, you lose the stretch in the posterior lower leg. Adequate flexibility in the posterior lower leg is important in the prevention of Achilles tendon problems.

6. Static stretches may be performed as a part of warm-up, preferably following a general warm-up movement such as running.

7. Greatest extensibility will be noticed in muscles and connective tissue after they have been warmed by exercise or other means.

8. Performing flexibility exercises before a strength or cardiovascular function work-out helps to prevent strains and other forms of muscle and connective tissue problems. Performing these exercises after the work-out reduces muscle soreness, and helps to stretch muscles that actually may have been shortened by the work-out. Thus, it is important to engage in flexibility exercises both *before* and *after* other forms of exercise.

THE FLEXIBILITY PROGRAM

Choose at least one exercise from each area and hold in a static position for 20 to 30 seconds. Relax and repeat the stretch. Try to relax the muscle being stretched. Do not bounce. The stretch should be done slowly.

Neck Area

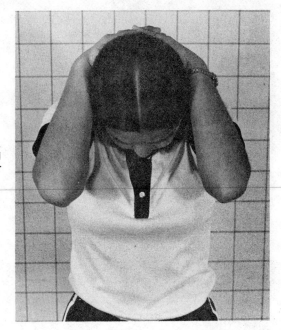

Figure 6–1. Posterior Neck Muscles. Gradually press down and hold. You should feel a stretching of the muscles in the posterior neck area.

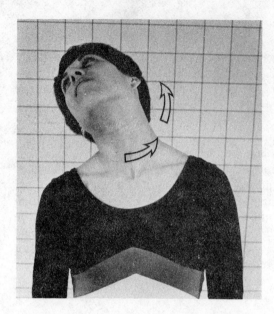

Figure 6–2. Neck (all areas). Slowly move the neck in a large circular pattern. (Avoid this exercise if you have any evidence of neck injury.)

Anterior Upper Chest Area

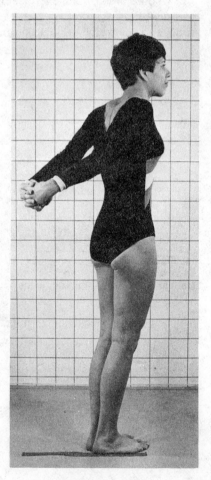

Figure 6–3. Raise arms in back and hold. This exercise also is conveniently done while holding a large ball between the hands.

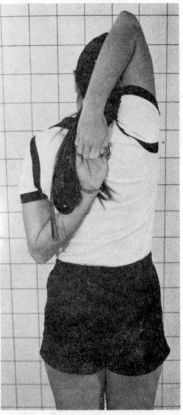

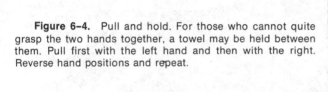

Figure 6-4. Pull and hold. For those who cannot quite grasp the two hands together, a towel may be held between them. Pull first with the left hand and then with the right. Reverse hand positions and repeat.

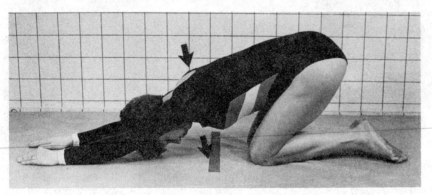

Figure 6-5. Lower shoulder joint to floor and hold.

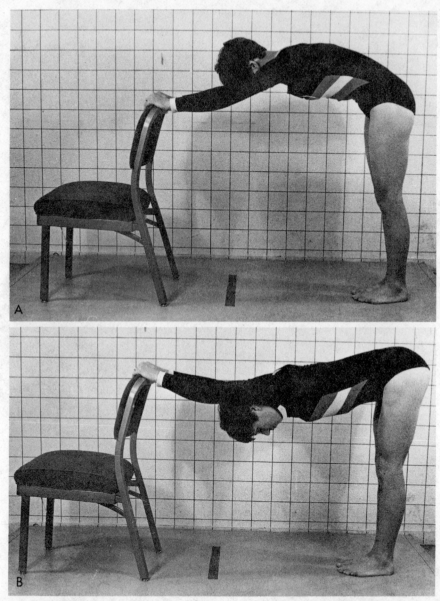

Figure 6-6. This is a modified position for the exercise in Figure 6-5. Start in the position shown in A. Bend forward at the waist and lower the head between the arms as far as possible *(B)*. If the exercise is done properly, you should feel the stretch in the anterior shoulder area and across the chest.

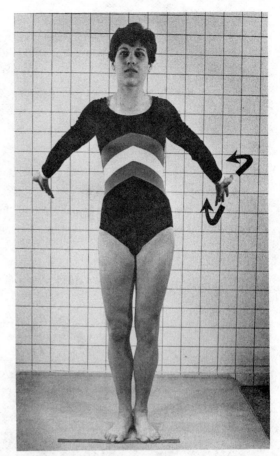

Figure 6–7. Push arms as far back as possible, then slowly move arms in a large circular pattern.

Upper Back Area (Shoulder Muscles)

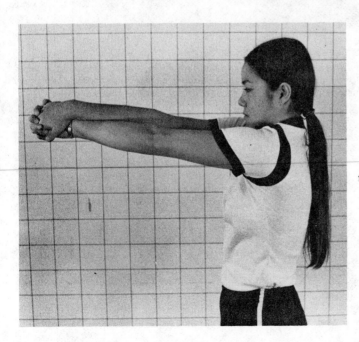

Figure 6–8. Reach arms as far forward as possible and hold.

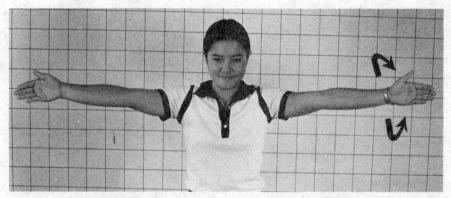

Figure 6–9.   Hold arms slightly in front of the body, then slowly move arms in a large circular pattern.

Upper Back Area (Trunk Muscles)

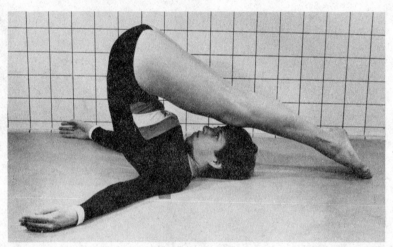

Figure 6–10.   Support body with shoulders, arms, and head on a mat. Move hips and back into a vertical position and hold. *Avoid this exercise if you are not comfortable with the position–especially position of the neck.* If the hamstrings are the limiting muscle group, flex the knees slightly.

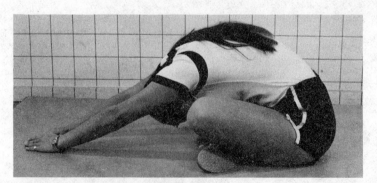

Figure 6–11.   Cross legs, lower head toward the floor, and hold. Allow the back to be rounded.

Middle and Low Back Areas

Note: The exercises shown in Figures 6–16*A*, *B*, 6–17, 6–18, and 6–19 also stretch the lower back as they stretch the posterior hip and thigh.

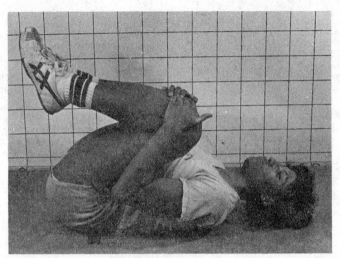

Figure 6–12.   Contract abdominal muscles, pull knees to chest, press low back to floor, and hold.

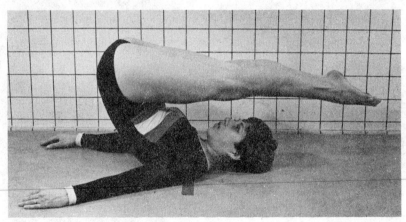

Figure 6–13.   Lie supine (flat on back) arms at side. Draw knees to chest, then straighten legs so that they are over the head and trunk, *parallel* to the floor *(do not allow the buttocks to go beyond the head).*

Trunk Area

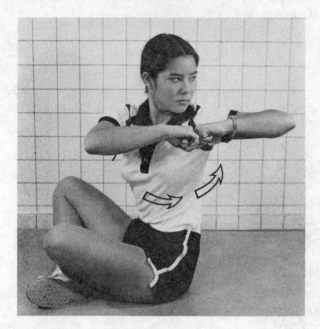

Figure 6–14. Slowly rotate trunk and hold. Repeat in opposite direction.

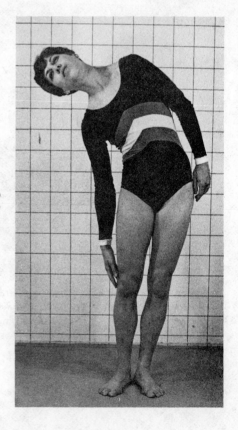

Figure 6–15. Lateral Trunk Flexion. Flex trunk to the side (lateral flexion) and hold. Repeat to the opposite side of the body.

Posterior Hip and Thigh Areas (Also Involves Low Back Area)

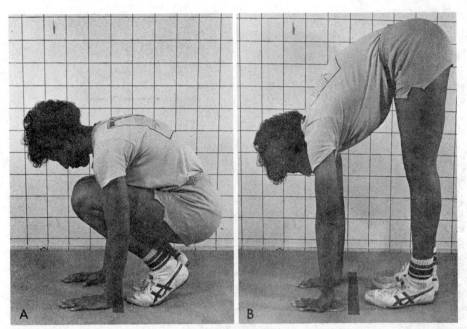

Figure 6–16. *A* and *B,* Cat Stand. Assume a flexed hip and knee position with the hands on the floor *(A).* Then attempt slowly to straighten the legs while the original position of the arms and hands is maintained. The abdominal muscles should be strongly contracted as the legs are straightened.

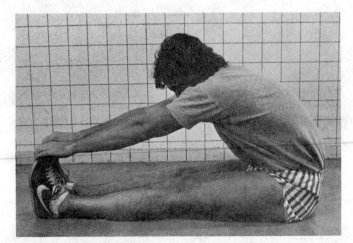

Figure 6–17. Place the hands on or near the feet. Keep the toes back toward the body to stretch the calf muscles also. Keep the back straight and attempt to place the chest on the thigh by bending forward at the waist. This exercise is similar to the one shown in Figure 6–16 except that it is in a nonweight-bearing position. Less stress is placed on the low back. Therefore, when convenient, the sitting position is preferred.

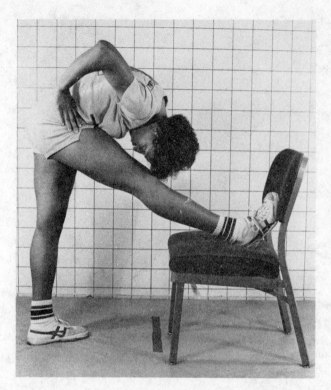

Figure 6–18. Stand with one foot supported on a bench or chair. Keep the leg straight. Bend the trunk forward trying to touch the head to the knee. Keep hands on hips. Repeat with the opposite leg.

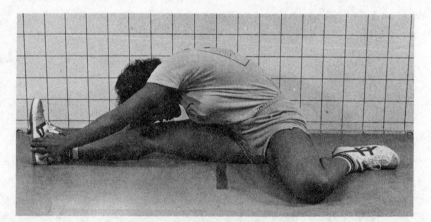

Figure 6–19. The Hurdler's Stretch. Sit on the floor with one leg bent to the side, with the inside of the ankle touching the floor. Try to pull the head to the knee of the straight leg by grasping the foot and pulling with the arms. Change leg positions and repeat with the other leg. (This exercise can also provide an additional exercise for Area H. The anterior thigh muscles of the bent leg may be stretched by inclining the trunk slowly backward as far as possible while maintaining the leg position shown (Fig. 6–23).)

Anterior Hip and Thigh Area

Note: The exercise shown in Figure 6–29 also may be used to stretch the anterior hip area.

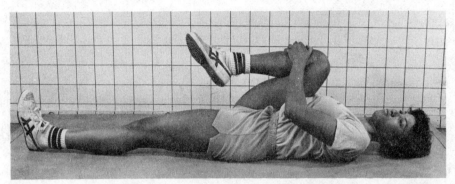

Figure 6–20.   Lie flat on the back. Draw one knee up to the chest and pull it tightly down with the hands. Slowly return to the original position. Repeat with the other knee. Make an effort to keep the straight leg in contact with the floor throughout the stretch. (This exercise also may be done in the standing position by pulling the knee up tightly to the chest while keeping the other leg straight.)

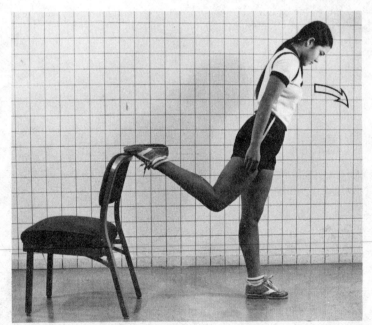

Figure 6–21.   Hook foot on a table, bench, or chair. Lean forward and hold to feel stretch in anterior thigh area. Repeat with the opposite leg.

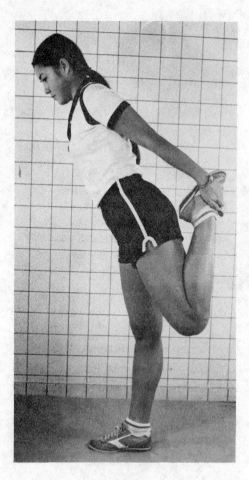

Figure 6–22. Similar to Figure 6–21. Flex knee and grasp ankle behind body. Stretch anterior hip and thigh by pulling up on the leg as you lean forward slightly. This exercise also may be done while lying on the side. Grasp the foot of the top leg in the manner shown, and slowly pull up and back on it.

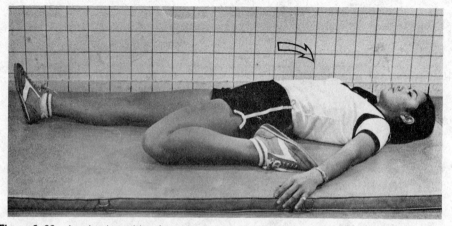

Figure 6–23. Lay back position from the hurdler's stretch (Fig. 6–19). From the hurdler's stretch position, incline the trunk slowly backward as far as possible while maintaining the leg position shown.

Medial and Lateral Hip Area

Note: The exercises shown in Figures 6–19 and 6–23 also may be used to stretch this area of the body.

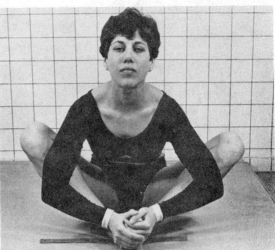

Figure 6–24. Lean forward and hold. Keep the back straight. (Mostly medial hip muscles.)

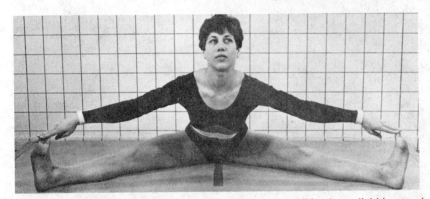

Figure 6–25. Lean forward and hold. Keep the back straight. (Mostly medial hip muscles.)

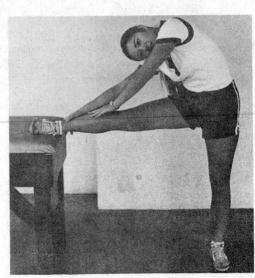

Figure 6–26. Move the trunk toward the raised leg and hold. Repeat to the other side of the body.

Posterior Lower Leg Area (Calf Muscles)

Note: It is very important to stretch the calf muscles *before* and *after* jogging or other activities involving running. This should prove very effective in preventing many of the common injuries to the lower leg, foot, and ankle.

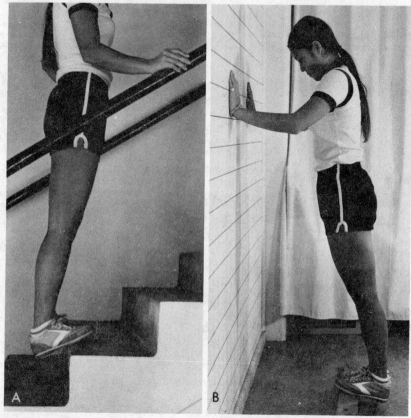

Figure 6–27. Heel Lowering. *A*, Lower heels over edge of stair and hold. *B*, This exercise may be performed with a thick piece of wood or smilar object placed under the front portion of the foot. In both cases, alternately rise up on toes and lower heels as far as possible.

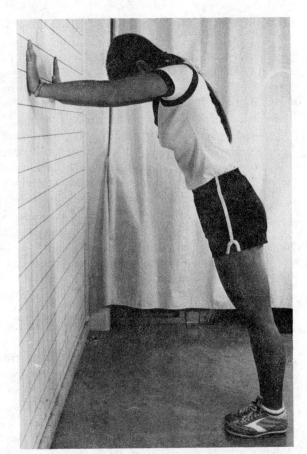

Figure 6-28. Lean forward with a straight trunk and hold. Heels must remain on the floor. Move feet as far away from the wall as possible, but keep heels on floor and back straight.

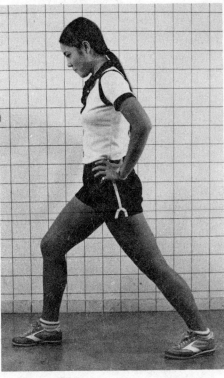

Figure 6-29. Flex forward knee and lean forward slightly to feel stretch in calf of the straight leg. Feet must remain flat on the floor with toes pointing straight ahead. (This exercise also stretches the anterior hip area of the rear leg.)

LEARNING OBJECTIVES

After studying the concepts and exercises for Chapter 6, students should be able to:

1. Define flexibility.

2. Explain why flexibility is important to movement.

3. Identify the common "problem areas" for flexibility (areas in most individuals especially needing additional flexibility).

4. Explain why some body areas have more flexibility than others.

5. Explain the specific goal of flexibility exercise for most persons.

6. Identify and explain any male–female differences in flexibility.

7. Explain the reasons why static stretching is preferred over ballistic.

8. Explain why the muscle being stretched should be relaxed, not contracting.

9. Explain why it is better not to evoke the stretch reflex in a flexibility exercise.

10. Explain reciprocal innervation (review Chapter 2 for an explanation of this concept).

11. Explain how reciprocal innervation can be used to relax the muscle being stretched.

12. Indicate how the Golgi tendon organ can be used to help maintain relaxation in the muscle being stretched.

13. Indicate when the Golgi tendon reflex mechanisms would be most effective in aiding flexibility exercises.

14. Indicate how long one should hold a stretching exercise.

15. Tell how much stretch is best for flexibility exercises.

16. Identify and explain the proper position of the toes when doing stretching exercises for the lower legs.

17. Explain when stretching exercises should be performed.

18. Demonstrate at least one flexibility exercise for the muscles in each of the following body areas:

    a. posterior neck.

    b. anterior chest.

    c. posterior leg (hamstrings).

    d. anterior leg (quadriceps femoris).

    e. posterior lower leg (calf).

    f. medial leg.

    g. upper back.

    h. lower back.

    i. lateral trunk (waistline area).

REFERENCES

1. American Alliance for Health, Physical Education, and Recreation: *AAHPERD Health-Related Physical Fitness Test Manual*. Washington, D. C., The Alliance, 1980.

2. Clarke, H. H. (ed.): Joint and Body Range of Movement. *In Physical Fitness Research Digest*. Washington, D.C., President's Council on Physical Fitness and Sports, Series 5, No. 4, 1975.

3. Cureton, T. K.: Flexibility as an aspect of physical fitness. Res. Q. Am. Assoc. Health Phys. Educ. (Suppl.) *12*:382, 1941.

4. de Vries, H. A.: *Physiology of Exercise*. Dubuque, Iowa, Wm. C. Brown Co., 1974.

5. Holt, L. E.: *Scientific Stretching for Sport*. Halifax, Nova Scotia, Canada, Sport Research Ltd., 1976.

6. Hupprich, F. L., and Sigerseth, P. O.: The specificity of flexibility in girls. Res. Q. Am. Assoc. Health Phys. Educ. *21*:26, 1950.

7. Kirchner, G., and Glines, D.: Comparative analysis of Eugene, Oregon, elementary school children using the Kraus-Weber test of minimum muscular fitness. Res. Q. Am. Assoc. Health Phys. Educ. *28*:16, 1957.

8. Laubach, L. L., and McConville, J. T.: Relationships between flexibility, anthropometry, and the somatotype of college men. Res. Q. Am. Assoc. Health Phys. Educ. *37*:241, 1966.
9. Leighton, J. R.: On the significance of flexibility for physical educators. J. Health Phys. Educ. Recr. *31(8)*:27, 1960.
10. Massey, B. H., and Chaudet, N. L.: Effects of systematic, heavy resistive exercise on range of joint movement in young male adults. Res. Q. Am. Assoc. Health Phys. Educ. *27*:41, 1956.
11. Mathews, D. K., Shaw, V., and Bohnen, M.: Hip flexibility of college women as related to length of body segments. Res. Q. Am. Assoc. Health Phys. Educ. *28*:352, 1957.
12. Mathews, D. K., Shaw, V., and Woods, J. B.: Hip flexibility of elementary school boys as related to body segments. Res. Q. Am. Assoc. Health Phys. Educ. *30*:287, 1959.
13. Phillips, M., Bookwalter, C., Denman, C., McAuley, J., Sherwin, H., Summers, D., and Yeakel, H.: Analysis of results from the Kraus-Weber test of minimum muscular fitness in children. Res. Q. Am. Assoc. Health Phys. Educ. *26*:314, 1955.
14. Tyrance, H. J.: Relationships of extreme body types to ranges of flexibility. Res. Q. Am. Assoc. Health Phys. Educ. *29*:349, 1958.
15. Wickstrom, R. L.: Weight training and flexibility. J. Health Phys. Educ. Recr. *34(2)*:61, 1963.

Recommended Supplementary Reading

16. Anderson, R.: The perfect pre–run stretching routine. Runner's World *13(5)*:56, 1978.
17. Ryan, A. J.: Yoga and fitness. J. Health Phys. Educ. Recr. *42(2)*:26, 1971.

Chapter 7

Psychological Aspects of Exercise Participation and Training

INTRODUCTION

To determine many of the physiological adaptations to chronic and acute exercise that have been discussed in previous chapters, one needs to quantify physical *performance* such as weight lifted, number of repetitions executed, distance run, and/or speed, duration, and intensity of the exercise. The performance-based approach to exercise prescription outlined in previous chapters is a concession to our recognition that the human organism is *biological* in nature. It is also a reflection of the relative degree to which our society has been able to advance explanations regarding the responses to, and effects of, exercise. In the area of physiological responses to exercise, a large and fairly well defined body of knowledge has accumulated over the past two to three decades. It is important to realize, however, that although performance is mainly *physiological* in nature (i.e., primarily dependent on the body's ability to metabolize foodstuffs and deliver oxygen to the working muscles), it is also quite dependent on the integration of these processes by the central nervous system, and therefore is also *psychological* in nature. In a more correct sense, we are *psychobiological* organisms. In effect, "the body has a head"—a fact recognized as early as the classic civilizations of ancient Athens

186

where education was directed toward achieving an optimal blend of development of mind, body, and spirit.

Although the subdiscipline of sport and exercise psychology is still in its infancy as compared with exercise physiology, great strides have been made over the past few years in identifying and assessing many of the psychological correlates of exercise. Through the work of dedicated sport psychologists, it has become increasingly apparent that psychological traits and states often are equally as important in determining exercise behavior and outcomes as are physiological phenomena. There also appear to be many desirable psychological alterations in the individual that may be derived from exercise participation. This chapter presents and discusses the current knowledge regarding psychological benefits of exercise, along with psychological characteristics that may affect exercise behavior.

STRESS

Perhaps no concept more clearly illustrates the interface of physiological and psychological processes in the behavior of man than does *stress*. Marathon running, channel swimming, 30-kilometer cross-country skiing, even the 12-minute run, all are stress-producing. Mid-term and final exams, job interviews, and first dates are stress-producing too—and *not* in a different way, as initially might be expected. The causes of stress (stressors) may be quite different and either physiological or psychological in nature, but the stress reaction, regardless of the cause, is the same in each instance. Therefore, stress is considered to be a generalized organismic reaction to situational demands. Simply stated, the reaction can be conceptualized easily in terms of the classic fight/flight response that results in acute (immediate) increases in metabolic preparedness during a threatening situation.

However, it is important to realize that stress may be chronic (long-term) as well as acute, and that the precipitators of stress may be imagined as well as real. For example, a single exercise bout might be stressful in an acute sense, whereas an entire training program might represent chronic stress. Similarly, apprehension and worry over the anticipated outcome of an important examination might be manifest only the night before the test, or could have begun three weeks earlier. As further illustration, the primary stressor during the 12-minute run is the actual work being done, and is thus physiological. However, psychological stressors also might be evoked by: (1) anxiety over performing poorly and being evaluated negatively; or (2) negative affect (emotion) resulting from an unfavorable attitude toward running or a dislike for the perceptual consequences of intense exercise.

The biochemical changes that accompany stress are outlined in Figure 7–1. Certain other physiological alterations also accompany acute exercise stress. These include increased activity of the sympathetic nervous system, which results in increases of circulating epinephrine and norepinephrine; increased heart rate; increased breathing rate and intensity; increased body temperature; increased sweating; and increased oxygen consumption. Interestingly, this same physiological arousal also characterizes anxiety—an imaginary stressor.

Since much of the previous discussion in this text has focused on adaptations to exercise demands, it is useful also to view such adaptations with regard to stress. Hans Selye, the most noted authority on stress, has proposed a conceptual model for viewing stress that complements nicely the SAID principle previously introduced in Chapter 2. Selye's General Adaptation Syndrome (GAS) characterizes stress in three stages:

1. The *alarm reaction,* during which the stressor is perceived, alerts the Reticular

STRESS RESPONSE

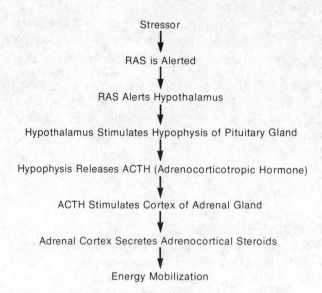

Stressor

↓

RAS is Alerted

↓

RAS Alerts Hypothalamus

↓

Hypothalamus Stimulates Hypophysis of Pituitary Gland

↓

Hypophysis Releases ACTH (Adrenocorticotropic Hormone)

↓

ACTH Stimulates Cortex of Adrenal Gland

↓

Adrenal Cortex Secretes Adrenocortical Steroids

↓

Energy Mobilization

Figure 7–1. Outline of the succession of neurophysiological and biochemical changes that characterize the stress response. (RAS is the Reticular Activating System of the brain.)

Activating System (RAS) in the central nervous system. This mechanism controls alertness or attention of the cerebral cortex, and is responsive to somatic (body) disturbances as well as sights, sounds, smells, tastes, and even the cortex itself, e.g., a thought.

2. Once a stressor is detected, the *resistance* stage is evoked, during which body systems attempt to adapt to and combat the stressor. This stage is characterized by the physiological arousal previously outlined.

3. If resistance is inadequate to offset the stressor, *exhaustion* occurs and the stress syndrome is complete.

During exercise training, chronic adjustments in the ability to tolerate the same stressor with a less pronounced stress reaction clearly illustrates the SAID principle. In terms of stress, the specific adaptation refers to a reduced physiological arousal to a specific work intensity, duration, or frequency. This can be illustrated by increases in maximal oxygen consumption and anaerobic threshold (Chapter 5), which permit subsequent work at the same absolute intensity to be less stressful than it was before training. In fact, the purpose of cardiovascular training is to impose a progressively increasing exercise stressor to evoke adaptations in the heart and lung systems during the resistance phase of the GAS in a chronic sense. In this context, an individual who is physically fit is able to tolerate a greater exercise stressor. Moreover, maximal oxygen consumption determined by graded work on a motor-driven treadmill or estimated by the 12-minute run is simply a measure of the ability to resist the stressor of increasingly intense physical work.

Thus, the body has the ability to adapt to a stressor. However, there are individual differences in resistance capacity prior to exhaustion, and physical injury or emotional collapse result from *excessive* amounts of unrelieved stress. It should be noted, however, that some degree of stress is desirable for effective biological functioning, and that each individual probably has an optimal level of stress which facilitates maximal performance. If stress is viewed on a continuum, such as presented in Figure 7–2, too little stress can be likened to a state of quiescence or sleep in which the RAS is inactive, whereas too much stress may result in exhaustion. From a standpoint of performance, Selye considers each of these extremes undesirable and refers to them as *Distress,* while the remainder of the stress continuum lies within an optimal range of *Eustress.*

From the standpoint of health or wellness, a key consideration is the fact that optimal habitual exercise may be viewed both as a potential mode of adaptation to a physiological stressor and as a coping strategy in the management of psychological stressors such as anxiety. An appreciation of this fact is quite important, since it has been estimated that 30 to 70 per cent of the illness treated by physicians in general practice has its origin in unrelieved stress. It is important to recognize that exercise can be either a negative *or a* positive factor in the adaptation to stress, both from a physiological and/or a psychological perspective. The remainder of this chapter is devoted to discussion of various stress-producing or stress-relieving aspects of exercise participation.

EXERCISE AND MENTAL HEALTH

Physical educators and other health professionals traditionally have advocated that involvement in regular physical activity enhances the psychological well-being of the participant. Reductions in tension and increases in self-esteem have been commonly proposed as such positive psychological effects of exercise. Although in the past these claims generally have been supported only by intuition, common sense, or perhaps the "vested interests" of their proponents, recent research by exercise scientists has provided considerable evidence which indicates that these *beliefs* concerning the psychological benefits of physical activity are indeed well supported.

Anxiety

A series of studies at the University of Wisconsin has indicated that *state* anxiety (temporary feelings of tension and apprehension) can be reduced significantly following a single vigorous exercise session, and that *trait* anxiety (a general tendency to be anxious) can be reduced after chronic (long-term) involvement in an exercise training program. Also, other studies in California have shown that tension decreases following both short bouts of physical activity and full-fledged conditioning programs. When one considers that approximately 10 to 15 million Americans suffer from symptoms associated with

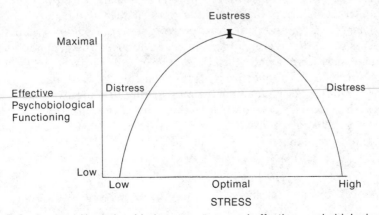

Figure 7–2. Inverted U relationship between stress and effective psychobiological functioning. Areas of distress and eustress are shown. (Adapted from Selye, H.: *The Stress of Life*. New York, McGraw-Hill Book Co., 1976.)

anxiety and tension, the significance of physical exercise as a successful "coping strategy" for major mental health problems becomes quite apparent.

Depression

Up to 15 million Americans are beset each year with symptoms of depression, which, along with anxiety, represents the most prominent mental disorder in our society. Several studies have revealed that regular endurance-type activity, such as running or jogging over a period of at least six weeks, is effective in reducing or alleviating symptoms of moderate depression. Also, such exercise appears to be an equally effective, and certainly less expensive, alternative to psychotherapy in the treatment of nonpsychotic depression. Furthermore, participants typically report that they "feel better" following exercise, and the prevalence of this phenomenon generally has approached 85 per cent of those involved.

Several factors have been proposed as possible mechanisms for observed reductions in depression, and these have included: (1) enhanced feelings of mastery; (2) distraction from physical symptoms; (3) relief of symptoms; and (4) consciousness alteration. However, exercise also produces certain biochemical changes that do not occur in traditional depression therapy settings. Most specifically, blood levels of norepinephrine are known to increase with vigorous exercise. Since depressed patients typically are deficient in brain norepinephrine, acute exercise may influence depression through subtle alterations of this hormone in the brain.

Psychotic Disorders

In addition to the effectiveness of physical activity in the management of anxiety and depression, it also has been implicated in the treatment of psychotic disorders. Schizophrenia, for example, which is often characterized by detachment from reality and absence of emotion, is generally known to vary in severity with the degree of physical fitness. That is, as the severity of psychosis increases to pathological levels, the measured capacity to do physical work (including cardiovascular and muscular endurance) is less. Although evidence does not indicate that a causal relationship exists, it is a common clinical observation that reduced psychosis and increased physical working capacity take place concurrently. In addition, it is quite common to observe actual pathological changes in muscle cell structure of psychotic patients, and these are apparently reversible as the severity of the disorder is reduced. Also, abnormal levels of creatine phosphokinase (an enzyme which is involved in anaerobic metabolism and which is present in abnormally high concentrations following incidents of muscle tissue damage, e.g., heart attack) are often found in the musculature of acutely psychotic patients. Such findings as these provide considerable support for the view that psychotic disorders are complexly psychobiological in nature, and once again suggest that physical activity may play a significant therapeutic role in the maintenance of desirable mental health.

Mental Health Aspects of Habitual Exercise and Athletics

Individuals whose lifestyles are characterized by vigorous physical activity consistently demonstrate psychological profiles which, from a standpoint of mental health, are more desirable than those of the average person. World class athletes, for example, participating in a variety of sports at the national and international level, characteristically present what has been referred to by William P. Morgan, a world-renowned sport psychologist, as the "iceberg" profile of mood states. In this profile (Fig. 7–3), the typical elite athlete scores *below* the "surface" on tension, depression, anger, fatigue, and confusion, and *above* the "surface" on vigor. Each of these psychological characteristics is related to mental health, and although they may reflect necessary psychological requirements for athletic success, these findings also may be viewed as support for the positive influence of habitual exercise on psychological wellness.

In fact, several of these variables, most specifically tension, depression, fatigue, and vigor, have been found to be altered favorably with regular exercise for nonathletic groups also. Since the activity in these programs has involved several different types or modes of exercise (e.g., running, weight-training, rowing, and racquetball), it appears that physical activity settings per se may be responsible for the observed psychological improvements, and not any one specific type of exercise. It should be noted that these changes have occurred for individuals scoring within the normal range on the variables

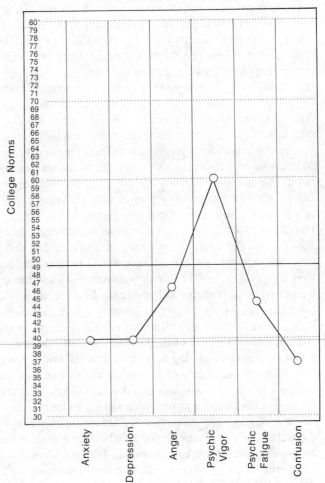

Figure 7–3. Typical "iceberg" profile of mood states characterizing world class athletes as compared to college norms. (Adapted from Morgan, W. P.: Prediction of Performance in Athletics. *In* P. Klavora (ed.) Toronto: *Proceedings of the Applied Sciences Symposium of the Canadian Society for Psychomotor Learning and Sport Psychology Congress, 1979.*)

PROFILE OF MOOD STATES

discussed, and consequently provide additional support for the previously discussed "feeling better" phenomenon in persons not necessarily clinically depressed or anxious.

Psychological Correlates of the "Training Dosage"

A word of caution is necessary concerning the *amount* of exercise that is desirable. There is some evidence suggesting that participants in running programs are most *satisfied* when exercising 30 minutes, three days per week, at 75 to 85 per cent of their maximal heart rate, but little evidence is available regarding the *optimal* frequency, duration, and intensity required to achieve the psychological effects previously discussed. It is interesting, however, that the *preferred* amount just mentioned is nearly identical to the optimal values required for physiological training effects to occur in the average person (Chapter 5). At any rate, it is quite possible that *too much exercise* can have undesirable consequences. Both the overtrained or "stale" athlete and the clinically depressed patient illustrate a syndrome of overstress and exhaustion, namely: (1) reductions in appetite, body weight, libido, sleep, and psychic vigor; (2) psychomotor retardation; (3) confusion; (4) chronic fatigue; (5) increased perception of effort; and (6) increased activity by the sympathetic nervous system, resulting in elevated resting and exercise heart rates and slower recovery from exercise stress. In extreme cases, an actual *reduction* in maximal oxygen consumption occurs.

For the recreational exercise enthusiast or the "hobby jogger," similar problems may arise if the exercise duration or intensity is too great for the individual's capacity. For example, habitual exercise recently has come to be considered as a "positive" addiction, owing to many of the benefits previously discussed which relate to physiological and psychological wellness. However, in the isolated individual for whom increasingly larger amounts of exercise are required to obtain the same feeling of well-being, it may in fact be a "negative" addiction much like heroin dependence or alcoholism. As illustration, consider a jogger who begins running 10 miles a week only to discover that 20, then 40, and finally, 100+ miles per week are necessary to obtain the same "feeling better" sensation obtained initially. In some instances, such exercise "addicts" are known even to quit employment or school, neglect families, and essentially "drop out" of society to make time for their running habit. Often, the physiological or orthopedic integrity of such individuals cannot accommodate their psychological needs, and stress injuries that force withdrawal may lead to neurotic disturbances. Although this illustration may appear somewhat contrived, similar incidents are not uncommon among running cultists. In fact, for the exerciser with latent competitive tendencies, running, weight-training, racquetball, etc. may become an achievement endeavor, and success (as measured by distance run, pounds lifted, games won, or even calories expended) may be internalized as a vital part of self-concept. In itself this is not necessarily undesirable, but in the case of the *injured* "addict" deprivation may even further compound a neurotic episode owing to forced "withdrawal" from vital exercise reinforcements.

Although such negative consequences can and do occur, there is little need for concern in the average individual who wishes to embark on a training program. The previous illustration was provided simply to increase awareness of a potential, although not widespread, negative effect of obsessive exercise behavior. It serves to emphasize the fact that obsessive behavior may be detrimental in the exercise situation just as it may be with sex, food intake, gambling, drinking alcoholic beverages, pursuit of monetary gain, etc. As long as: (1) exercise amount remains well within biological capacities (as determined by medical examination and an exercise tolerance test); (2) exercise stress is not sufficient to result in injury; and (3) exercise behavior does not become excessively goal-oriented, there should be little reason for undesirable psychological consequences to arise.

EXERCISE AND ONE'S PERCEPTION OF EFFORT AND SELF

It has been emphasized previously that cardiovascular adaptations to exercise stress are dependent on frequency, duration, and intensity of the activity. Although cardiac frequency (heart rate) and caloric expenditure are excellent indices of optimal training intensity, another easily monitored indicator of exercise demand relates to an individual's perception of effort, i.e., how intense does the work *feel*? Another type of exercise perception relates to the way in which a person views personal characteristics. This self-perception is an important aspect of self-esteem (or the attitude individuals have toward themselves), and will be discussed as another psychological effect of involvement in physical activity.

Perceived Exertion

An abundant literature on perceptual responses to exercise indicates that the normal individual (one who is not anxious, neurotic, or depressed) is quite capable of accurately perceiving the metabolic demands of work. In other words, sensory inputs from a variety of bodily sensations, including (1) the frequency and intensity of breathing, (2) accumulation of lactic acid in the working muscles, (3) body temperature, (4) muscular and joint aches and pains, and (5) heart rate, etc., all are integrated in the central nervous system to provide a subjective estimate of exercise intensity that closely resembles the actual metabolic cost (oxygen consumption) of the work. In fact, Gunnar Borg of Sweden has proposed a model for predicting actual exercise heart rate from verbal ratings of *perceived exertion*. (Remember, heart rate is the best physiological predictor of oxygen consumption.) This model states that the rating of perceived exertion (RPE) on a scale from 6 to 20 (Fig. 7–4), multiplied by a factor of 10, corresponds to actual heart rate at that particular work intensity, i.e., RPE × 10 = HR. For example, if work is perceived at an intensity of 15, predicted heart rate according to Borg's model would be 150.

It is noteworthy that submaximal ratings of perceived exertion using Borg's scale have actually been found to predict more accurately maximal working capacity than submaximal heart rate—the conventionally used physiological predictor (Fig. 7–5). This

PERCEIVED EXERTION SCALE

Figure 7–4. Borg's category rating scale for perceived exertion during exercise. Note that in this model, a rating of very, very light, i.e., 6, corresponds to what is generally considered to be an average resting heart rate of 60 beats/minute, and a rating of very, very hard work, i.e., 20, corresponds to an average maximum heart rate of 200 beats/minute. (From Borg, G. A. V.: Perceived exertion: a note on "history" and methods. Med. Sci. Sports 5:90, 1973.)

6	
7	Very, Very Light
8	
9	Very Light
10	
11	Fairly Light
12	
13	Somewhat Hard
14	
15	Hard
16	
17	Very Hard
18	
19	Very, Very Hard
20	

9:00

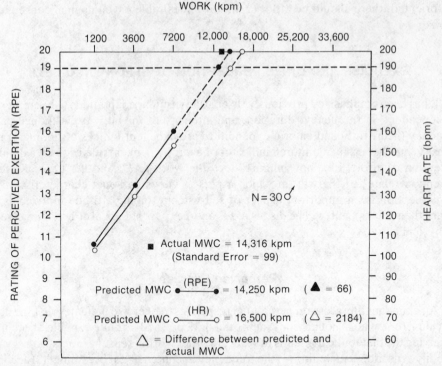

Figure 7-5. Plots of submaximal heart rate and ratings of perceived exertion used to predict actual maximal working capacity. (MWC). (Adapted from Morgan, W. P. and Borg, G. A. V.: Perception of effort and the prescription of physical activity. *In* T. Craig (ed.) *Mental Health and Emotional Aspects of Sports.* Chicago. Copyright 1976, American Medical Association.)

is not surprising, since RPE is based on sensory information from many other body systems involved in supplying energy for work, apart from just heart rate. In other words, heart rate is merely a part of RPE and, logically, no part should be a better predictor than the whole.

One implication of perceived exertion for cardiovascular training is clear in that, during the beginning stages of an exercise program in particular, individuals should attempt to "read" their bodies as means for regulating intensity. This reading will closely follow the actual metabolic stress being placed on the cardiovascular system, and so, if intensity *feels* too difficult, it probably is, and should be reduced slightly. Sedentary individuals just beginning exercise can obtain significant cardiovascular improvements without working far outside their "comfort zone." In fact, the beginning exerciser should avoid intense work of short duration that exceeds about 50 to 70 per cent of maximum. Such work provokes anaerobic metabolism in the untrained person, and results in the accumulation of lactic acid in the working muscles. Lactic acid is a primary cause of muscular fatigue and pain, and has been implicated as a major factor that increases the perception of effort. Also, circulatory adjustments for very intense work may be quite abrupt, and blood may be shifted away from the gastrointestinal organs to increase supply to the working muscles. This redistribution of blood together with accumulating lactic acid may result in nausea or "pain in the side," conditions which, although not physiologically damaging, are perceptually very undesirable for the nonmasochist! Although these responses sometimes occur in an "all-out" exercise effort such as the 12-minute run test, they are not necessary for cardiovascular adaptations to take place and, because of their aversive influence on effort perception, they should be avoided during initial training by maintaining work intensity at moderate levels.

However, perception of effort should be used to avoid "getting into trouble," e.g., being injured, and *not* as an excuse for avoiding optimal physiological training intensity. Cardiovascular overload often necessitates working slightly above one's comfort zone, but substantial training effects *can occur* in the untrained *without pain*. Effort perception is equally important for the experienced exerciser, especially when working in extreme environmental conditions such as intense heat and high humidity. Bodily perceptions of skin temperature and muscular pain can signal early detection of dehydration and heat stress, which may necessitate lower intensity or cessation of work.

Changes in perceived exertion can also be used to monitor progress in a conditioning program. Significant reductions (approximately 20 per cent) in effort perception have been observed consistently following endurance training, and these reductions generally have mirrored the actual physiological changes that have occurred. In other words, after training, the same work intensity *feels* easier because it now *is* easier, owing to increases in metabolic capacity. Also, with training, the intensity relative to maximal capacity at which an individual can work without large increases in lactic acid levels is increased, and subsequently perception of effort at higher intensity is reduced.

However, there are days when the track just seems longer, and the hills are definitely steeper! These are the days when the body probably just isn't metabolically or biochemically equipped for a vigorous work-out, and the average individual should adjust work intensity accordingly. In this regard, breathing rate and intensity have been found to be primary cues in perceived exertion, and a reasonable "rule of thumb" for regulating the intensity of a work-out is to run or otherwise exercise at a pace that will permit a comfortable conversation with an exercising companion.

Appendix A–12 is provided to give students practice in rating perceived exertion and, combined with Appendix A–9, may help them determine their conditioning threshold for cardiovascular function exercise.

Self-perception

Research consistently has demonstrated an increase in self-perception of physical ability following involvement in exercise training programs, and these findings are in agreement with certain theoretical expectations. Also, the increases have occurred for individuals experiencing cardiovascular improvements as well as for those with no training effects, and therefore mere involvement in an exercise program may be sufficient for improvement of self-concept. For many people these self-perceptions may produce an increase in self-esteem, which in this regard may be considered a desirable psychological consequence of physical activity. Of course, if an individual becomes too goal-oriented, or establishes training or fitness objectives which are unattainable or unrealistic, and subsequently attributes failure to reach these to internal and stable factors such as lack of ability, there also exists the possibility of reduced self-esteem. Therefore, it is quite important to attempt to establish training goals (i.e., how much should I improve?) which are within metabolic limits of initial fitness levels at the outset of a training program (Chapter 5).

FACTORS MOTIVATING EXERCISE INVOLVEMENT AND ADHERENCE TO A PROGRAM

Proximity

As noted previously, the value of vigorous physical activity in the management of coronary disease and mental health is well documented, and exercise generally is accepted in the health-related sciences as an effective therapeutic agent in the maintenance of both physiological and psychological wellness. Alarmingly, however, nearly 50 per cent of American adults do not participate in physical activity of a vigorous nature. In addition, 50 per cent of those who *do* begin an exercise program typically discontinue their participation within six months. Thus, initial involvement in exercise, and adherence to a program once it has been initiated, represent major concerns when viewing physical activity in a therapeutic or preventive medicine context.

Surprisingly, little research evidence is available regarding factors that may influence exercise involvement. College professors who elected to participate in an exercise program at the University of Wisconsin in 1967, and who were still involved in 1974, were found to reside in offices significantly closer to the exercise facility than were those professors who initially had elected not to take part. A similar finding was also obtained by Finnish researchers, who observed proximity to the exercise facility to be a major determinant of exercise involvement for business executives. Consequently, it appears that accessibility of the exercise setting, or the "convenience" with which an individual can exercise in a "traditional" environment, is quite important in the involvement process.

Instrumental Value of Physical Activity

It is reasonable to assume that the probability of a person becoming involved in a certain activity is enhanced if that involvement offers a desirable consequence. If the exercise can provide an outcome which is valued, an individual is more likely to exercise. Since physical activity is multimodal (i.e., has a variety of forms such as running, swimming, tennis, racquetball, biking, etc.), it would seem to have the potential to offer something to everyone. In this regard, Kenyon has proposed a conceptual model (Kenyon Attitude Toward Physical Activity Scale) for viewing involvement. It consists of six values that may be realized through participation in physical activity. These include involvement as: (1) a social experience; (2) health and fitness; (3) the pursuit of vertigo (e.g., through activity that involves risk or extreme excitement, such as parachuting or white water canoeing); (4) an aesthetic experience; (5) catharsis, e.g., reduction in tension or anxiety; and (6) an ascetic experience, i.e., the discipline or regimentation of training. It appears reasonable that many values of physical activity that people perceive may fall within one of these broader categories.

The most apparent motive for involvement in an exercise program is the attainment of health and fitness, but it is quite reasonable to expect that additional instrumental values also might be important, and that anticipation of these values being satisfied through participation might influence involvement. For example, social reinforcement through affiliation with other exercisers may be quite important to one individual, and relief of tension (catharsis) or the satisfaction of "staying with" a training regimen (ascetic value) may be important to another. The key consideration from a standpoint of involvement is that participants choose a type of exercise or an exercise setting that allows their most important values to be realized. In other words, they should not restrict involvement to a single "physiologically best" mode or type of activity, to the exclusion of other modes that might better satisfy important psychological values. This is especially important since, from either a physiological or psychological training standpoint, many exercise modes can be quite effective as long as: (1) they are rhythmic in nature; (2) they involve a large muscle mass; and (3) the intensity, duration, and frequency of the activity approximates the optimums previously discussed (Chapter 5).

Adherence Patterns

Although the benefits of habitual physical activity from a standpoint of physiological and psychological wellness are well supported, compliance with exercise participation represents a major problem in most exercise programs. Adult fitness programs typically have reported adherence rates of only 40 to 65 per cent, and these figures indicate a substantial drop-out percentage of those who voluntarily enter an exercise program. Also, there is a remarkable similarity in drop-out rates for participants in a variety of other therapeutic settings. Interestingly, the relapse rates following treatment for major addictions such as smoking, alcoholism, and drug dependence all follow curves similar to those representing adherence to voluntary exercise programs across several months (Fig. 7–6). These curves are characterized by a rapid and substantial decrease in the percentage of participants during the initial three to six months, an asymptote at this point, and a fairly stable plateau across the next 12 to 15 months. This similarity suggests that common factors may operate to influence adherence or therapeutic compliance in general.

Self-motivation

It may be that certain people simply do not have the will power to persist in a treatment program or, in this case, an exercise program. In fact, research has indicated that an individual's self-motivation is substantially related to adherence behavior, and that self-motivation scores, combined with certain measures of body composition (body weight and percentage fat), are predictors with 80 per cent accuracy of whether or not a person will drop out of or adhere to an actual exercise program. The participant prone to drop out has been found to be heavier, fatter, and less self-motivated than the adherer at

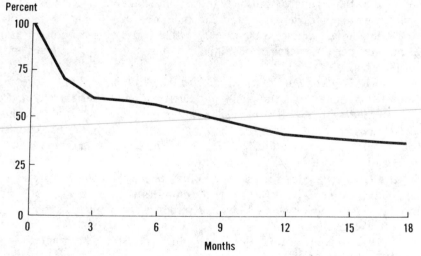

DROPOUT CURVE REPRESENTING ADHERENCE IN
PROGRAMS OF HABITUAL PHYSICAL ACTIVITY

Figure 7–6. Typical adherence pattern showing percentage of original participants still exercising at various points in an 18-month conditioning program.

the outset of involvement. Furthermore, this self-motivation trait has been observed as the only one of several seemingly relevant psychological variables to be significantly related to exercise adherence.

Related studies have suggested that the attitudes that "significant others" (spouse, friends, etc.) have toward an individual's exercise behavior, as well as a person's social stability, exert an influence on adherence to exercise. Surprisingly, however, neither the *participant's* attitude toward physical activity nor previous exercise behavior has been found to be related to adherence to an exercise program. Appendix A–13 provides an exercise whereby readers may calculate a rough estimate of the strength of their likely adherence to an exercise program. It is based on the above discussion.

Strategies to Support Involvement and Adherence

Individuals with low self-motivation are more inclined to drop out of an exercise program, and need to be particularly aware of factors that may affect their tendency to do so. The following "strategies" are proposed to help facilitate participation by those people who have trouble staying with a training program.

Proximity 1. Find a place to exercise that is *conveniently* located so that getting to and from work-outs is not a hardship. Remember, you can run anyplace!

2. Decide whether it is more enjoyable to exercise alone, with another person, or in a group, and plan your work-outs accordingly.

3. Don't allow yourself to become totally committed to only a single type of exercise or a single exercise setting. Change is important in terms of motivation, and it makes you feel better too!

4. Avoid becoming excessively goal-oriented. Training objectives are important, but there may be other aspects of exercise that are more important for *you*.

5. Don't expect *too* much. Training objectives should be realistic and individualized. Not everyone has the same genetic potential, and not everyone can reach the same fitness level, but everyone *can* improve.

6. Be patient! Fitness takes time. Think in terms of months, not days.

7. Keep a daily exercise record. When you are feeling discouraged, it is sometimes buoying to know that you have improved more than you thought. Remember, however, fitness increases reach a plateau as you become more fit.

8. During initial training sessions, stay within your "comfort zone." Remember, for the untrained person, exercise doesn't have to hurt in order for the heart and lungs to increase their capacities.

9. If you are not one of those who like to push to their limits, choose an activity (large muscle, rhythmic) that you can *enjoy* participating in consistently, and don't be overly concerned with exercise intensity. Although exercise heart rate and caloric expenditure are important training considerations, the most important factor is staying with your program. Training effects *result from* involvement, and do not have to be the primary goal or purpose for your participation.

10. If you really want to exercise, but nothing seems to enable you to stay with your program, think of some activity that you really enjoy or that you *have* to do. Then make a promise to yourself that you won't allow yourself to do the preferred activity unless you have already exercised.

11. Be proud of yourself for staying with your conditioning program. Fifty per cent of the population can't do that!

RELAXATION AND MEDITATION

A basic premise of this chapter is that vigorous exercise is effective in reducing anxiety—one of contemporary man's most prominent health disorders. However, it should be mentioned that certain relaxation and meditational techniques have been shown to be equally effective in this regard. Of course, exercise offers the added benefit of controlling risk factors related to cardiovascular disease and other physical health problems which relaxation techniques probably do not, and in this respect it is more desirable from an over-all health standpoint. In fact, rhythmic endurance-type exercise involving at least 60 per cent of total muscle mass (e.g., running) has an inherent relaxation effect on the circulatory system, resulting in reduced peripheral blood pressure and less work for the heart than more static forms of exercise (e.g., weight-lifting). Also, as mentioned previously, vigorous exercise of both an acute and a chronic nature is known significantly to reduce muscular tension—a prime factor in relaxation.

From a standpoint of *feeling states,* however, relaxation effects that are independent of exercise may be equally as effective as physical activity in the reduction of tension and anxiety. Support for this comes from at least two recently reported studies. In one of these, subjects either: (1) exercised vigorously by walking on a motor-driven treadmill at 70 per cent of their maximal capacity; (2) sat quietly and read in a reclining chair; or (3) practiced Benson's relaxation response for 20 minutes. The latter technique combines several aspects of meditational practices found in both eastern and western cultures, and consists of: (1) resting comfortably in a quiet environment; (2) maintaining a passive state of mind; and (3) repeating a word or phrase at a constant cadence. (Appendix A–14). Interestingly, in this study, subjects in each group experienced a significant reduction in state anxiety (Fig. 7–7). This would indicate that exercise, meditation/relaxation, and simple "time-out" therapy are *all* effective in the temporary relief of anxiety symptoms.

Figure 7-7. Comparison of the effects of vigorous exercise, noncultic meditation, and simple rest on state anxiety. (From Bahrke, M. S., and Morgan, W. P.: Influence of acute physical activity and non-cultic meditation on state anxiety. Cognitive Therapy and Research 2:323, 1978. Plenum Publishing Co., New York.)

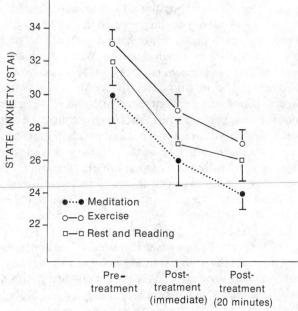

At first glance, these findings might appear somewhat incongruous, since exercise and meditation represent opposite ends of the arousal continuum. Anxiety is typically accompanied by increased activity of the sympathetic nervous system (e.g., increases in heart rate, catecholamine secretion, body temperature, breathing rate, and oxygen consumption), and exercise produces a similar physiological arousal. Meditation has an opposite, quiescent effect. However, both decrease anxiety!

Two common aspects of exercise and meditation may help to explain this finding. Each condition represents a *change in arousal.* Therefore, it may be that increases or decreases in arousal are unimportant in the relief of anxiety, but rather that a change in arousal or "arousal jag" is the essential factor. Also, both exercise and meditation provide a distraction or opportunity to "get away" from a situation or thought that may be the cause of anxiety, and this aspect, of course, is also a characteristic of simple rest. Under certain conditions, getting out of the dorm room or library or "away from the books" for a quiet afternoon in the park may be equally as effective from a standpoint of psychological health as a vigorous exercise session or the practice of transcendental meditation. However, it must be re-emphasized that physiological adaptations resulting from habitual physical activity offer added potential for the maintenance of cardiovascular health, more than that provided by meditation and simple rest.

ERGOGENIC PHENOMENA

In the introduction to this chapter, it was noted that exercise prescription tradition-ally has been based on physical performance, and such performance is primarily depen-dent on the ability of *physiological* systems to provide the energy for muscular work. However, in order to appreciate the biological adaptations to stress that typically accom-pany an exercise training program, it is necessary also to understand the relative contri-bution to performance of certain *psychological* factors.

Numerous accounts of "supramaximal" feats of muscular strength and endurance have appeared in the popular literature, and often have been simultaneously accepted as truths by the lay public and rejected as myths by the "scientific" community. There is ample evidence that such events do occur, but that they should not necessarily be considered as superhuman in nature. When considering the expression of human strength and endurance, the *capacity* or ability to do work must be addressed, but so must *willingness* or motivation. In other words, it is essentially impossible accurately to assess an *actual* physical performance "maximum" because of motivational limitations. Also, motivational influence on performance cannot be considered merely "psychological," i.e., conscious desire, but it is often psychobiological in nature. For example, a variety of experimental treatments, including hypnotic suggestion, ingestion of amphetamines, injections of Adrenalin (epinephrine), simple shouting, or being startled by an unex-pected gunshot, have been shown to increase previous "maximal" strength by as much as 30 per cent. These conditions probably do not alter the tensile strength of the muscle fibers involved, but it is likely that they influence mechanisms of the central nervous system that control strength expression.

Other, similar increases in muscular and cardiovascular endurance have been noted, and may be related to a similar but unknown mechanism. For example, two researchers several years ago reported the case study of a professional football player whose "maxi-mal" endurance while bench-pressing a 47-lb barbell was assessed at 130 consecutive repetitions, which certainly represents a performance beyond that of the average person off the street! However, under subsequent hypnotic suggestion, he was able to overcome fatigue plateaus or "sticking points" during the bench press, and increased his "maximum'' to 233 repetitions! An additional increase to *350* repetitions was later obtained in a normal waking state, and the investigators considered this performance increase as representing a "psychological breakthrough." Certainly, no physiological changes could account for this increase, as insufficient time for training had elapsed. The football player eventually revealed that continuing the exercise had become quite ego-involving, "a matter of life or death," and that he just wouldn't allow himself to stop.

It should be emphasized at this point that hypnosis per se apparently does not produce performance gains above those that can be realized following *suggestion* in the waking state. Sufficient evidence is available to add some credence to the adage: "if you think you can, you can"—within physiological limits. Also, artificially-induced fitness increases obtained through suggestion are often as great as those typically reported in actual strength and endurance training programs, and such findings again illustrate the difficulty in assessing true performance maximums.

Several studies using placebo treatments, such as an innocuous capsule or pill or a pseudo-training technique, have also shown significant increases in both muscular strength and endurance. Placebo is a Latin word meaning "as you please," and these findings also support physical performance as being quite sensitive to factors of a psychological nature.

Furthermore, a variety of cognitive strategies are known to influence endurance performance in activities such as running. Anthropological reports have indicated that Tibetan monks trained in the meditational art of Lung Gom (swiftness of foot) were capable of running a distance of 300 miles across rugged terrain at high altitude in a 30-hour period. The meditation strategy they employed included: (1) trance-like visual fix on an object in the distance; (2) the synchronization of running stride with breathing rate; and (3) the repetition of a *mantra* or religious chant. The veracity of such anecdotal accounts, of course, is open to question. However, implementation of a similar meditational technique called "dissociation" has been found to increase running endurance at 80 per cent of maximal capacity by approximately 30 per cent in laboratory settings. Also, the typical marathon runner is known to adopt a similar dissociative approach to overcome pain while running, and this generally involves simply thinking about something else, rather than attending to bodily sensations relating to the perception of effort or pain.

Additional support for the influence of motivation on physical performance is evidenced by the finding that attitude toward physical activity is the best psychological predictor of endurance time while running at 80 per cent of maximal aerobic power. Even 18 per cent of performance on the 12-minute run test, which is an easy and practical way to estimate aerobic power or cardiovascular function, can be accounted for by motivational factors such as attitude. This latter finding serves as an excellent illustration of the relationship between motivation and capacity in the determination of an individual's maximal strength and endurance. For example, actual or true aerobic power can be assessed by measuring the amount of oxygen which the heart and lungs can deliver to working muscles, and this is done by analysis of expired gases during work on a motor-driven treadmill or other ergometric device (Chapter 5, Fig. 5–2). This procedure represents a true cardiovascular *maximum* because aerobic power is defined by a physiological plateau in oxygen consumption, and therefore motivation to perform is not a factor. Thus, even though an individual is still performing work, no additional oxygen is extracted at the tissue level, and a true *capacity* has been determined. Conversely, when employing the 12-minute run as an *estimate* of actual aerobic power, cardiovascular endurance is not defined physiologically but rather is based on performance of running speed. This obviously is quite dependent on *willingness* to exert an all-out effort. For this reason, even though the 12-minute run *can* provide a very close approximation of actual cardiovascular function, it can never supply an *exact* measure of maximal capacity. This is yet another confirmation of the strong interaction between physiological and psychological variables in an exercise setting.

LEARNING OBJECTIVES

After studying the material in Chapter 7, students should be able to:

1. Describe the difference between *state* and *trait* anxiety, and indicate the influence of acute and chronic physical activity on each.

2. Understand the effect that vigorous exercise has on neuromuscular tension.

3. Indicate the prevalence in modern society of anxiety and depression as mental disorders, e.g., how many Americans suffer from symptoms of each?

4. Describe the influence of chronic physical activity such as jogging on nonpsychotic depression, and provide four explanations for this effect.

5. Briefly discuss the mediating role that norepinephrine may play between vigorous exercise and reductions in depression.

6. Recognize typical symptoms of schizophrenia, and describe the relationship between the severity of psychotic disorders and at least two measures of physical fitness.

7. Understand the relationship between psychosis and muscle pathology, and specifically indicate the common influence on creatine phosphokinase levels that accompanies anaerobic work, heart attack, and psychotic disorder.

8. Illustrate the "iceberg" profile, describe its psychological components, and discuss its implications for mental health in athletics and other physical activity.

9. Recognize the "feeling better" phenomenon and indicate its prevalence among exercise participants.

10. Indicate the exercise training (1) intensity, (2) frequency, and (3) duration with which participants are most *satisfied*. Compare these *psychological* "dosages" with recommended *physiological* "dosages."

11. Describe symptoms of "staleness" or overtraining in athletics that are identical to symptoms of clinical depression, and briefly discuss the implications of "negative addiction" in exercise.

12. Explain the meaning of perceived exertion and how it can be measured. Also, describe five physiological variables that serve as cues to the individual's subjective estimation of actual metabolic work intensity.

13. Illustrate Borg's model for the relationship between ratings of perceived exertion and heart rate, and explain why this model should be expected to be accurate.

14. Explain how and why both heart rate and RPE can be used by the participant to monitor exercise intensity, and discuss the relative accuracy of each in the prediction of physical working capacity.

15. Provide a general "rule of thumb" for the use of body perception in regulating exercise intensity on the basis of breathing rate and intensity.

16. Explain why RPE decreases at a given exercise intensity as cardiovascular conditioning progresses.

17. Indicate one instance in which involvement in an exercise training program might *not* be associated with increases in self-perception of physical ability and self-esteem.

18. Estimate the percentage of American adults who are involved in physical exercise, and the percentage of those who become involved but subsequently drop out.

19. Describe the curve representing adherence rates in formal exercise programs, and compare this curve with those representing compliance with medical treatment programs for alcoholism, drug addiction, etc.

20. List from Kenyon's model the six instrumental values that physical activity may have for the individual.

21. Discuss the importance of *not* limiting exercise participation to only one mode or form in terms of Kenyon's instrumental value model and the psychological aspects of exercise involvement.

22. List those factors which have been reported in the research literature to be related to exercise involvement and adherence.

23. Indicate in what way self-motivation scores and body composition are related to adherence to exercise.

24. Briefly discuss the inherent relaxation effect that exercise has on the circulatory system, and describe the type of exercise required to produce this effect.

25. Indicate how effective ratings of self-motivation and body composition are in correctly identifying those persons who will and those who won't adhere to an exercise program.

26. Describe Benson's relaxation response and compare its effectiveness in the reduction of anxiety with that of vigorous exercise and rest.

27. Briefly discuss the relationship between *capacity* and *willingness* in determining physical performance "maximums."

28. Provide two different explanations for the observation that both exercise and meditation can *reduce* anxiety—since anxiety often is equated with arousal, and since meditation and exercise represent opposite ends of the arousal continuum (i.e., meditation decreases arousal and exercise increases arousal).

29. Compare the effectiveness of hypnosis vs. mere suggestion in a normal waking state as an ergogenic aid.

30. Briefly discuss the influence of placebos on the expression of both muscular strength and endurance.

31. Explain dissociative strategies as a meditation technique in the increase of endurance.

32. Explain why determination of actual aerobic power cannot be influenced by motivation, whereas indirect determination of aerobic power in the 12-minute run can be.

33. Indicate what percentage of performance in the 12-minute run can be accounted for by motivational factors such as attitude toward physical activity.

REFERENCES

1. Akiskal, H. S., and McKinney, W. T., Jr.: Overview of recent research in depression. Arch. Gen. Psychiatry *32*:285, 1975.
2. Baekeland, F., and Lundwall, L.: Dropping out of treatment: a critical review. Psychol. Bull. *82*:738, 1975.
3. Bahrke, M. S., and Morgan, W. P.: Influence of acute physical activity and non–cultic meditation on state anxiety. Cognitive Ther. Res. *2*:323, 1978.
4. Benson, H.: *The Relaxation Response.* New York, William Morrow & Co., 1975.
5. Blythe, P.: *Stress Disease.* New York, St. Martin's Press, 1973.
6. Borg, G. A. V., and Noble, B. J.: Perceived Exertion. *In* J. Wilmore (ed.) *Exercise and Sport Sciences Reviews.* New York, Academic Press, 1974.
7. Cafarelli, E., and Noble, B. J.: The effect of inspired carbon dioxide on subjective estimates of exertion during exercise. Ergonomics *19*:581, 1976.
8. de Vries, H. A.: Immediate and long term effects of exercise upon resting muscle action potential level. J. Sports Med. Phys. Fitness *8*:1, 1968.
9. Dishman, R. K.: Aerobic power, estimation of physical ability, and attraction to physical activity. Res. Q. Am. Assoc. Health Phys. Educ. *49*:285, 1978.
10. Dishman, R. K., Ickes, W., and Morgan, W. P.: Self-motivation and adherence to habitual physical activity. J. Appl. Social Psychol. in press, 1980.
11. Docktor, R., and Sharkey, B. J.: Note on some physiological and subjective reactions to exercise and training. Percept. Mot. Skills *32*:233, 1971.

12. Ekblom, B., and Goldbarg, A. N.: The influence of training and other factors on the subjective rating of perceived exertion. Acta Physiol. Scand. *83*:399, 1971.
13. Fischman, D. A., Meltzer, H. Y., and Poppel, R. W.: Disruption of myofibrils in the skeletal muscles of psychotic patients. Arch. Gen. Psychiatry *23*:503, 1970.
14. Greist, J. H., Klein, M. H., Eischens, R. R., and Faris, J. W.: Antidepressant running: running as a treatment for non-psychotic depression. Behav. Med. June, 1978, p. 19.
15. Hanson, M. G.: Coronary Heart Disease, Exercise, and Motivation in Middle-Aged Males. Unpublished Doctoral Dissertation, University of Wisconsin, 1976.
16. Ikai, M., and Steinhaus, A. H.: Some factors modifying the expression of human strength. J. Appl. Physiol. *16*:157, 1961.
17. Johnson, W. R., and Kramer, G. F.: Effects of stereotyped non-hypnotic, hypnotic and post-hypnotic suggestions upon strength, power, and endurance. Res. Q. Am. Assoc. Health Phys. Educ. *32*:522, 1961.
18. Kenyon, G. S.: A conceptual model for characterising physical activity. Res. Q. Am. Assoc. Health Phys. Educ. *39*:566, 1968.
19. Little, J. C.: The athlete's neurosis—a deprivation crisis. Acta Psychiatr. Scand. *45*:187, 1969.
20. Meltzer, H. Y., and Engel, W. K.: Histochemical abnormalities of skeletal muscle in acutely psychotic patients, part II. Arch. Gen. Psychiatry *23*:492, 1970.
21. Meltzer, H. Y., and Moline, R.: Muscle abnormalities in acute psychoses. Arch. Gen. Psychiatry *23*:481, 1970.
22. Morgan, W. P.: Hypnosis and Muscular Performance. *In* W. P. Morgan (ed.) *Ergogenic Aids and Muscular Performance*. New York, Academic Press, 1972.
23. Morgan, W. P.: Psychological factors influencing perceived exertion. Med. Sci. Sports *5*:97, 1973.
24. Morgan, W. P.: Exercise and Mental Disorders. *In* A. J. Ryan, and F. L. Allman, Jr. (eds.) *Sports Medicine*. New York, Academic Press, 1974.
25. Morgan, W. P.: Staleness in Athletes—Physical or Mental? Invited Lecture, Research Institute of Applied Physiology, Cumberland College of Health Sciences, Sydney, N.S.W., Australia, 1976.
26. Morgan, W. P.: Psychological Consequences of Vigorous Physical Activity and Sport. *In* M. Gladys Scott (ed.) *The Academy Papers*. Iowa City, American Academy of Physical Education, 1976.
27. Morgan, W. P.: Involvement in Vigorous Physical Activity with Special Reference to Adherence. Proceedings, College Physical Education Conference, Orlando, Fla., 1977.
28. Morgan, W. P.: Anxiety reduction following acute physical activity. Psychiatr. Ann. 1979.
29. Morgan, W. P., and Coyne, L. L.: The Effect of Experimenter Oriented Autosuggestion on the Expression of Muscular Strength and Endurance. Paper presented at the Annual Session of the American Congress of Physical Medicine and Rehabilitation, Philadelphia, 1965.
30. Morgan, W. P., Hirota, K., Weitz, G., and Balke, B.: Hypnotic perturbation of perceived exertion: ventilatory consequences. Am. J. Clin. Hypn. *18*:182, 1976.
31. Morgan, W. P., and Johnson, R. W.: Psychologic characterization of the elite wrestler: a mental health model. (Abstr.) Med. Sci. Sports *9*:55, 1977.
32. Morgan, W. P., and Pollock, M. L.: Physical Activity and Cardiovascular Health: Psychological Aspects. *In* F. Landry (ed.) Proceedings, International Congress of Physical Activity Sciences, Quebec City, 1977.
33. Morgan, W. P., Roberts, J. A., Brand, F. R., and Feinerman, A. D.: Psychological effect of chronic physical activity. Med. Sci. Sports *2*:213, 1970.
34. Nadel, E. R., and Horvath, S. M.: Physiological responsiveness of schizoid adolescents to physical stress. Int. J. Neuropsychiatry *3*:191, 1967.
35. Nagle, F. J., Morgan, W. P., Hellickson, R. O., Serfass, R. C., and Alexander, J. F.: Spotting success traits in Olympic contenders. Physician and Sports Med. *3*:31, 1975.
36. Pitts, F. N.: The biochemistry of anxiety. Sci. Am. *220*:69, 1969.
37. Selye, H.: General adaptation syndrome and diseases of adaptation. J. Clin. Endocrinol. Metab. *6*:117, 1946.
38. Selye, H.: *The Stress of Life*. New York, McGraw-Hill Book Co., 1976.
39. Sime, W. E.: A comparison of exercise and meditation in reducing physiological response to stress. (Abstr.) Med. Sci. Sports *9*:55, 1977.
40. Teraslinna, P., Partanen, T., Koskela, A., and Oja, P.: Characteristics affecting willingness of executives to participate in an activity program aimed at coronary heart disease prevention. J. Sports Med. Phys. Fitness *9*:224, 1969.
41. Vendsalu, A.: Studies on adrenaline and noradrenaline in human plasma. Acta Physiol. Scand. *49*:57, 1960.
42. Wallace, R. K., and Benson, H.: The physiology of meditation. Sci. Am. *226*:84, 1972.

Chapter 8

Exercise and Diet in Weight Control

INTRODUCTION

Estimates show that 40 per cent of all Americans are overweight. Although many people would not consider weight control an exercise-dependent component of physical fitness, it is an exercise-related topic and extremely relevant to physical fitness, performance, and health. Most overweight individuals did not suddenly awake one morning in their obese state, but instead gradually accumulated the excess calories—"creeping obesity." Typical overweight Americans are approximately 20 per cent over their ideal weight, and became that way by a gradual accumulation of excess calories. Actually, the amount is small; for example, only 20 excess Calories per day adds 2 lbs of fat per year, and in 20 years an individual is 40 lbs overweight. Thus, we are not describing "gluttons," but rather average Americans who eat slightly more than they need and who gradually become overweight.

Nutritionists explain how easy the weight control formula is—simply balance "calories in" with "calories out!" "Calories in" come from the food we eat; "calories out" are a result of our basal metabolism plus the energy expended in all the physical activities in which we engage. In order to lose weight, one must decrease the food intake and/or increase the energy demands of physical activity.

Energy of the body is defined as the force or power that enables the body to carry on life-sustaining activities, and is derived from the breakdown of foodstuffs that release energy in the form of body work and heat. This energy value of foods is expressed in *kilogram calories* (kcal). A kcal is expressed as the amount of heat required to raise 1 kilogram of water 1 degree Centigrade, and sometimes is referred to as "Calorie"—the same Calories used in most food caloric charts, exercise cost charts, etc. The caloric value of foods is measured as the heat produced when a known amount of food is dried and burned in a sealed combustion chamber surrounded by water. A sensitive thermome-

205

ter records the heat produced, and thus the energy value of the food expressed in calories. The caloric values of foods differ, but the caloric value of the three basic energy nutrients is well established and rounded off as follows: 1 gm of carbohydrate yields 4 kcal; 1 gm of protein yields 4 kcal; and 1 gm of fat yields 9 kcal. One lb of stored fat in the body represents 3500 kcal. Thus, to gain or lose 1 lb of fat, there must be a 3500-kcal excess or deficit, respectively.

For those who prefer the metric system, the unit of energy measure is the *"joule"* *(J)*. One kcal equals 4184 joules (4.184 kJ); thus, a 2000 kcal diet is expressed as 8400 kJ. The converted energy value per gram of carbohydrate is 17 kJ; for protein, 17 kJ; and for fat, 38 kJ.

BASIC NUTRIENTS

Energy Nutrients

A brief review of the six basic nutrients may be helpful. Proteins, fats, and carbohydrates are the basic energy sources used in various ways by the body, which needs differing amounts of each. The major problem for the dieter is to have good sources of proteins and complex carbohydrates without high amounts of fats and simple sugars.

Protein makes up more than one-half of the human body, and is essential in the diet for the synthesis of body protein for tissues. Dietary protein is broken down by the body into amino acids, of which 23 are needed. Of these 23, 10 are not readily synthesized by the body and must be included in the diet; these are called the *essential* amino acids. They are found in high-quality protein foods such as cheese, eggs, fish, meat, milk, poultry, and whole grain cereal. Protein constitutes about 14 per cent of the calories in the average American's diet, and usually ranges from 10 up to as much as 20 per cent of the calories. The recommended amount of dietary protein is about 0.9 gm per kg of body weight per day. Additional protein for athletes is not recommended; the old notion that athletes require great amounts of protein is false. Since amino acids are so important to the body's build-up of muscle, bone, and other important agents such as enzymes and hormones, calories from protein generally are not used as an energy source unless other sources of energy are unavailable. The protein content of some typical foods is shown in Figure 8–1.

The body's primary sources of energy are carbohydrates and fats. Exercise of short duration uses carbohydrates as almost the total fuel. Work of longer duration uses both carbohydrates and fats as fuel. As aerobic work increases in duration, the amount of fat used as the fuel for exercise increases. Submaximal exercise lasting an hour uses about 60 per cent fat and 40 per cent carbohydrate as exercise fuels.

About one-half of our calories are taken in as *carbohydrates*, which are mainly starches and sugars derived from plants. Carbohydrates are quickly digested and stored by the liver and muscle in the form of glycogen, as our short-term energy storage system. When immediate energy is needed for exercise, the glycogen is converted to glucose and used as a primary fuel. Recently, terms such as "glycogen loading" have been popularized by endurance athletes who are lowering levels of muscle glycogen several days before competition by long-duration exercise and eating diets rich in carbohydrates. As the muscles replace their glycogen supply, the glycogen fuel is available for work. Carbohydrate content of some typical foods is shown in Figures 8–2 and 8–3.

The other primary fuel for exercise is *fat*. As carbohydrate (glycogen) represents the body's short-term storage system, fat represents long-term storage. If you were suddenly forced to go two weeks without food, the body's fat supply would allow you to survive. The average American's diet is high in fat from which come about 40 per cent of the

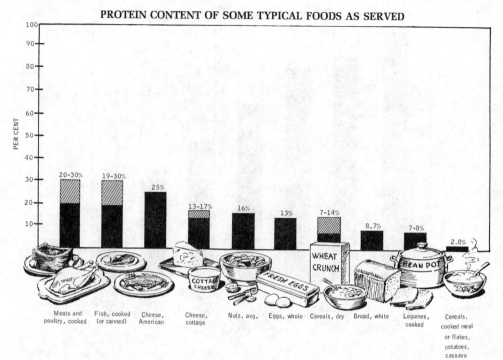

Figure 8–1. (From Briggs, G. M., and Calloway, D. H.: *Bogert's Nutrition and Physical Fitness* (10th ed.). Philadelphia, W. B. Saunders Co., 1979, p. 102.)

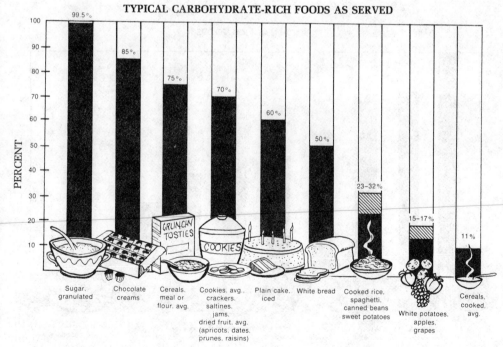

Figure 8–2. (From Briggs, G. M., and Calloway, D. H.: *Bogert's Nutrition and Physical Fitness* (10th ed.). Philadelphia, W. B. Saunders Co., 1979, p. 58.)

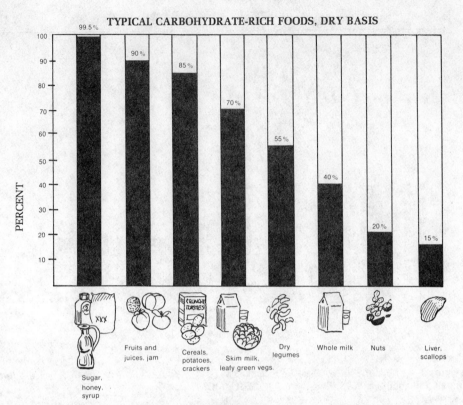

Figure 8–3. (From Briggs, G. M., and Calloway, D. H.: *Bogert's Nutrition and Physical Fitness* (10th ed.). Philadelphia, W. B. Saunders Co., 1979, p. 58.)

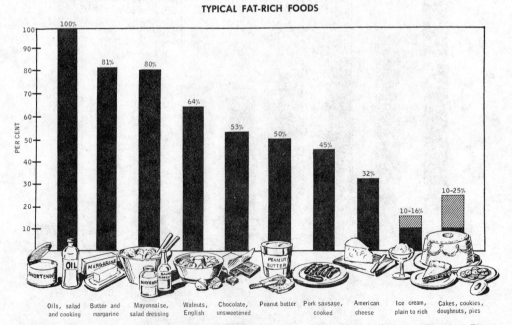

Figure 8–4. (From Briggs, G. M., and Calloway, D. H.: *Bogert's Nutrition and Physical Fitness* (10th ed.). Philadelphia, W. B. Saunders Co., 1979, p. 72.)

calories. The Food and Nutrition Board of the National Research Council suggests 25 per cent as a much healthier percentage of dietary fat. Fats are digested into their basic forms of fatty acids (FA) and glycerol, which are absorbed into the cells of the small intestine. In these cells the basic forms are reconverted into triglycerides (three fatty acids and one glycerol), which is the form of fat storage. Fatty acids that attach to other compounds are important to body structures; examples include lipoproteins (FAs and protein), glycolipids (FAs and carbohydrates), phospholipids (FAs and phosphoric acid), and cholesterol. These large molecules are transported by the lymph and blood systems to membrane structures and fat storage cells throughout the body. Typical fat-rich foods are shown in Figure 8–4.

Other Nutrients

Besides the three basic energy components in our food, water, vitamins, and minerals are also essential to health. _Water_ constitutes about 40 to 60 per cent of total body weight and is the fluid medium for the body. Water _inside_ the cell is referred to as intracellular (about 62 per cent), and _outside_ the cell as extracellular (about 38 per cent). Food, oxygen, and waste products essentially move in a water medium. Beside its function as the body's fluid base, water is very important in the regulation of body temperature. Because of water's important cooling function and its importance to exercise, guidelines for water replacement during exercise are presented later in this chapter.

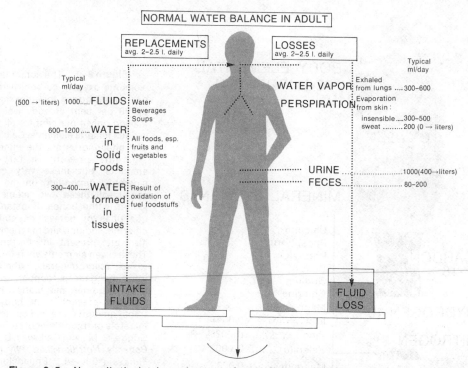

Figure 8–5. Normally the intake and output of water from the body are approximately in balance. If much water is drunk, the volume of urine excreted increases. If water intake is low or the amount lost in perspiration is high (with exercise or in hot weather), the urine will be reduced in volume. With fever, vomiting, or diarrhea, there is excessive loss of water. Any excessive loss should be made up by taking more fluids so that body stores of water are not depleted. (From Briggs, G. M., and Calloway, D. H.: _Bogert's Nutrition and Physical Fitness_ (10th ed.). Philadelphia, W. B. Saunders Co., 1979, p. 240.)

The major sources of water are the fluids we drink, water contained in the foods we eat, and water produced by the chemical reactions as we metabolize foods. Sources of water loss include, in descending order of amount lost under normal conditions, urine, sweat, water vapor in expired air, and that in fecal material (see Fig. 8–5).

Vitamins are organic substances which are needed in small amounts to perform specific bodily functions. A deficit in a vitamin normally required by the body results in the cells of the body being unable to perform some normal function, and in a set of symptoms associated with the specific vitamin deficiency. The major vitamins are reviewed briefly in Appendix B. Although recommended daily allowances are available for the various vitamins, a simple but sound approach is to eat a balanced diet from the basic food groups to insure that appropriate vitamins are present in the diet (Table 8–1).

Analysis or separation of the human body into basic elements would reveal at least 31 known chemical elements, of which 24 are believed to be essential (Fig. 8–6). These elements can be described basically as nonmetals of which the main elements are oxygen (65 per cent), carbon (18 per cent), hydrogen (10 per cent), and nitrogen (3 per cent), and the 22 metallic elements called *minerals*. The most abundant minerals of the body are calcium, phosphorus, sodium, potassium, chlorine, sulfur, and magnesium. Other minerals are described as "trace elements," and include iron, zinc, selenium, manganese, iodine, copper, fluorine, and chromium. Minerals are essential to the body and help to regulate many of its vital processes. The "Recommended Daily Dietary Allowances" include suggested daily amounts for various vitamins and minerals.

However, the simplest way to approach sound nutrition is to include the recom-

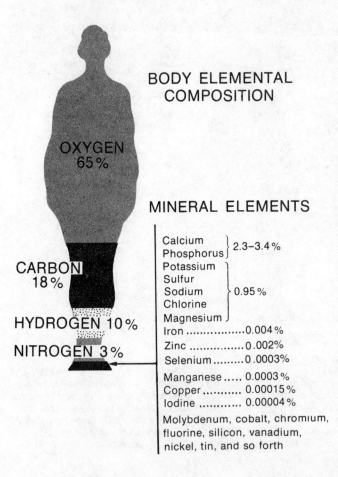

BODY ELEMENTAL COMPOSITION

OXYGEN 65%

MINERAL ELEMENTS

Calcium ⎫
Phosphorus ⎬ 2.3–3.4%

Potassium ⎫
Sulfur
Sodium ⎬ 0.95%
Chlorine
Magnesium ⎭

Iron 0.004%
Zinc 0.002%
Selenium.........0.0003%

Manganese..... 0.0003%
Copper........... 0.00015%
Iodine 0.00004%

Molybdenum, cobalt, chromium, fluorine, silicon, vanadium, nickel, tin, and so forth

CARBON 18%

HYDROGEN 10%

NITROGEN 3%

Figure 8–6. The nonmetallic elements oxygen, carbon, hydrogen, and nitrogen together make up 96 per cent of body weight, leaving only 4 per cent for all the various mineral elements. Calcium and phosphorus are the mineral elements present in largest amounts, but these vary considerably, depending on the reserves of these two elements stored in the bones. Substantial quantities of potassium, sulfur, chlorine, sodium, and magnesium also are present in the body. These seven elements are referred to as macrominerals, whereas iron, manganese, copper, zinc, cobalt, iodine, and many other elements present in the body in trace amounts are called trace minerals or trace elements. (From Briggs, G. M., and Calloway, D. H.: *Bogert's Nutrition and Physical Fitness* (10th ed.). Philadelphia, W. B. Saunders Co., 1979, p. 237.)

FAT SOL- A, D, E, K

Table 8–1. A DAILY FOOD GUIDE*

Review of the Four Basic Food Groups

Milk Group (8-ounce cups)

> 2 to 3 cups for children under 9 years
> 3 cups or more for children 9 to 12 years
> 4 cups or more for teenagers
> 2 cups or more for adults
> 3 cups or more for pregnant women
> 4 cups or more for nursing mothers

Meat Group

> 2 or more servings. Count as one serving:
> 2 to 3 ounces lean, cooked beef, veal, pork, lamb, poultry, or fish (without bone)
> 2 eggs
> 1 cup cooked dry beans, dry peas, or lentils
> 4 tablespoons peanut butter

Vegetable–Fruit Group (½ cup serving, or 1 piece fruit, etc.)

> 4 or more servings per day, including:
> 1 serving of citrus fruit, or other fruit or vegetable as a good source of vitamin C, or 2
> servings of a fair source
> 1 serving, at least every other day, of a dark-green or deep yellow vegetable for
> vitamin A
> 2 or more servings of other vegetables and fruits, including potatoes

Bread–Cereals Group

> 4 or more servings daily (whole grain, enriched, or restored). Count as 1 serving:
> 1 slice bread
> 1 ounce ready-to-eat cereal
> ½ to ¾ cup cooked cereal, corn meal, grits, macaroni, noodles, rice, or spaghetti

*"Daily Food Guide" in Consumers All Yearbook of Agriculture, 1965, U.S. Department of Agriculture, Washington, D.C., p. 394.

mended portions of the four basic food groups. Since these are so important to diet, they are reviewed in Table 8–1. For other important dietary goals, see Chapter 3, p. 51.

ENERGY NEEDS OF THE BODY

How many kcal do we need per day? Although a precise answer to this question is extremely difficult, many average estimates are available. The energy needs are based essentially on the activity or exercise requirements and on the *basal metabolic rate* (BMR). The BMR is defined as the energy needs of the body at complete rest in a fasting state, i.e., the energy necessary to sustain life. Although BMR can be measured by *direct* calorimetry, an expensive process in which the individual is placed in a chamber that measures all the heat produced by the body, a simpler technique is *indirect* calorimetry, in which respiratory gases are measured to determine the amount converted into kcal of heat produced per square meter of body surface area per hour, and expressed as caloric expenditure. Since this indirect method is well suited for both resting and active individuals, most measurements are based on this technique.

BMR is influenced by a number of factors, one of which is body size and composition. Tall, thin persons with large body surface areas experience greater heat loss than short, muscular individuals; thus, the BMR of tall persons is greater. Muscle tissue uses more energy than fatty tissue; thus the BMR of muscular athletes is about 5 per cent greater than average. Fat persons have lower BMR per weight than muscular persons of the same weight. The BMR of women generally is 5 to 10 per cent lower than that of men, possibly owing to the greater accumulation of fat and lower lean body mass in women—difference in body compositon (see Chapter 1).

Other factors influencing BMR include age, amount of sleep, function of the endocrine glands, state of nutrition, and fever. BMR is greatest during periods of rapid growth in early childhood, and secondly in the growth spurt associated with puberty. In adulthood, BMR declines slowly with increasing age at approximately 2 per cent per decade. Therefore, if the diet remains constant, the individual will gain weight (see Fig. 8–7). As a result, nutritionists have recommended reducing the daily caloric intake of older persons. One such estimate recommends that daily caloric allotment be reduced as follows: by 2.5 per cent in each ten-year period between ages 20 and 40; by 5 per cent between ages 40 and 50; by 7.5 per cent between ages 50 and 60; by 10 per cent between ages 60 and 70; and by 12.5 per cent after age 70. A simplified approximation is to reduce caloric consumption by 5 per cent for each decade past 25 years of age. Thus, by age 35, we are eating only 95 per cent of our caloric allotment at age 25. By 45 years of age, we are reduced to 90 per cent, by 55 years to 85 per cent, etc. As we grow older, we actually must eat less to maintain the desired balance.

The secretions of the endocrine glands help to regulate metabolic rate. Inadequate

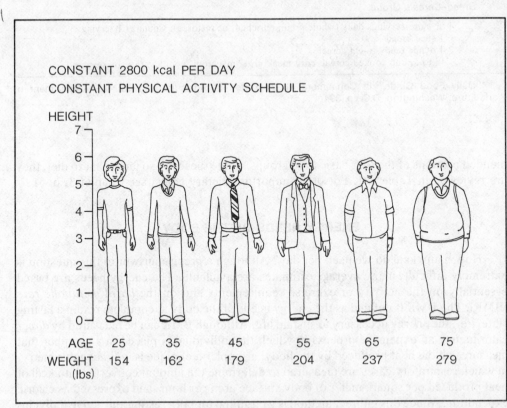

Figure 8–7. The reference man age 25 is in perfect caloric balance at 154 lbs eating 2800 kcal per day. If he continues to eat this amount until he is 75 years old, he will gradually become overweight and eventually obese. These figures do not take into account any reductions in activity or work level that normally accompany aging.

thyroxine from the thyroid gland may cause BMR to drop as much as 30 to 50 per cent, whereas overproduction may double it. The male sex hormones increase BMR by 15 to 20 per cent, and the female hormones by slightly less. The growth hormone may increase BMR up to 20 per cent. Hormones such as epinephrine and norepinephrine from the adrenal glands also influence BMR, as do the hormones cortisol and insulin.

Since sleep lowers BMR by 10 to 15 per cent, the amount of sleep is relevant. Climatic conditions also have been shown to affect BMR, with individuals in tropical areas exhibiting as much as 10 to 20 per cent lower BMR. In addition, infections, certain diseases, and fever increase BMR about 7 per cent for each additional degree of increased body temperature.

With so many factors influencing BMR, it is understandable why individuals vary in BMR and why average estimates are not totally accurate. With these influencing factors, we can begin to appreciate that weight control efforts are far from equal among individuals. Because of these obvious variations, caloric consumption during activity and caloric allowances are based on the *"reference man and woman."* Both are 22 years of age (weight added after this age is most likely to be fat), live in a temperate climate, experience light activity, and weigh 70 kg (154 lbs) (man) and 58 kg (128 lbs) (woman).

It has been estimated that basal metabolic needs account for 50 to 70 per cent of the total daily caloric requirement for sedentary and moderately active individuals. Of course, the more physically active a person is, the lower this percentage. The standard allowance for individuals of average height and weight is 1 kcal per kg of body weight per hour for the male, and 0.9 kcal per kg per hour for the female. The 24-hour requirement for our reference male would thus be 1680 kcal (24 hrs × 70 kg), and for the reference female 1253 (24 hrs × 0.9 x 58 kg).

In addition to BMR, physical activity has the next greatest influence on energy balance (Appendix A–15). Because of its large, varying influence, it is best to make a closer estimate of kcal consumed in activity where possible. A simplified procedure for estimating the energy expenditure of physical activity is provided in Appendix A–17.

Appendix A–15 makes the effect of physical activity on daily caloric need obvious. If we add physical activity needs to BMR, our reference man ranges from 2034 kcal in light activity days to 4536 kcal on days of very heavy activity. The reference woman ranges from 1574 kcal in light activity to 2427 in heavy activity. A very heavy estimate is not available for women.

Another extremely simple estimate of daily kcal requirement is 13 and 15 kcal per pound of ideal body weight for the sedentary and moderately active individual, respectively (use Table 8–2 and/or Appendix A–16 for an estimate of ideal body weight). Thus, for a sedentary reference man, this formula would yield 154 lbs times 13 kcal, or an estimate of 2002 kcal per day. The sedentary reference woman, at 128 lbs times 13 kcal, needs 1664 kcal per day. Similar estimates for the moderately active reference man and woman would be 2310 and 1920 kcal/day, respectively.

In addition to the numerous factors affecting BMR, and the very significant effects of level of activity on the daily caloric requirement, the old "heredity and environment" argument is of special interest in weight control. Statistics indicate that one's chances of becoming obese are less than 10 per cent if neither parent is obese. If only one parent is obese, the chances of obesity jump to 40 per cent, and if both parents are obese they soar to 80 per cent. The reasons for these statistics are not so well defined, and probably are combinations of both the genetic or inherited traits and one's learned environmental traits.

Consider your environmental factors. If neither parent is obese, the chances are your eating "models" are very appropriate to your body size and lifestyle. If only one parent is obese, you still have one valid model. If both parents are obese, you probably

Table 8–2. IDEAL WEIGHTS FOR MEN AND WOMEN*

According to Height and Frame, Ages 25 and Over
(Weight in Pounds, in Indoor Clothing)

	Height (with shoes on 1-inch heels)		Small** Frame	Medium Frame	Large Frame
	Feet	Inches			
	5	2	112–120	118–129	126–141
	5	3	115–123	121–133	129–144
	5	4	118–126	124–136	132–148
	5	5	121–129	127–139	135–152
	5	6	124–133	130–143	138–156
Men	5	7	128–137	134–147	142–161
	5	8	132–141	138–152	147–166
	5	9	136–145	142–156	151–170
	5	10	140–150	146–160	155–174
	5	11	144–154	150–165	159–179
	6	0	148–158	154–170	164–184
	6	1	152–162	158–175	168–189
	6	2	156–167	162–180	173–194
	6	3	160–171	167–185	178–199
	6	4	164–175	172–190	182–204

	Height (with shoes on 2-inch heels)		Small Frame	Medium Frame	Large Frame
	Feet	Inches			
	4	10	92– 98	96–107	104–119
	4	11	94–101	98–110	106–122
	5	0	96–104	101–113	109–125
	5	1	99–107	104–116	112–128
	5	2	102–110	107–119	115–131
Women	5	3	105–113	110–122	118–134
	5	4	108–116	113–126	121–138
	5	5	111–119	116–130	125–142
	5	6	114–123	120–135	129–146
	5	7	118–127	124–139	133–150
	5	8	122–131	128–143	137–154
	5	9	126–135	132–147	141–158
	5	10	130–140	136–151	145–163
	5	11	134–144	140–155	149–168
	6	0	138–148	144–159	153–173

*Excerpted from *Build and Blood Pressure Study,* Society of Actuaries, October, 1959.
**Use Table 8–3 to get an estimate of frame size.

have learned eating practices from your parents which are conducive to fatness: how much you eat, what types of foods you prefer, how often you eat, how often you snack, etc. These considerations place heavy emphasis on your learned dietary practices.

On the other hand, the identical twin studies of Jean Mayer, and the mounting evidence concerning fat cell number, point more toward the genetic make-up and to the very early eating practices. Mayer, who has studied sets of identical twins reared under very different and completely separate environmental situations, reports an astonishing similarity in the body size and composition of these individuals.

Excess calories are stored in the body as adipose tissue or in fat cells, which are specialized cells for storing fat. Individuals differ in the size and number of their fat cells. In the last decade, scientists have developed a relatively simple test for determining the number and size of fat cells. By taking a needle biopsy of adipose tissue, the fat cells can be isolated, sized, and counted in a high-precision automatic cell counter. These improved methods for determining how many fat cells a person has, and how large the cells are, have led to some interesting studies. Obese people have approximately three times as many fat cells as the nonobese, and the fat cells of obese persons have greater quantities of fat per cell. As an adult gains or loses fat, the number of fat cells remains constant, but the size of the cells changes according to the amount of fat being stored. Individuals with large numbers of fat cells appear to be predisposed to fatness.

Since the number of fat cells is constant for the adult, yet very important to body fatness, the critical question is, when are these cells formed and can their number be altered? Evidence indicates that there are three critical stages for increasing the number of fat cells: (1) the last three months of pregnancy; (2) the first year of infancy; and (3) during the adolescent growth spurt. The control of fatness at these three stages appears to be particularly critical to the number of fat cells we have, and thus to our future fatness (see also Chapter 1).

Age is another important factor in weight control, probably because it reflects many other changes that are taking place. For example, in describing BMR and fat cell number, two growth-related increases were noted: one in early years and another in adolescence. The recommended reduction in BMR for each decade in adulthood was described on p. 212. Additionally, if we examine height and weight tables for the adult population, we will notice the increase in weight with increasing age. Additional weight after maturity is almost always fat unless a large increase in muscle tissue has been associated with a heavy strength-building program. There is no physiological rationale for becoming fatter as you grow older, but there probably are a number of reasons why the increases commonly occur.

1. By adulthood most dietary practices are well established, and these "habits" are difficult to change.

2. BMR is gradually slowing down; thus, you must eat slightly less to maintain your weight (see p. 212 for an explanation).

3. Most American adults become less active as they grow older; thus, they must reduce their caloric consumption to account for reduced activity.

4. "Creeping obesity" is a gradual accumulation of fat over a long period of time, which is difficult to detect and become alarmed about.

In essence, adults must gradually eat less and/or exercise more to insure the proper balance of calories to maintain "ideal" weight. To avoid "creeping obesity," adults should set a firm, realistic ideal weight, weigh daily either naked or in the same clothes, and make changes when this value is exceeded even by a small amount such as 5 lbs. Note that normal day-to-day fluctuation in body weight is about 2 to 3 lbs, and that dehydration associated with intense exercise may exceed this. These fluctuations are normal and should not trigger any dietary changes, except in the case of weight loss by dehydration; water should be drunk to replace necessary body fluids. The authors know of no uncontrollable physiological reasons why adults should become fatter as they grow older.

HOW FAT IS FAT?

Since fat is a normal, healthy energy reserve, we all need some fat storage. The critical question is "how much?" A precise, scientific answer is not available, but there is a great deal of scientific information to help us as individuals to answer this question. Obviously, all attempts to measure fat in living persons must be indirect. Appendix A–16 is designed to help answer the question of *"how much fat?"*

Possibly the simplest test of fatness is to stand naked in front of your mirror and closely examine your physique. If you "look fat," the chances are you are overweight.

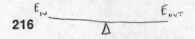

Table 8–3. DETERMINATION OF RELATIVE FRAME SIZE OF THE HUMAN BODY*

Frame size is easily determined from ankle circumference, which should be measured with a tape measure at the smallest point above the two bones that protrude on each side (external and internal malleolus). The tape measure should be pulled as tight as possible. Frame size is classified as follows:

Sex	Small Frame	Medium Frame	Large Frame
Male	<8"	8 to 9¼"	>9¼"
Female	<7½"	7½ to 8¾"	>8¾"

*Adapted from Johnson, P. B., Updyke, W., Schaefer, M., and Stolberg, D. C.: *Sport, Exercise and You.* New York, Holt, Rinehart, and Winston, 1975, p. 57.

Another simple estimate is to compare your height and weight to height and weight tables or norms. Table 8–2 is based on the weight of a large number of people as reported to large insurance companies. In these tables, insurance actuaries have devised desirable weights, *not* the actual weights. These desirable weights are derived from people showing the lowest mortality rates, and such individuals happen to be *below* the "average" weights.

Check Table 8–3 to get an estimate of frame size for use in Table 8–2. Keep in mind that there are no clear definitions of frame size. Therefore, the total procedure is a rough estimate of frame size and desirable weight.

Another common problem with height and weight tables is that normally no adjustment is made for the amount of muscle tissue, which is actually heavier than fat. Muscular individuals will be "overweight" when compared with these tables, but not necessarily "overfat." Strong individuals with much muscle development will appear fatter than they actually are. For this reason, it is desirable to estimate fatness by some method other than total body weight alone.

Another method of estimating fatness is a "scientific pinch." Since much of the body fat is subcutaneous, i.e., just under the skin and overlying the muscles, the thickness of a "pinch" of skin and fat can be used as a good indicator of total body fatness. This procedure is easily illustrated by pinching the skin on the back of the hand, the back of the upper arm, and the abdomen near the waistline. The different thickness of these sites is due to the different amounts of underlying fat. As a rough estimate, pinch the skin and fat on the back of the arm over the triceps muscle, at the lower tip of the shoulder blade on the back, and over the abdomen. The thickness of these folds should *average* not more than about ¾-inch.

The thickness of the fatfold can be measured more accurately with skinfold calipers.* The better ones measure the thickness of the fatfold while exerting a constant pressure (10 gm/mm²) to the fold. The fatfold should be firmly grasped between the thumb and forefinger at a distance of 1 cm from the measurement site. The depth of the fold is determined by the amount of fat present. As the caliper is applied, the fold should be slightly released so that most of the tension is on the caliper surface, not the fingers (see Fig. A–16 *c* to *f*). The thickness of the fold is read in millimeters from the caliper dial. Normally, three measurements at each site are taken and averaged. To assess fat loss, the thickness of folds can be taken before and after an exercise and/or dietary program, and folds from several sites can be used to predict total body fat and percentage body fat. By measuring the skinfold or fatfold at specified sites, a prediction equation can be used to

---

*A number of skinfold calipers are commercially available; see Appendix A–16 for recommendations.

calculate the specific gravity or body density, and thus the percentage of fat on the body (Fig. A–16 g and h). The best skinfold sites for predicting total fatness are dependent on the fat patterning of the person measured.

Fat patterning appears to be an individual trait which is highly influenced by the inherited genetic pattern, by sex, and by age. Before puberty, the fat patterning of boys and girls is quite similar, but at puberty boys tend to put on fat in the upper torso and stomach and girls tend to accumulate fat around the hips and upper thighs. After puberty, the average young female has approximately twice as much fat as the average young male. Males, who usually mature later than females, have a longer growing period, and also at puberty males experience a rapid growth in lean body mass. Thus females have a larger amount of fat and a smaller lean body mass, making the fat percentage considerably higher than in the male (Fig. 1–5). This smaller over-all body size, the smaller lean body mass, and the high percentage of fat are generally believed to account for many performance differences between men and women. For these reasons, the best predictive skinfold sites for each sex are usually different.

Predictive equations from skinfolds are derived from measuring numerous skinfold sites over a large group of people of the same sex, and about the same age and fatness. The same people then are weighed under water to determine their body density or specific gravity. This figure is employed to calculate the percentage body fat, using data from cadavers of known body density and percentage body fat. The best predictive sites for skinfolds are determined mathematically, and a skinfold formula is derived. The greatest accuracy in predicting percentage fat from skinfold measurements occurs when the person to be measured is the same sex and age as the sample of people from which the prediction equation was derived, and has similar fat patterning. Thus, these formulae are better suited to some individuals than others. A second problem in accuracy with skinfold measurement is that of measurement error. The measurement procedures must be carefully standardized and practiced before reliable results can be expected. For those individuals who have access to skinfold calipers, prediction equations recommended for young men and for young women are included in Appendix A–16. Readers are encouraged to obtain an estimate of their percentage fat and ideal weight as calculated by this method.

DIET VS. EXERCISE FOR WEIGHT REDUCTION

The Disadvantages of Diet Alone

Since it is possible to be totally inactive and still maintain an ideal weight simply by controlling diet, why is the role of exercise so highly emphasized in most healthy weight control programs? Certainly, one reason is that there are many other health benefits from exercise, such as good muscle tone, cardiovascular endurance, strength, and flexibility. Another compelling reason is that, for most people learning a lifestyle conducive to health and slimness, the combination of sensible diet and exercise is much easier to maintain than weight control by exercise or diet alone.

A common excuse for omitting the exercise in a weight control program is often: "Exercise makes me more hungry!" Actually, exercise does not always stimulate the appetite and may even suppress it. Dr. Lawrence Oscai, a nutrition expert, has summarized research in this area, and concluded that exercise of long duration performed on a regular basis in occupations such as lumberjacking does stimulate the appetite sufficiently to account for the increased caloric requirement. He reported caloric expenditures among lumberjacks and farm laborers to be approximately double the requirements for office workers. Conversely, more vigorous exercise of shorter duration did not appear to stimulate the appetite. A 1-hour exercise program consisting of 45 minutes of jogging and light calisthenics three days a week did not increase the appetite of middle-aged men, although it improved their exercise tolerance. Thus, it appears that this exercise myth should be recognized as such, and placed alongside other such myths.

If regular exercise is included as a part of the weight control program, the individual can essentially consume more calories per day. This greater consumption, nutritionally speaking, is often an advantage, especially in those who do not regularly consume many calories. Although thousands of calories per day do not insure adequate nutrients from the diet, the chances of getting better nutrition increase as number of calories increases. It takes a very nutritionally sophisticated individual to get a balanced diet from 1000 kcal per day, and most of us have very little knowledge of nutrition.

What Type of Exercise Is Best for Weight Control?

In Chapter 5 on cardiovascular fitness, the importance of duration, intensity, and frequency of exercise was emphasized. In the weight control chapter, the emphasis is on the total amount of work accomplished per day. Why not walk to school or work every morning instead of riding? Why not take the most distant space in the parking lot, not the closest? Why not walk up three flights of stairs instead of taking the elevator? Why not begin that cardiovascular fitness program? Small changes in attitude such as these can really make a difference in total calories stored per day, especially over a long period of time.

Many individuals initiating an exercise program begin by saying where they would, and would not, like to lose weight. Surely you can guess the body areas for yourself. Everyone would like to *"spot reduce,"* i.e., reduce this area, but not that area. We sometimes feel that if we do sit-ups, we will lose weight in the stomach area, but not the breasts or some other area. Unfortunately, that is not the way the body works. Fat patterning is individual, but affected by age, sex, and heredity. Diet and exercise can change the amount of fat and the muscle tone, but not the patterning. The last fat you gained will be the first you lose. How would you look if you gained 20 lbs? Find someone in your family with a body type who is overweight, and the chances are your fat patterning will be similar. Problem areas for men appear to be the stomach area and upper torso, and for women the stomach area and lower torso, i.e., the hips and thighs. There is no scientific evidence that we can substantially change our patterning by exercising a specific body area; you can improve the appearance of an area by increased muscle tone in a specific area, but the fat pad is still the same. For example, if a person with little muscle strength does side waist bends for the lateral trunk and waistline area, the waist measurement initially may be smaller owing to improved muscle tone. Additional exercise specifically aimed at this area will maintain strength and tone, but is not likely to show greater reductions in girth without over-all weight loss. Spot reducing is another myth, one in which many of us would like to believe, but one not well-founded in body composition research literature.

If you cannot spot reduce a body area, can you "vibrate" or "bump" it off? This question has been studied by application of vibration of the most vigorous type with belts placed around the abdomen of 13 men, some of whom were markedly overweight. The results indicated that 15 minutes of vigorous vibration used the equivalent of 1/23 of an ounce of fat more than simply sitting at rest. No changes in blood fats were seen. It was concluded that the belt vibrator is not to be taken seriously as a device for removing or shifting fat deposits—another myth for our shelf. In summary, an effortless form of exercise has not been found. To consume kcal, you must oxidize food, and work is required for this process.

This same work principle applies to "sweating pounds off." Body dehydration (loss of body water) results in considerable weight reduction, but fortunately this condition is easily corrected. Simply drink water to replace the fluids, and thus the pounds. The use of the sauna or steam bath for healthy individuals may be a relaxing experience, but is not a valuable weight reduction aid. Exercising in such environments places an increased stress on the cardiovascular system, and definitely should be avoided. Exercising in rubberized suits or any clothing designed to retain body heat is only good for temporary weight loss, and is considered very dangerous from the viewpoint of heat exhaustion. Exercise under these conditions should be avoided. Ample water should be ingested before all exercises, especially those of an endurance nature, and drinking water during and after the exercise is recommended in order to delay dehydration and performance decrements which accompany general fatigue, and as a means of maintaining lower body temperature.

Ingesting salt tablets, salty foods, or much solid food prior to exercise in hot environments is not recommended, because the higher concentration of salt and/or foodstuff in the stomach actually draws water into the gut area away from the blood and muscle tissue that need the water so badly. Unless an extreme amount of exercise is conducted in hot environments, most individuals maintain adequate salt by using a moderate amount in the diet. Ingestion of some foods rich in potassium *is* recommended. However, dietary salt supplements simply are not needed in almost all exercise conditions, and are detrimental to performance when administered immediately before exercise.

Nathan Smith, in his book, *Food for Sport,* recommends adding salt to the normal diet if rates of water loss per work-out exceed 5 to 10 lbs. He cautions against using high concentrations of salt as in tablets, or an excessive amount of fluids containing salt. The abuse of salt tablets should be recognized as the result of another misconception concerning exercise. Furthermore, heat stress studies have shown that salt tablets often do not dissolve sufficiently while passing through the gastrointestinal tract. X-ray photographs have shown visible remains of salt tablets ingested as long as six hours before the photographs were taken.

Drinking adequate water before and during exercise in hot environments is especially important to health and performance. Dr. David Costill, Director of the Human Performance Laboratory at Ball State University, who summarized studies showing improved athletic performance with ingesting of water during performance, discussed the value of water replacement during exercise, and gave the following "guidelines for the drinking athlete." Although these were intended for the endurance athlete, the individual performing endurance exercise in a hot environment has much to gain from them. Remember, when exercising in hot and/or humid environments, that a headache may well be the first warning sign of heat problems. Those who develop a headache when exercising in such environments should stop the exercise and drink plenty of cold water. Without symptoms of excessive heat or dehydration, the following guidelines can be adapted to exercise in these environments.

1. The drink should be:
   a. Hypotonic (few solid particles per unit of water).
   b. Low in sugar concentration (less than 2.5 g per 100 ml of water).
   c. Cold (roughly 45–55°F or 8–13°C).
   d. Consumed in volumes ranging from 100 to 400 ml (3 to 10 ounces*).
   e. Palatable (the drink should not have a strong flavor).

---

*8 ounces = 1 cup.

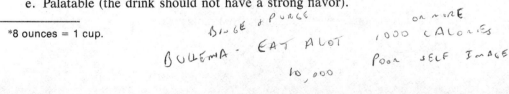

2. Drink 400–600 ml (13.5 to 20 ounces) of water or similar drink 30 minutes before the start of exercise.

3. During the exercise, 100 to 200 ml (3 to 6.5 ounces) of fluid should be taken at 10 to 15 minute intervals throughout the activity.

4. Following the exercise, modest salting of foods and the ingestion of drinks with essential minerals can adequately replace the electrolytes lost in sweat.

5. The exercise participant should keep a record of his/her morning body weight (taken immediately after rising, after urination, and before breakfast), to detect symptoms of a condition of chronic dehydration.

6. Drinks are of significant value in exercise lasting more than 50 or 60 minutes."[6]

Many scientists study the effects of regular exercise on body composition: i.e., how much exercise does it take for most people to lower their percentage body fat? Many individuals see little weight change in an exercise program, but, if body fat is estimated, it is clear that fat is being lost and lean body mass is being gained. These changes are especially true for men, who more easily attain changes in lean body mass. General agreement from exercise studies is that regular work-outs of a 300- to 500-kcal energy expenditure level are necessary for significant body composition changes. For the average person, a 300- to 500-kcal work-out translates into 3 to 5 miles per day. To those who have never experienced a jogging program, a mile seems a long distance, but to those who have gradually increased their distance through a successful jogging program, 5 miles does not seem very far. A good weight control program might be a minimum of 30 minutes of jogging, or 45 minutes to 1 hour of brisk walking.

How many kcal are stored in a pound of fat? The average estimate is 3500 kcal. If your arithmetic is anything at all, you have already decided that a 500-kcal deficit per day is needed just to lose 1 lb of fat a week—a 1000 kcal deficit for 2 lbs per week. At this point, someone usually recalls a friend or relative who once lost 7 to 10 lbs in one week, or a pro football lineman who lost 8 lbs in one work-out. Remember that the average daily weight fluctuation is 2 to 3 lbs—hardly 2 to 3 lbs of fat. By now it should be evident that a pound of body weight is quite different from a pound of fat. The largest causes of weight fluctuation appear to be first, body water, and second, the presence or absence of food in the gut. Dehydration of body water following exercise is responsible for large amounts of temporary weight loss, and water loss is the basis for the often amazing initial weight loss associated with low carbohydrate diets. Since 3 gm of water are stored with 1 gm of carbohydrate, loss of carbohydrate stores in the body results in a dramatic weight loss. As a normal diet is resumed, carbohydrate stores are replenished and the weight regained. These types of diet are not recommended from a health viewpoint.

Most nutritionists agree that the maximal recommended weight loss should not exceed 2 lbs of fat per week, which is a fairly stringent 1000 kcal-per-day reduction. One lb per week is much more realistic—after all, that is a 500-kcal reduction per day and 52 lbs of fat per year. A ten-week combined diet and exercise program is a 10- or 20-lb reduction of fat, and in addition to the new, slimmer "you" there is an improved state of physical fitness and some established new dietary practices that improve your chances of maintaining what you have accomplished. It has been estimated that 90 per cent of all those who manage to lose weight on a "crash diet" regain it. By using a more gradual approach combining both diet reduction and increased physical activity, you will be more likely to accomplish permanent weight loss and also learn new, healthy diet and exercise habits.

The recommended type of exercise program is one of continuous aerobic activity such as jogging, swimming, cycling, Nordic skiing, or other continuous activity-type sports. Use a kcal-per-minute-type chart such as in Table A–17 a to estimate the caloric consumption of various sports. Remember that, unless these charts have kcal per lb, they are based on the "reference man and woman" explained on p. 213. If you are larger than the reference person, allow slightly more; if smaller, allow less. Caloric expenditure in an activity is directly dependent on intensity, duration, and frequency, or in short the total amount of work performed. Table 8–4 has been included as an estimate of cost per minute and per mile of various running speeds and different body sizes. If you will take a few minutes to study the chart, you will see that speed of running or jogging is not very

Table 8–4. CALORIC COST OF RUNNING*

| Body Weight | | \multicolumn{11}{c}{Running Time in Minutes per Mile} |
lbs	kgs	6:00	6:30	7:00	7:30	8:00	8:30	9:00	9:30	10:00	10:30	11:00
100	45.5	65 / 10.9	64 / 10.0	64 / 9.2	64 / 8.5	63 / 7.9	62 / 7.3	62 / 6.9	61 / 6.4	61 / 6.1	60 / 5.7	59 / 5.4
110	50.0	72 / 12.0	72 / 11.0	71 / 10.1	71 / 9.4	69 / 8.7	68 / 8.1	68 / 7.6	67 / 7.1	67 / 6.7	66 / 6.3	65 / 5.9
120	54.5	79 / 13.1	78 / 11.9	77 / 11.0	77 / 10.2	75 / 9.4	74 / 8.8	73 / 8.2	73 / 7.7	72 / 7.2	71 / 6.8	70 / 6.4
130	59.1	85 / 14.2	84 / 13.0	83 / 11.9	83 / 11.0	82 / 10.2	81 / 9.5	80 / 8.9	79 / 8.3	79 / 7.9	78 / 7.4	77 / 6.9
140	63.6	92 / 15.3	90 / 13.9	90 / 12.8	89 / 11.9	88 / 11.0	87 / 10.2	86 / 9.6	85 / 8.9	85 / 8.5	83 / 7.9	82 / 7.3
150	68.2	98 / 16.4	97 / 15.0	97 / 13.8	96 / 12.8	94 / 11.8	93 / 10.9	92 / 10.3	91 / 9.6	91 / 9.1	89 / 8.5	88 / 8.0
160	72.7	104 / 17.4	103 / 15.9	103 / 14.7	102 / 13.6	101 / 12.6	99 / 11.7	98 / 10.9	97 / 10.3	97 / 9.7	96 / 9.1	95 / 8.6
170	77.3	111 / 18.5	111 / 17.0	109 / 15.6	108 / 14.5	107 / 13.4	105 / 12.4	104 / 11.7	103 / 10.9	103 / 10.3	102 / 9.7	100 / 9.1
180	81.8	117 / 19.6	116 / 17.9	116 / 16.5	114 / 15.2	113 / 14.2	112 / 13.2	112 / 12.4	109 / 11.5	109 / 10.9	107 / 10.2	106 / 9.7
190	86.4	124 / 20.7	124 / 19.0	123 / 17.5	122 / 16.2	119 / 14.9	118 / 13.9	117 / 13.0	116 / 12.2	115 / 11.5	113 / 10.8	112 / 10.2
200	90.9	130 / 21.8	129 / 19.9	129 / 18.4	127 / 16.9	126 / 15.7	124 / 14.6	123 / 13.7	122 / 12.8	121 / 12.1	120 / 11.4	118 / 10.7
210	95.5	137 / 22.9	137 / 21.0	135 / 19.3	134 / 17.9	132 / 16.5	131 / 15.4	130 / 14.4	128 / 13.5	127 / 12.7	125 / 11.9	124 / 11.3
220	100.0	144 / 24.0	143 / 22.0	141 / 20.2	140 / 18.7	138 / 17.3	137 / 16.1	136 / 15.1	134 / 14.1	133 / 13.3	131 / 12.5	130 / 11.8
230	104.5	150 / 25.0	149 / 22.9	147 / 21.0	146 / 19.5	145 / 18.1	143 / 16.8	141 / 15.7	140 / 14.7	139 / 13.9	138 / 13.1	135 / 12.3
240	109.1	157 / 26.2	156 / 24.0	154 / 22.0	153 / 20.4	151 / 18.9	150 / 17.6	148 / 16.4	146 / 15.4	145 / 14.5	143 / 13.6	142 / 12.9
250	113.6	163 / 27.3	162 / 24.9	160 / 22.9	159 / 21.2	158 / 19.7	156 / 18.3	155 / 17.2	152 / 16.0	151 / 15.1	149 / 14.2	147 / 13.4
260	118.2	170 / 28.4	169 / 26.0	167 / 23.9	166 / 22.1	163 / 20.4	161 / 19.0	160 / 17.8	159 / 16.7	157 / 15.7	155 / 14.8	153 / 13.9
270	122.7	176 / 29.4	175 / 26.9	174 / 24.8	172 / 22.9	170 / 21.2	168 / 19.8	167 / 18.5	164 / 17.3	163 / 16.3	161 / 15.3	160 / 14.5

Units = kcal.
Top value = Total cost per mile in kcals.
Bottom value = Cost per minute in kcals running at the speed shown.

*This chart is courtesy of Terry L. Baylor, Ph.D., Director of the Adult Fitness Cardovascular Program at The University of Texas, Austin. The values were calculated from formulae presented in the following articles: Costill, D. L., and Fox, E. L.: Energetics of marathon running. Med. Sci. Sports 1:81, 1969; and Harger, B. S., Miller, J. B., and Thomas, J. C.: The caloric cost of running: its impact on weight reduction. J.A.M.A. 228:482, 1974.

important to the total cost of running a mile, but that body size *is* very important. You also should realize that this chart is a conservative estimate. It was calculated mostly from competitive male distance runners who probably are quite efficient at running. Estimates are that individuals who run inefficiently probably use about 5 to 7 per cent more calories. The Table is applicable to both males and females. Runners who are running in hot or cold environments, with more or heavier clothing, or across difficult running surfaces will use slightly more calories than estimated in the chart. The rule of thumb is 100 kcal per mile, but you can see from the chart that this varies considerably with body weight.

It also should be noted that this chart is not appropriate for walking. A separate regression equation is needed for computing the kcal used during walking. Unlike running, the speed of the walk is much more important to the cost of walking a mile. For a 130-lb man or woman to run a mile in 6 minutes, it costs 85 kcal, and in 8 minutes it costs 82, only 3 kcal less; a 160-lb person requires 104 and 101 kcal to run the same speeds of 6- and 8-minute miles respectively. For walking, the cost of walking a slow mile is considerably less than that of walking a fast mile. Thus, speed is very important to the caloric cost of walking, but not very important to the caloric cost of running. With these comments in mind, a realistic caloric estimate for walking 3 to 4 mph is roughly 70 per cent of the running value shown in Table 8–4 for an 11 minutes-per-mile pace.

Although any amount of exercise is helpful in maintaining a caloric balance, at least three exercise periods per week, of at least 20 minutes' duration, and intense enough to expend at least 300 kcals, have been suggested as the threshold amount of exercise for changing body composition (significant fat loss). Work-outs of 200 kcal have also been reported to affect body composition favorably if done at least four times per week. Often, persons in a beginning running program who accomplish a goal of being able to jog for 30 minutes without stopping will ask the question, "Is it better to work on increasing speed of running or increasing distance?" The answer from a weight control viewpoint is very clearly to increase distance, not speed. *Small increases in speed have practically no effect on caloric cost of the mile.*

Are these types of exercise duration practical for the average American? The answer again is a definite "yes" for anyone who has gradually developed a cardiovascular fitness program. Many individuals may need to begin by walking short distances, and older people may take longer to attain improved performance, but this type of aerobic exercise is a realistic goal of all normal individuals. The common mistake of most beginning runners is that they expect too much, too soon. Americans seem to want crash diets and crash exercise programs. Neither leads to a lifestyle of health and fitness. You gradually become overweight and out of shape, and it takes time and effort to reverse the process. Slow down and be patient. Regularity and duration are critical and, of course, intensity must be appropriate to fitness level. Most beginning runners need to slow down to a point at which they are not so out of breath that they cannot converse during the entire exercise period, and then increase its duration. These types of exercise are easier to perform, result in less muscle soreness, have fewer injuries, and are easier on exercise motivation (i.e., it is easier to come back tomorrow or the next day).

Recognize the benefits of exercise but do not overestimate them. Although it is true that you must run approximately 35 miles to lose 1 lb of fat, there is another approach. An exercise program that includes 35 miles per week means 1 lb of fat per week. In 10 weeks you are 10 lbs lighter, in 20 weeks, 20 lbs lighter. You can see that the adoption of such a program for half a year means 26 lbs by exercise alone, or 52 lbs a year. If you combine this program with a 500 kcal-per-day dietary intake deficit, this results in 104 lbs a year. The effects of the regular habit of aerobic exercise are enormous. Combine these effects with some wise caloric choices, and you are developing a lifestyle of fitness and slimness. One approach is to start with a dietary analysis. Appendix A–18 is provided for con-

BLOOD   DOPING

ANABOLIC   STEROIDS — USED TO INCREASE MUSCLES A
ILLEGAL

venience in doing the analysis. Appendix C, which includes samples of highly nutritious diets at several caloric levels, may be used for making wise dietary choices. A rational exercise program is the capstone to a functional personal health plan.

Dr. Jean Mayer, a very well-respected professor of nutrition while at Harvard University, and now President of Tufts University, clearly recognized the important role of exercise in weight control. In one of his books he concluded his chapter on "Exercise and Weight Control" with a comment on inactivity. Our chapter is concluded with the following quote from the section, "Comment," in Dr. Mayer's book.

"I am convinced that inactivity is the most important factor explaining the frequency of "creeping" overweight in modern Western societies. Natural selection, operating for hundreds of thousands of years, made men physically active and resourceful, well-prepared to become hunters, fishermen or agriculturalists. The regulation of food intake was not designed to adapt to the highly mechanized sedentary conditions of modern life, just as animals were not created to be caged. Adapting to these conditions without developing obesity means either that the individual will have to step up his activity or that he will be mildly or acutely hungry all his life. The first solution is difficult, especially as present conditions in the United States—particularly in cities—offer little inducement to walking and often have poorly organized facilities for adult exercise. Even among the young, highly competitive sports for the few are emphasized at the expense of individual sports which all could learn and continue to enjoy after the high school and college years are over. But if stepping up activity is difficult, it is well to remember that the alternative

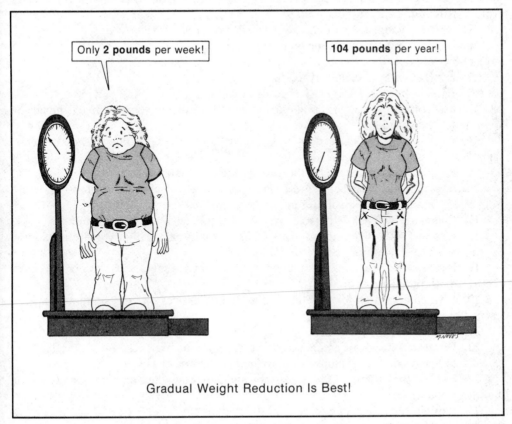

Figure 8–8. The effects of small changes in diet and exercise when practiced over long periods of time make large differences in body weight.

(lifetime hunger) is so much more difficult that relying on it for weight control programs will only continue to lead to fiascoes of the past. Strenuous exercise on an irregular basis is obviously not advocated for untrained obese persons. However, a reorganization of one's life to include regular exercise adapted to one's physical potentialities is a justified return to the wisdom of the ages."[17]

LEARNING OBJECTIVES

After completing a study of Chapter 8, students should be able to:

1. Define the terms calorie and kilocalorie.
2. List the nutrient that has the greatest caloric value per gram.
3. Tell how many kilocalories are stored in 1 lb of fat.
4. Explain which basic nutrient is usually the body's primary fuel for exercise of short duration; which nutrient becomes more important as a fuel in exercise of longer duration; and which basic nutrient is not used as a body fuel unless others are unavailable.
5. Name some good sources of high quality protein; of fat; of carbohydrates.
6. Explain why protein is important to the body.
7. Discuss whether athletes require more protein than the recommended daily allowance for all persons.
8. List the approximate percentage of the day's calories that should come from protein; from fat; from carbohydrates.
9. Define glycogen, and indicate where it is stored.
10. List the components of the four basic food groups and explain how they are used in planning the diet.
11. Explain what is meant by BMR.
12. Explain how BMR usually is measured.
13. List some of the factors that explain why the BMR of some people is higher or lower than that of others.
14. Explain why adults need to change their diet as they get older if they keep the same level of physical activity.
15. Explain what is meant by the "reference man and woman."
16. Explain what has the greatest single influence on caloric consumption, apart from BMR. Indicate how much difference it can make (see Appendix A–15).
17. Calculate their BMR plus activity level estimate of caloric expenditure.
18. List the rule of thumb in terms of kcal per lb as a daily estimate of caloric expenditure in a moderately active individual.
19. Indicate their chances of being obese if neither parent is obese; if one parent is obese; if both parents are obese.
20. Give an argument for genetic or inherited influences on body composition; for learned or environmental influences.
21. Define "creeping obesity."
22. Discuss methods of estimating fatness, and compare these for themselves.
23. Indicate what determines an individual's pattern of fat.
24. Explain the differences between men and women in their amount of body fat; in their lean body mass.
25. Explain the effect of exercise on the appetite.
26. Explain what type of exercise is best for weight control.
27. Explain what is known about "spot reduction" with exercise.

28. Explain the weight loss effect of exercising in a rubber suit, and indicate any possible hazards of the practice.

29. Explain the recommended practices in regard to drinking cold water and taking salt tablets in connection with exercise.

30. Explain how much exercise per day and per week is necessary before significant body composition changes are noticed.

31. Explain the difference between a pound of fat and a pound of body weight.

32. Tell how much fat loss per week is a realistic goal.

33. Explain the best way to analyze their diet.

34. Explain the relationships between body weight and speed of running and the caloric cost of running a mile.

35. Make an estimate of the caloric cost of walking.

36. Say whether speed or distance is more important for weight loss in a jogging program.

REFERENCES

1. American College of Sports Medicine: The recommended quantity and quality of exercise for developing and maintaining fitness in healthy adults. Med. Sci. Sports *10*:vii, 1978.
2. Briggs, G. M., and Calloway, D. H.: *Bogert's Nutrition and Physical Fitness*. 10th ed. Philadelphia, W. B. Saunders Co., 1979.
3. Burke, E. J.: Work Physiology and the Components of Physical Fitness in the Analysis of Human Performance. *In* E. J. Burke (ed.) *Toward an Understanding of Human Performance*. Ithaca, New York, Mouvement Publications, 1977.
4. Buskirk, E. R.: Diet and health. Postgrad. Med. *61*:229, 1977.
5. Clark, H. H. (ed.): Exercise and Fat Reduction. In *Physical Fitness Research Digest*. Washington, D. C., President's Council on Physical Fitness and Sports, Series 5(2), April, 1975.
6. Costill, D. L.: Fluids for Athletic Performance: Why and What Should You Drink During Prolonged Exercise. *In* E. J. Burke (ed.) *Toward an Understanding of Human Performance*. Ithaca, New York, Mouvement Publications, 1977.
7. Deutsch, R. M.: *Realities of Nutrition*. Palo Alto, CA, Bull Publishing Company, 1976.
8. Hernlund, V., and Steinhaus, A. H.: Do mechanical vibrators take off or redistribute fat? Am. Correct. Ther. J. *11*:96, 1957.
9. Hirsch, J., and Gallian, E.: Methods for the determination of adipose cell size in man and animals. J. Lipid Res. *9*:110, 1968.
10. Hirsch, J., and Han, P. W.: Cellularity of rat adipose tissue: effects of growth, starvation, and obesity. J. Lipid Res. *10*:77, 1969.
11. Johnson, P. R., Zucker, L. M., Cruse, J. A. F., and Hirsch, J.: Cellularity of adipose depots in the genetically obese Zucker rat. J. Lipid Res. *12*:706, 1971.
12. Katch, F. I., and McArdle, W. D.: *Nutrition, Weight Control, and Exercise*. Boston, Houghton Mifflin Co., 1977.
13. Knittle, J. L., and Hirsch, J.: Effect of early nutrition on the development of rat epididymal fat pads: cellularity and metabolism. J. Clin. Invest. *47*:2091, 1968.
14. Krause, M. V., and Hunscher, M. A.: *Food, Nutrition and Diet Therapy*, 5th ed. Philadelphia, W. B. Saunders Co., 1972.
15. Leithead, C. S., and Lind, A. R.: *Heat Stress and Heat Disorders*. Philadelphia, F. A. Davis Co., 1964.
16. Mathews, D. K., and Fox, E. L.: *The Physiological Basis of Physical Education and Athletics*. Philadelphia, W. B. Saunders Co., 1976.
17. Mayer, J.: *Human Nutrition: Its Physiological, Medical and Social Aspects*. Springfield, Ill., Charles C Thomas, 1972.
18. Oscai, L. B.: The Role of Exercise in Weight Control. *In* J. H. Wilmore (ed.) *Exercise and Sport Sciences Reviews*, Vol. 1, 1973.
19. Oscai, L. B., Babirak, S. P., Dubach, F. B., McGarr, J. A., and Spirakis, C. N.: Exercise or food restriction: effect of adipose tissue cellularity. Am. J. Physiol. *227*:901, 1974.
20. Oscai, L. B., Spirakis, C. N., Wolff, C. A., and Beck, R. J.: Effects of exercise and of food restriction on adipose tissue cellularity. J. Lipid Res. *13*:588, 1972.
21. Pollock, M. L., Wilmore, J. H., and Fox, S. M.: *Health and Fitness Through Physical Activity*. New York, John Wiley & Sons, 1978.
22. Sloan, A. W., and Weir, J. B. D. V.: Nomograms for prediction of body density and total body fat from skinfold measurements. J. Appl. Physiol. *28*:221, 1970.

23. Smith, N. J.: *Food for Sport*. Palo Alto, CA, Bull.Publishing Co., 1976.
24. Smith, N. J.: Gaining and Losing Weight in Athletics. *In* E. J. Burke (ed.) *Toward an Understanding of Human Performance*. Ithaca, New York, Mouvement Publications, 1977.
25. Stare, F. J., and McWilliams, M.: *Living Nutrition,* 2nd ed. St. Louis, C. V. Mosby Co., 1977.
26. Wagner, B.: Nutrition in Athletics. *In* E. J. Burke (ed.) *Toward an Understanding of Human Performance*. Ithaca, New York, Mouvement Publications, 1977.
27. Williams, S. R.: *Nutrition and Diet Therapy,* 2nd ed. St. Louis, C. V. Mosby Co., 1973.
28. Young, C. M.: Body fatness in normal young women, N.Y. State J. Med. *61*:1928, 1961.
29. Young, C. M.: Body composition and body weight: criteria of overnutrition. Can. Med. Assoc. J. *93*:900, 1965.

Appendix A–1

What Is Your Cardiovascular Risk?

The purpose of RISKO is to give you an estimate of your chances of suffering heart attack.

The game is played using Table A–1*a* by marking squares which—from left to right—represent an increase in your RISK FACTORS. These are medical conditions and habits associated with an increased danger of heart attack. *Not all risk factors are measurable enough to be included in this game.*

RULES. Study each RISK FACTOR and its row. Find the box applicable to you and circle the number in it. For example, if your age is 37, circle the number in the box labeled 31–40. After checking out all the rows, add the circled numbers. This total—your score—is an estimate of your risk.

IF YOU SCORE:
6–11—Risk well below average.
12–17—Risk below average.
18–24—Risk generally average.
25–31—Risk moderate.
32–40—Risk at a dangerous level.
41–62—Danger urgent. See your doctor now.

HEREDITY. Count parents, grandparents, brothers, and sisters who have had heart attack and/or stroke.

WEIGHT. Use Table 8–2 and/or Appendix A–16 to determine standard weight.

TOBACCO SMOKING. If you inhale deeply and smoke a cigarette way down, add one to your classification. Do *not* subtract because you think you do not inhale or smoke only a half-inch on a cigarette.

Table A–1a. CARDIAC RISK INDEX

1. Age	10 to 20	21 to 30	31 to 40	41 to 50	51 to 60	61 to 70
	1	2	3	4	(6)	8
2. Heredity	no known history of heart disease	1 relative over 60 with cardiovascular disease	2 relatives over 60 with cardiovascular disease	1 relative under 60 with cardiovascular disease	2 relatives under 60 with cardiovascular disease	3 relatives under 60 with cardiovascular disease
	1	(2)	3	4	6	8
3. Weight	more than 5 lbs below standard weight	−5 to +5 lbs standard weight	6–20 lbs overweight	21–35 lbs overweight	36–50 lbs overweight	51–65 lbs overweight
	0	(1)	2	3	5	7
4. Tobacco Smoking	nonuser	cigar and/or pipe	10 cigarettes or less a day	20 cigarettes a day	30 cigarettes a day	40 cigarettes or more a day
	0	1	2	(4)	6	10
5. Exercise	intensive occupational and recreational exertion	moderate occupational and recreational exertion	sedentary work and intense recreational exertion	sedentary work and moderate recreational exertion	sedentary work and light recreational exertion	complete lack of all exercise
	1	2	3	5	(6)	8
6. Cholesterol or % Fat in Diet	cholesterol below 180 mg%	cholesterol 181–205 mg%	cholesterol 206–230 mg%	cholesterol 231–255 mg%	cholesterol 256–280 mg%	cholesterol 281–330 mg%
	no animal or solid fats in diet	10% animal or solid fat in diet	20% animal or solid fat in diet	30% animal or solid fat in diet	40% animal or solid fat in diet	50% animal or solid fat in diet
	1	2	(3)	4	5	7
7. Blood Pressure	100 upper reading	120 upper reading	140 upper reading	160 upper reading	180 upper reading	200 or over upper reading
	1	2	(3)	4	6	8
8. Sex	female under 40	female 40–50	female over 50	male	stocky male	bald stocky male
	1	2	3	(5)	6	7

Total Score ____29____

RISKO is reprinted courtesy of Michigan Heart Association. © Michigan Heart Association.

EXERCISE. Lower your score one point if you exercise regularly and frequently.

CHOLESTEROL OR SATURATED FAT INTAKE LEVEL. A cholesterol blood level determination is best. If you can't get one from your doctor, then estimate honestly the percentage of solid fats you eat. These are usually of animal origin—lard, cream, butter, and beef and lamb fat. If you eat much of this, your cholesterol level probably will be high. The U. S. average, 40 per cent, is too high for good health. Use Appendices A–19, C, and D to aid in this determination.

BLOOD PRESSURE. If you have no recent reading but have passed an insurance or industrial examination, the chances are you have an upper reading of 140 or less. See Chapter 5 for a discussion of blood pressure.

SEX. This line takes into account the fact that men have between six and ten times more heart attacks than women of child-bearing age.

Discussion of Your Coronary Risk Factors

A. What was your over-all point value? In what risk category did that place you? If you score above 24, it is suggested that you seek medical consultation regarding these factors.

B. What areas of risk represent your greatest problem?

C. In what areas of risk do you score particularly low?

D. What specific steps can you take to reduce your coronary risk?

Appendix A-2

Type A or Type B

Certain behavior characteristics appear to be linked to greater risk of coronary heart disease. Before reading any of the explanation of this risk factor in Chapter 3, students should answer the following questionnaire concerning their behavior.

Cardiac Risk Behavioral Pattern Questionnaire

Respond to the following questions with YES or NO answers.

1.	I have an intense sustained drive to get ahead.	Yes__	No__
2.	I'm anxious to reach my goals, but I'm uncertain what those goals are.	Yes__	No__
3.	I feel a need to compete and win.	Yes__	No__
4.	I have a persistent desire for recognition.	Yes__	No__
5.	I always seem to be involved in too many things at once.	Yes__	No__
6.	I'm always racing the clock, constantly on edge, have deadlines.	Yes__	No__
7.	I have a need to speed things up, get things done faster.	Yes__	No__
8.	I'm extraordinarily alert mentally and physically.	Yes__	No__
	Total	__	__

From Friedman, M., and Rosenman, R. H.: Association of specific overt behavior patterns with blood and cardiovascular findings. J.A.M.A. *169*:1286, 1959.

Discussion of Behavior Characteristics

A. Count the number of "yes" responses to the above questionnaire. The "yes" response is linked to Type A behavior, which represents a greater risk for coronary heart disease.

B. Read the section in Chapter 3 related to stress as a coronary risk factor.

C. What specific changes can you make in your behavior that will change some of your "yes" answers to "no" answers?

Appendix A–3

Testing Muscular Strength

A convenient method for testing specific muscular strength in both males and females is determination of the one repetition maximum (1 RM). The specific muscle group to be tested is selected, and then individuals are given a series of trials to determine the maximal weight they can lift just once for that particular lift. Since most persons are largely inexperienced in weight-training, the test is conducted largely through trial and error. The test should start with a weight that can be lifted comfortably, then keep adding weight until a weight is found that can be lifted *correctly* just one time. If the weight can be lifted more than once, more weight needs to be added until a true 1 RM is reached.

One RMs can be obtained for any basic weight-training exercise. However, for most individuals, determination of 1 RM for the exercises listed in Table A–3*a* will provide a good assessment of basic strength.

Since the resistances to be overcome in 1 RM testing are relatively heavy for each individual, it is important that proper safety procedures be followed. It is very important to learn to exhale *during the resistance*

Table A–3*a*. OPTIMAL STRENGTH VALUES FOR VARIOUS BODY WEIGHTS (BASED ON THE 1-RM TEST)*

Body Weight (lb)	Bench Press Male	Bench Press Female	Shoulder Press Male	Shoulder Press Female	Biceps Curl Male	Biceps Curl Female	Leg Press Male	Leg Press Female
80	70	60	55	40	40	30	160	120
100	85	70	70	50	50	35	200	150
120	105	85	80	60	60	40	240	180
140	125	100	95	65	70	50	280	210
160	145	115	110	75	80	60	320	240
180	160	125	120	85	90	65	360	270
200	180	140	135	95	100	70	400	300
220	200	155	150	105	110	75	440	330
240	225	170	160	115	120	85	480	360

*Data in pounds; obtained on Universal Gym apparatus, applicable ages 17–30. Adapted from Pollock, M. L., Wilmore, J. H., and Fox, S. M., III: *Health and Fitness Through Physical Activity*. New York, John Wiley & Sons, 1978.

phase of the exercise (i.e., when the weight is lifted) so that one is not working with a closed glottis (see p. 72). Other safety precautions are listed on p. 73, Chapter 4. See Figures 4–23, 4–28*B*, 4–29, and 4–78 for illustrations of the exercises in Table A–3*a*.

Various dynamometers (grip, back and leg, cable tensiometer, etc.) can also be used to test strength. However, they are usually found in laboratories and typically are not available to most persons, especially once they leave the college or university setting. Also, these devices usually measure isometric strength, and not the type of dynamic strength used in sport and other forms of physical activity and measured by the 1 RM testing procedure.

Appendix A-4

The Sit-Up Test

(1) Minimum Abdominal Strength Test
(2) One-Minute Speed Sit-Up

FITNESS COMPONENT MEASURED: ABDOMINAL MUSCULAR STRENGTH AND ENDURANCE

Note: The sit-up exercise, even when performed with the knees flexed, depends on action from both the abdominal muscles (trunk flexors) and the iliopsoas (hip flexors). The range of motion of the flexed knee sit-up is approximately 90° (supine to erect sitting position). The first 45° of movement is primarily trunk flexion and requires strong activity within the abdominal muscles. The second 45° of movement is hip flexion, and requires action primarily from the hip flexors. The iliopsoas is *least active* during the flexed knee sit-up with the feet *unsupported*.

Supporting the feet during the sit-up provides an anchor for the hip flexors. *In this situation, it is possible for some persons with very weak abdominal muscles to perform sit-ups by employing an arched back and reverse action of the hip flexors.* Therefore, before testing on the 1-minute speed sit-up, a screening test for minimal abdominal muscular strength should be utilized.

MINIMUM ABDOMINAL MUSCULAR STRENGTH SIT-UP

Test Description

Starting Position:
1. Lie on back, preferably on a gym mat (or dry grass).
2. Cross arms on chest and place hands on opposite shoulders.
3. Bend knees, feet flat and slightly apart; heels should be no more than 18 inches from the buttocks. This is called the "hook lying" position.

Performance: 1. With head flexed forward, curl up and touch both elbows to the thighs (Fig. 4–57a).

2. Return to the starting position with middle of the back touching the mat. Keep head up and chin down throughout.

3. During the action, maintain feet, elbow, knee, and hand position throughout, with middle of the back touching the mat following each sit-up. *The heels should remain in contact with the mat throughout the sit-up.*

4. Repeat continuously five times (no resting allowed between sit-ups).

Inability to do five consecutive sit-ups in this manner indicates a lack of minimal abdominal strength. The individual failing this test should begin a conditioning program for this area of the body, using the strength and endurance exercises in Sections C 9 and 10, Chapter 4, and the flexibility exercises of Section IV, E, F, and G, Chapter 6 (see table of contents for each chapter).

For those who can complete the five consecutive sit-ups as above, the degree of strength and muscular endurance can be further quantified by the 1-minute speed sit-up.

ONE-MINUTE SPEED SIT-UP. The starting position and sit-up action for this test are exactly the same as in the minimal abdominal muscular strength sit-up *except* that the feet are supported by a partner or similarly anchored (see Fig. 4–60), and the person being tested attempts to complete as many sit-ups as possible in one minute.

Scoring: 1. A *rest* between sit-ups *is allowed,* if needed, before the one minute is up.

2. Record the number of valid sit-ups in the 1-minute period.

Equipment: 1. A gym mat.

2. An accurate watch or clock.

ADMINISTRATIVE SUGGESTIONS FOR SIT-UP TESTS

1. The supervising tester acts as the timer.
2. Partners should count and record each other's score. The *supervising tester and/or the partner must carefully observe to assure that the sit-ups are being done correctly.*
3. Several pairs can be tested at once.
4. In order to obtain an optimal score, the individual should perform to a near-maximal rate continuously throughout the 1-minute period.
5. An individual's score is most valid and reliable if the movement is performed with a rounded back throughout—curling up and down, thus maintaining a round spine. A straight or arched back accentuates the action of the hip flexors.

Table A–4a may be used to evaluate performance on the 60-second timed sit-up.

Table A–4a.   SIXTY-SECOND TIMED SIT-UP PERFORMANCE
STANDARDS

Sex and Age	Poor	Low	Average	Good	Excellent
Males					
17–29	0–35	36–41	42–47	48–50	51+
30–39*	0–26	27–32	33–38	39–43	44+
40–49	0–22	23–27	28–33	34–38	39+
50–59	0–16	17–21	22–28	29–33	34+
60–69	0–12	13–17	18–24	25–30	31+
Females					
17–29	0–28	29–32	33–35	36–42	43+
30–39*	0–22	23–28	29–34	35–40	41+
40–49	0–18	19–23	24–30	31–34	35+
50–59	0–12	13–17	18–24	25–30	31+
60–69	0–10	11–14	15–20	21–25	26+

*Values for ages 30 and over are estimated since no specific norms exist for
these age-groups.

REFERENCES

1. AAHPERD: *AAHPERD Health-related Physical Fitness Test Manual.* Washington,
      D.C., American Alliance for Health, Physical Education, Recreation, and
      Dance, 1980.
2. Kendall, H. O., Kendall, F. P., and Wadsworth, G. E.: *Muscles: Testing and Func-
      tion.* Baltimore, Williams & Wilkins Co., 1971.
3. Pollock, M. L., Wilmore, J. H., and Fox, S. M., III: *Health and Fitness Through
      Physical Activity.* New York, John Wiley & Sons, 1978.

Appendix A–5

Circuit Weight-Training

It has been shown that, when approximately two-thirds of a maximal number of repetitions are performed against a fixed resistance, both strength and muscular endurance tend to be developed at an optimal rate for most purposes. This procedure was introduced as circuit training by R. E. Morgan and G. T. Adamson in England. It is a form of interval training for increasing strength and muscular endurance. The objective as the program progresses is to do increasing amounts of work in a given time or the same work in a shorter time.

Commonly, the procedure involves a sequence of five to ten exercises that impose resistances that are arbitrarily established. At the outset of the training program, an effort is made to achieve a maximal number of repetitions for each exercise. Once this has been established, the maximal number is reduced by *one-third* for each exercise. The object is then to complete a *circuit* of all the exercises in a progressively diminishing amount of time. To further increase the demands, the procedure can be intensified periodically by increasing the number of repetitions and/or the amount of resistance appropriately.

As an example for one exercise, suppose double biceps curls (Fig. 4–21) has been included in a circuit for elbow flexion work, and 55 lbs of resistance has been arbitrarily established. Further suppose an individual can perform 21 repetitions with the 55 lbs. This would then be reduced to 14 repetitions, and this number would be performed each time through the circuit. A circuit generally is performed three times during a work-out period. To intensify the exercise in the circuit, the time to complete the circuit would be decreased periodically, or the number of repetitions would be increased, or the resistance would be increased beyond 55 lbs. Alternatively, a combination of the above intensification procedures might be used.

Although any group of exercises may be included in a circuit, a sequence of eight essential exercises are recommended, purposely arranged in order to allow for distributed effort of body segments and all-around body development, and illustrated in Figure A–5a. These exercises have been described previously in Chapter 4.

Where possible, it is recommended that the Universal Gym or similar apparatus be used as the exercise device. It has the advantage

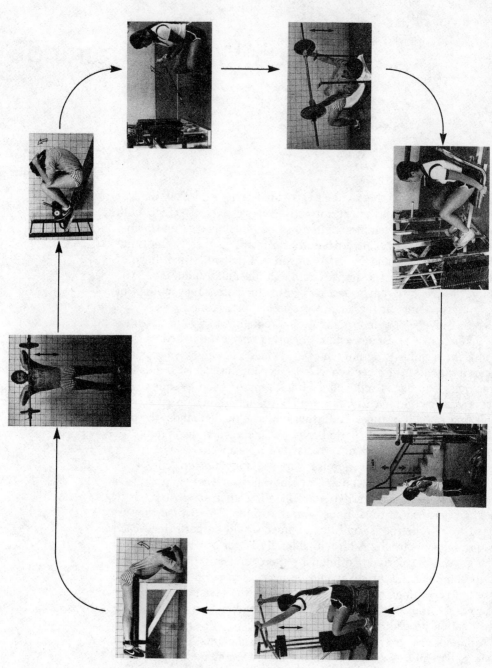

Figure A–5 a.   Recommended Circuit Training Stations. Circuit training application of these eight stations will train all the large muscle groups of the body. The circuit should be followed in a clockwise order as indicated. If time and space are limited, a five-station circuit composed of loaded sit-up, back raise, leg press, shoulder press, and biceps curl is recommended.

Table A–5a. ARBITRARY INITIAL STARTING WEIGHTS AND RECORDING FORMAT
FOR EIGHT ESSENTIAL CIRCUIT TRAINING EXERCISES

Week	Upright Row	Loaded Sit-Up	Biceps Curls	Bench Press	Leg Press	Lat Pulls	Shoulder Press	Back Raise
Example	16/50 30:60	20/25 30:60	12/50 30:60	10/100 30:60	14/200 30:60	16/100 30:60	8/50 30:60	20/15 30:60
1	/	/	/	/	/	/	/	/
2	/	/	/	/	/	/	/	/
3	/	/	/	/	/	/	/	/
4	/	/	/	/	/	/	/	/
5	/	/	/	/	/	/	/	/
6	/	/	/	/	/	/	/	/
7	/	/	/	/	/	/	/	/
8	/	/	/	/	/	/	/	/

of safety over free weights, and resistance can be changed quickly from
one student to the next without wasting time. If a Universal Gym is not
available, other forms of exercise can be used (see Chapter 4).

In the blocks under each exercise in Table A–5a, the number left
of the slash mark refers to the number of repetitions, and the number
right of it to the resistance. The lower number is the work:rest ratio.
In the example (160-lb college male), 16 repetitions of upright rowing
would be done with a resistance of 50 lbs. The numbers 30:60 refer to
30 seconds allowed for the exercise and 60 seconds for rest.

RECOMMENDED STARTING RESISTANCE.   The following resistances are recommended as starting points for each of the exercises.

Exercise	Recommended Starting Resistance as a Percentage and Proportion of Body Weight
Upright Rowing	33 (1/3)
Loaded Sit-Up	15 (1/7)
Double Biceps Curl	33 (1/3)
Bench Press	67 (2/3)
Leg Press	150 (1.5)
Latissimus Machine Pulldown	67 (2/3)
Shoulder Press	33 (1/3)
Back Raise	10 (1/10)

The resistances recommended above will not prove appropriate initially for some individuals, and adjustments will be necessary. On the maximal repetitions test with *each* of the exercises, the individual should be able to do *at least 12 repetitions but not more than 36.* If the maximal number of repetitions falls outside this range, adjustments should be made accordingly (more or less weight).

It is also recommended that the program start with 30 seconds for execution of the exercise followed by 60 seconds' rest. After the rest period, the individual should move immediately to the next exercise. With proper instruction under this system, students can work in groups of three at each station, changing stations at the end of each 1½-minute interval.

The individuals should go through the circuit three times, performing two-thirds of maximal repetitions at each station on the first two circuits. On the third circuit, the maximal number of repetitions should be performed at each station.

The time needed for the three circuits will be approximately 40 minutes. If time and space are limited, a five-station circuit composed of loaded sit-up, back raise, leg press, shoulder press, and biceps curls is recommended.

As strength and endurance improve, the individual should attempt to decrease the time taken for the circuit, especially the rest interval. Once an approximately 1:1 ratio has been achieved in work:rest, the resistance and number of repetitions can be increased. However, there are many possible variations, and students are encouraged to try whatever suits their inclination. The important factor is that strength and endurance continue to improve, or at least be maintained, if the latter is the objective.

EFFECTS OF CIRCUIT TRAINING ON OTHER COMPONENTS OF FITNESS.   The recommended circuit outlined above is designed to develop strength and muscular endurance. It would be expected to have minimal effect on other components of fitness, such as cardiovascular function. However, a circuit could be designed to include specific stations for other fitness components. Cardiovascular function could be emphasized, for example, by providing a running element between stations. In addition, the circuit presented here should develop additional strength, which would improve lean body mass. Also, there is a caloric expenditure! Intensive circuit training has been shown to result in expenditures of 125 to 200 Calories, depending on body weight, during a 20- to 30-minute session. If diet remains constant, this added expenditure of energy could have a significant impact on body fat percentage.

In regard to development of cardiovascular function, most studies have shown that the weight-training segment per se of the circuit has little, if any, value. However, recent investigations using intensive exercise where the work segment was twice the rest interval (i.e., 30 sec:15 sec), and resistance was set at about 50 per cent of individual one-repetition maximum for each station, have noted improvements in cardiovascular function. The level of intensity for this circuit (30 sec work:15 sec rest) is equivalent to jogging at 5 mph, cycling at 11.5 mph, or a vigorous game of volleyball or tennis.

Note: Even though some circuit weight-training programs have yielded moderate increases in maximal O_2 uptake, they cannot be considered equivalent to running in this regard. Studies with direct comparisons have shown running-type activities as definitely superior to circuit weight-training for the development of cardiovascular function.

REFERENCES

1. Allen, T. E., Byrd, R. J., and Smith, D. P.: Hemodynamic consequences of circuit weight training. Res. Q. Am. Assoc. Health Phys. Educ. *47*:299, 1976.
2. Falls, H. B., Wallis, E. L., and Logan, G. A.: *Foundations of Conditioning*. New York, Academic Press, 1970.
3. Gettman, L. R., Ayres, J. J., Pollock, M. L., and Jackson, A.: The effect of circuit weight training on strength, cardiorespiratory function, and body composition of adult men. Med. Sci. Sports *10*:171, 1978.
4. Girandola, R. N., and Katch, V.: Effects of nine weeks of physical training on aerobic capacity and body composition in college men. Arch. Phys. Med. Rehab. *54*:521, 1973.
5. Wilmore, J. H., et al.: Energy cost of circuit weight training. Med. Sci. Sports *10*:75, 1978.
6. Wilmore, J. H., et al.: Physiological alterations consequent to circuit weight training. Med. Sci. Sports *10*:79, 1978.

Appendix A-6

Step Test Response to Submaximal Exercise

Step tests provide a convenient procedure for assessing circulatory response to exercise. The test described in this appendix is a modification of the Harvard Step Test developed in the early 1940s for evaluating the physiological condition of military personnel. This particular version is presented because it is simple, involves only moderate exercise, and may be used conveniently, even in the home. It has been used in an epidemiological survey of an entire community, and provides percentile norms for several different ages in both males and females.

Equipment Needed:
1. An 8-inch bench or step (many stair steps are approximately this height).

Table A-6a. PERCENTILE NORMS OF A STEP TEST USED IN THE TECUMSEH, MICHIGAN, EPIDEMIOLOGICAL STUDY (8-INCH BENCH; 24 STEPS/MIN FOR 3 MINUTES; PULSE TAKEN 30 TO 60 SECONDS POSTEXERCISE)*

Percentile	Males			Females		
	17–19	20–29	30+	17–19	20–29	30+
95	34**	34	36	39	39	41
85	37	38	42	43	43	45
75	39	41	43	48	45	47
65	42	43	46	51	47	49
55	43	45	47	52	49	52
50	44	46	48	53	50	52
45	46	47	49	53	52	53
35	46	49	50	55	54	54
25	49	51	52	56	56	56
15	52	54	56	59	60	60
5	57	59	60	63	66	66

*Adapted from data presented in the reference below.
**Beats for the 30-second counting period.

2. A stopwatch or accurate wristwatch with second hand (any accurate clock with second hand may be used).
3. A metronome or other means for keeping cadence.

Procedure:
1. The person being tested steps up and down on the bench (step) at the rate of 24 complete ascents and descents/min (4-count sequence) for three minutes.
2. A pulse count is taken for 30 seconds, beginning 30 seconds after the exercise stops (30- to 60-seconds' postexercise count). (See p. 151 for pulse counting procedure.)
3. The count obtained during the 30-second period may be compared with the values in Table A–6*a* for a cardiovascular fitness rating (the 50th percentile is average).

REFERENCE

Montoye, H. J.: *Physical Activity and Health: An Epidemiologic Study of an Entire Community.* Englewood Cliffs, N.J., Prentice-Hall, 1975.

Appendix A–7

Maximal Oxygen Consumption Estimated From Step Test Performance

Several step test procedures allow estimates of maximal oxygen uptake from pulse rates taken in connection with the test procedure. The two presented here appear to provide for reasonably accurate estimates. It should be kept in mind that these procedures are not as valid or reliable as estimates of maximal oxygen uptake based on 12-minute run performance, but they often may be used more conveniently than the latter.

MALES: THE HELLER INSTITUTE TEST (Applicable to Ages 17 to 30).

Estimates of maximal oxygen uptake from this test have correlated r = 0.80 with estimates from the Astrand-Ryhming bicycle ergometer test. (See Appendix A–8 for references to the Astrand-Ryhming test.)

Equipment Needed:
1. Either a 15- or a 12-inch stepping bench.
2. A stopwatch, accurate wristwatch, or accurate clock with second hand.
3. A metronome or similar device for keeping cadence of the stepping.

Procedure:
1. The person being tested steps up and down on the bench at the rate of 25 complete ascents and descents/min (4-count sequence) for six minutes.
2. After the exercise stops, while subject remains standing, the pulse is counted for *10 seconds* during the period *5 to 15*

Table A–7a.   CLASSIFICATION OF FITNESS BASED ON RESULTS
OF THE HELLER INSTITUTE TEST (MALES)

Astrand Classification* of Fitness	Est. Max O$_2$ Uptake in ml/kg/min	15-Inch Bench 5–15-Second Pulse Count	12-Inch Bench 5–15 Second Pulse Count
Poor	<39	>26	>23
Low	39–43	25–26	22–23
Average	44–51	23–24	20–21
Good	52–56	21–22	18–19
High	>56	<21	<18

*See Table 5–2.

seconds postexercise. See p. 151 for pulse-counting procedures.

3. Scores (pulse counts) are evaluated using Table A–7a. See
   also Table 5–2.

FEMALES: THE QUEENS COLLEGE TEST (Applicable to Ages 17 to 30).

Estimates of max O$_2$ uptake from this test have correlated
$r = 0.75$ with actual max oxygen consumption measured in a laboratory
setting similar to Figure 5–2.

Equipment Needed:
1. A 16-inch stepping bench.
2. A stopwatch, accurate wristwatch, or accurate clock with
   second hand.
3. A metronome or similar device for keeping cadence of the
   stepping.

Procedure:
1. The person being tested steps up and down on the bench at
   the rate of 22 complete ascents and descents/min (4-count
   sequence) for three minutes.
2. After the exercise stops, subject remains standing, and a *15-
   second* pulse count is taken during the period *5 to 20 seconds
   postexercise.* See p. 151 for pulse-counting procedure.
3. Scores (pulse counts) are evaluated using Table A–7b. See
   also Table 5–2.

Table A–7b.   CLASSIFICATION OF FITNESS BASED ON RESULTS
OF THE QUEENS COLLEGE TEST (FEMALES)

Astrand Classification* of Fitness	Est. Max O$_2$ Uptake in ml/kg/min	Pulse Rate 5–20-Second Count
Poor	<28	>50
Low	29–34	43–49
Average	35–43	31–42
Good	44–48	25–30
High	>48	<25

*See Table 5–2.

REFERENCES

McArdle, W. D., Pechar, G. S., Katch, F. I., and Magel, J. R.: Percentile norms of a valid step test for college women. Res. Q. Am. Assoc. Health Phys. Educ. *44*:498, 1973.

Shapiro, A., Shapiro, Y., and Magaznik, A.: A simple step test to predict aerobic capacity. J. Sports Med. Phys. Fitness *16*:209, 1976.

Appendix A–8

Heart Rate Response to a Standardized Workload

This laboratory experience is provided to demonstrate establishment of a self-testing procedure utilizing any of several exercise modes and to illustrate a method whereby the progress of a conditioning program can be charted. The procedure illustrated here uses a simple bicycle ergometer as the exercise mode. The bicycle ergometer (Fig. A–8a) is an instrument for obtaining an accurate setting of workload that is repeatable from one exercise session to another.

Many schools, colleges, health clubs, and YMCAs and YWCAs are now providing these instruments as part of their exercise equipment. Many readers will have access to an ergometer. All that is needed in addition to the ergometer is a watch or clock with a second hand and someone to count the pulse (see p. 151 for suggestions on pulse-counting).

Testing Procedure
1. Select a convenient workload: about 300 to 600 kgm/min (50 to 100 watts) for females; 600 to 900 kgm/min (100 to 150 watts) for males.*
2. Begin riding the ergometer at the selected workload. Pedal at the rate of 50 to 60 revolutions/min. Remember that the work is a function of pedaling rate and resistance setting on the flywheel of the ergometer. If you are not familiar with setting the workload on the particular ergometer you are using, have someone who is familiar with it instruct you in its operation.
3. After about 1 minute of pedaling, count the pulse for 15 seconds and multiply by four to get a minute rate. Record in Table A–8a. Continue the ride, and count the pulse rate each successive minute until a steady-state (leveling off) of pulse rate is reached (about 4 to 5 minutes). If the pulse rates for minutes 4 and 5 are more than 8 beats apart, continue the ride for 1 to 3 more minutes until a leveling of pulse is reached. If the ride lasts for more than 6 minutes, the

---

*See glossary for kgm (kilogram-meters) and watts.

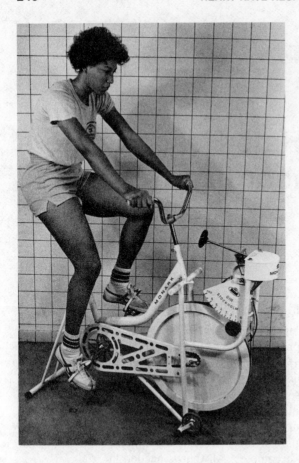

Figure A–8 *a*. The Monark Bicycle Ergometer.

Table A–8*a*. FORMAT FOR RECORDING HEART RATE RESPONSE TO AN ERGOMETER TEST

Date: _____; Time _____		Date: _____; Time _____	
Workload _____		Workload _____	
Minutes	*beats/min*	*Minutes*	*beats/min*
1	_____	1	_____
2	_____	2	_____
3	_____	3	_____
4	_____	4	_____
5	_____	5	_____
6	_____	6	_____
7	_____	7	_____
8	_____	8	_____
Average*	_____	**Average**	_____

*This should be the mean of the final two minutes' heart rates (beats/min).

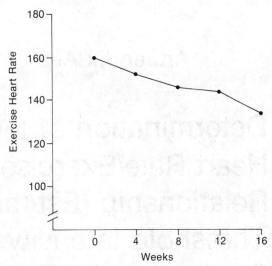

Figure A–8 b. Heart Rate Response to Standardized Work Over 16 weeks: 40-year-old male. Work was 900 kgm/min on a Monark bicycle ergometer. The test was repeated at four-week intervals.

average entered in Table A–8a should be the *last three* minutes of the ride. If the pulse rate does not reach 120 beats/min or more, the ride should be discontinued and the test repeated at a higher workload after full recovery is allowed (i.e., the heart rate returns to resting level).

4. The test may be repeated at intervals of two or more weeks as a guide to progress in the conditioning program. A simple graph constructed on standard graph paper will allow rapid determination of the rate of improvement. Figure A–8b illustrates how such a graph might appear over a 16-week period.

It is possible to estimate maximal oxygen uptake with some degree of accuracy from the ergometer test. Readers interested in the procedures for this should consult one of the following.

REFERENCES

1. Astrand, P.-O., and Rodahl, K.: *Textbook of Work Physiology*. New York, McGraw-Hill Book Co., 1977, pp. 344–358.
2. Baumgartner, T. A., and Jackson, A. S.: *Measurement for Evaluation in Physical Education*. Boston, Houghton Mifflin Co., 1975, pp. 190–195.
3. deVries, H. A.: *Laboratory Experiments in Physiology of Exercise*. Dubuque, Iowa, Wm. C. Brown Co., 1971, pp. 83–94.

If a bicycle ergometer is not available, conditioning progression can be charted using a graph similar to Figure A–8b with other modes of exercise. The individual may swim or run at constant and known speed, or may step up and down on a bench or skip rope at a measured cadence. The only requirement is that the exercise be steady-paced and repeatable. The rate should be moderate enough so that the exercise can be tolerated for 5 minutes without undue stress. At the end of the 5-minute period, the pulse is counted *immediately* for 10 seconds and *multiplied by six* to get a minute rate. The results are charted as in Figure A–8b.

Determination of Individual Heart Rate/Exercise Intensity Relationship (Estimation of Threshold Intensity for a Cardiovascular Training Effect)

One of the key elements in a cardiovascular function training program is the intensity of exercise. Threshold of intensity for a cardiovascular conditioning effect to occur is exercise that requires a heart rate response at about 75 per cent of the age-adjusted maximal heart rate (p. 151). This often requires an exercise effort much lower than one might suspect. This laboratory is designed to illustrate the relationship between heart rate and exercise of varying intensity, and to provide a convenient method for estimating the conditioning threshold.

Equipment Needed:
1. A 440-yard running track or other suitable running area where 55-yard intervals can be identified.
2. A stopwatch or wristwatch with accurate and easily readable second hand.
3. A loud whistle.

Procedure:
This exercise may be conducted as a class group with the instructor coordinating, or simply by two individuals working as partners.
1. Allow 5 minutes for counting the resting heart rate (see p. 151 for heart rate-counting procedures).
2. Two speeds of walking and four of running are given in Table A–9a.

Table A-9a. ELAPSED TIMES FOR DIFFERENT WALKS AND RUNS*

| | Walks | | Runs | | | |
| | (1) | (2) | (1) | (2) | (3) | (4) |
Elapsed Time	3 mph	4 mph**	5 mph	6 mph	6.67 mph	7.5 mph
1st 55 yds	0:37.5	0:28.0	0:22.5	0:19.0	0:17.0	0:15.0
2nd 55 yds	1:15.0	0:56.0	0:45.0	0:37.5	0:34.0	0:30.0
3rd 55 yds	1:52.5	1:24.0	1:07.5	0:56.5	0:51.0	0:45.0
4th 55 yds	2:30.0	1:52.0	1:30.0	1:15.0	1:07.5	1:00.0
5th 55 yds	3:07.5	2:20.0	1:52.5	1:34.0	1:24.0	1:15.0
6th 55 yds	3:45.0	2:48.0	2:15.0	1:52.5	1:41.0	1:30.0
7th 55 yds	4:22.5	3:16.0	2:37.5	2:11.5	1:58.0	1:45.0
8th 55 yds	5:00.0	3:44.0	3:00.0	2:30.0	2:15.0	2:00.0

Heart Rate

Response

Beats/Min†

*Times are in minutes and seconds.
**Some individuals may have difficulty walking 440 yards at this speed.
†If heart rate reaches 170 before all the runs are completed, there is no point in completing the more intense runs.

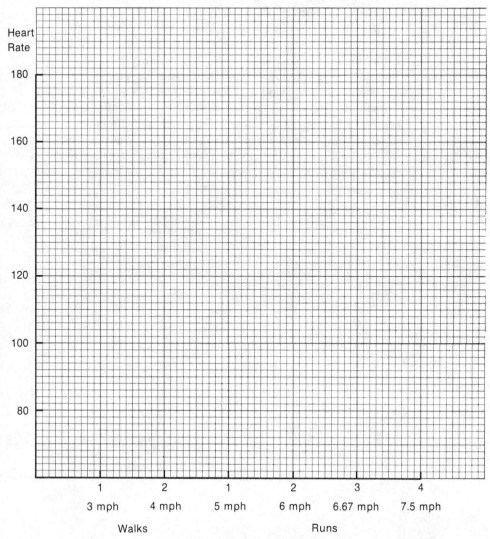

Figure A-9 a. Graph for Recording Heart Rate/Exercise Intensity Relationship.

3. The objective of the experiment is to complete one lap of the track at each of the speeds in Table A–9a (one lap of slow jogging around the track should be given as a warm-up). Sufficient rest should be allowed between all laps so that the heart rate recovers within 10 beats of the resting value obtained in 1 above.

4. The instructor or partner will give a whistle blast at each of the elapsed times called for in Table A–9a, as an aid in exact pacing. Remember, you must *keep with the pacing* or you will defeat the purpose of the exercise.

5. *Immediately* at the end of each walk or run, each individual will palpate the radial or temporal artery, and the instructor will give the commands "ready, count" as he starts the watch. At the end of 15 seconds of counting, the command "stop" is given. This 15-second count is multiplied by four and entered at the appropriate place in Table A–9a.

6. After all the laps have been completed, the data from Table A–9a may be used to complete the graph in Figure A–9a. Connecting each data point on the graph will give a curve of your individual heart rate/exercise intensity relationship. Using Table 5–4, calculate 75 per cent of your age-adjusted maximal heart rate (see p. 152 for exceptions to this). Draw a solid horizontal line across the graph of Figure A–9a at the value corresponding to 75 per cent of the age-adjusted maximal heart rate. This line represents your threshold of conditioning, and any exercise intensities above the line are sufficient to achieve a cardiovascular conditioning effect.

7. This exercise may be completed at periodic intervals in a training program to chart progress. The over-all response curve should decrease as conditioning improves, much in the manner of the illustration in Figure A–8b.

Appendix A–10

Interval Training

One of the most popular techniques in preparation for athletic competition is interval training, which allows for perhaps the most rapid gains in cardiovascular function. As the name implies, it is a series of repeated bouts of *exercise alternated with periods of relief.* Light or mild exercise usually constitutes the relief period. Interval training thus is intermittent in nature, alternating periods of high stress with ones of lower stress. The *average* heart rate thus can be kept at a threshold level for an entire work-out by alternately raising it above the threshold (work interval) and letting it drop below the threshold (relief interval). If the total work-out is long enough (20 to 30 minutes), this still meets the criteria for a training effect outlined in Chapter 5.

Because of the intermittent nature of the interval training procedure, an individual can exercise at a *greater intensity* and do *more total work* in a given time than with continuous exercise. At the same time, general strain on the body is no more, and in most cases even less, than with continuous exercise. When used properly, the intermittent relief intervals delay or prevent the accumulation of lactic acid in the muscles, and thus delay the onset of fatigue. Also, this type of exercise apparently invokes a greater stimulus for increase in stroke volume of the heart than that with continuous exercise. It has been shown (Fig. A–10*a*) that stroke volume is highest *not during exercise but during recovery from it.* With intermittent exercise, there are many recovery or relief intervals. Thus, the stroke volume reaches the maximum many times during an interval work-out instead of just once, as would be the case with a continuous exercise and only one recovery period. The repeated achievement of maximal stroke volume over several weeks of interval training provides a better stimulus for improving maximal stroke volume than that with continuous exercise because of the operation of the SAID principle (Chapter 2). By raising the stroke volume to higher levels, one is applying a more *specific* training effect to force adaptation than with continuous exercise. If the maximal stroke volume of the heart is improved, this improves the over-all capacity of the heart, the importance of which was discussed in Chapter 5.

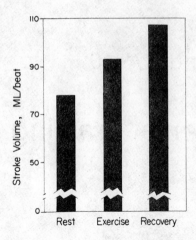

Figure A–10 a. The stroke volume is highest during the recovery period from exercise. During interval training, the stroke volume reaches its highest level many times because of the many relief (recovery) intervals. (From Fox, E. L., and Mathews, D. K.: *Interval Training.* Philadelphia, W. B. Saunders Co., 1974, p. 28.)

INTERVAL TRAINING TERMS

Work Interval. The portion of the interval that consists of the work effort. An example would be a 220-yard run at a prescribed time.

Relief Interval. The time between work intervals as well as between *sets* if more than one set of exercises is performed. The relief interval is *not a recovery period,* as the heart rate is not allowed to return to resting levels. The relief interval usually consists of walking or very light jogging, and usually is expressed in relation to the work interval as a work to rest ratio such as 1:½, 1:1, 1:2, etc. A ratio of 1:½ means the relief interval is one-half the length of the work interval.

Sets. A series of work and relief intervals is referred to as a set. Six 220-yard runs at a prescribed time with designated relief intervals is an example of a set. It might be followed by another set of 220-yard intervals or a set of intervals at another distance.

Training Time. The time taken to complete the work interval, e.g., 220 yards in 35 seconds; 35 seconds is the training time.

Repetitions. The number of work intervals in a set. In the above definition of set, 6 would be the number of repetitions.

Training Distance. The distance of the work interval.

Interval Training Prescription. This contains pertinent information concerning an interval training workout. For example, one set from a prescription might be written as follows:

Set 1:   8 × 220 at 0:35 (1:45)

Where   8   = number of repetitions

220   = training distance in yards

0:35   = training time in minutes and seconds

(1:45) = time of relief interval in minutes and seconds.

INTERVAL TRAINING VARIABLES. The training stimulus as applied through interval training is accomplished through manipulation of six variables:

1.   Distance of work interval.
2.   Time of the work interval.

3.   Number of repetitions of the work interval.
4.   Relief interval time.
5.   Type of activity during relief interval.
6.   Frequency of training per week.

CHOOSING THE WORK INTERVAL DISTANCE AND TIME.
Interval training is a technique to be used later in conditioning programs after a general base of conditioning is achieved. It is *not* recommended for use at the beginning of a conditioning program, especially in sedentary persons. Allow 6 weeks of other conditioning before using interval training. Also, the person unfamiliar with interval training will do best to stick with 220 and 440 yards as the basic training distances. Fred Wilt, former Olympic athlete and noted author on running, has provided a convenient method for determining the training time for the above distances. It involves determining the individual's best time for running 220 yards and 1 mile, with a running start in each case.

For 220-yard intervals add 5 seconds to the best time with a running start. This is the training time. For example, if you can run 220 yards at best effort in 32 seconds, your training time for intervals using this distance is 37 seconds.

For the training distance of 440 yards, the training time is 1 to 4 seconds *less* than one-fourth the time required to run a mile. For example, if you can run 1 mile in 7 minutes, the average time for each 440 yards is 105 seconds (420 seconds/4 = 105 seconds). Therefore, the training time should be between 101 and 104 seconds when 440 yards is used as the training distance.

The above method can also be applied to *swimming*. With swimming the training distances are *one-fourth* those used for running, i.e., 55 and 110 yards, and the training times are based on best times for 55 and 440 yards, respectively.

NUMBER OF REPETITIONS (AND/OR SETS) DURING A WORKOUT.   Optimal training effects can be achieved if the total number of repetitions and sets is sufficient to bring the total work interval distance of the workout up to 1½ to 2 miles each time.

RELIEF INTERVAL.   Beginners in the use of interval training should walk during the relief interval. They may progress to jogging later in the program. For 220-yard intervals, use a work:relief ratio of 1:3; for the 440-yard intervals, use 1:2.

FREQUENCY OF TRAINING.   Interval training applied two to three times per week for six to eight weeks is effective in making excellent improvements in cardiovascular function. If the individual wishes to work out more than three times per week, continuous running or some other forms of exercise should be used on those other days to help prevent overstress from one type of training (see Chapter 7).

TRAINING PROGRESSION.   As conditioning improves, the intensity of the interval program may be stepped up by:
1.   completing the work interval in a slightly shorter time.
2.   shortening the relief interval.

3. progressing to jogging during the relief interval.
4. combinations of the above.

SAMPLE INTERVAL TRAINING PROGRAM. The following is a sample interval training prescription for a 20-year-old college female who can run 1 mile in 9 minutes and 220 yards in 34 seconds:

220 yd time: $\dfrac{0:34}{A}$

1 mile time: $\dfrac{9:00}{B}$

Training Time 220 yds: $\dfrac{0:34}{A} + 5 = \dfrac{0:39}{C}$

Work:Relief Ratio, 1:3: $\dfrac{0:39}{C} \dfrac{(1:57)}{3 \times C}$

Training Time 440 yds: $\dfrac{540}{B}/4 = 135 - 4 = \dfrac{131}{D}$

Work:Relief Ratio, 1:2: $\dfrac{2:11}{D} \dfrac{(4:22)}{2 \times D}$

Set 1   4 × 440 at $\dfrac{2:11}{D} \dfrac{(4:22)}{2 \times D}$ = 1 mile distance

Set 2   4 × 220 at $\dfrac{0:39}{C} \dfrac{(1:57)}{3 \times C}$ = ½ mile distance

Total distance = 1½ miles

Table A–10a. FORMAT FOR DETERMINING A BEGINNING INTERVAL WORK-OUT PROGRAM USING 440- AND 220-YARD DISTANCES

220 yd best time (running start): $\dfrac{}{A}$

1 mile best time: $\dfrac{}{B}$

Training Time 220 yds: $\dfrac{}{A} + 5 = \dfrac{}{C}$

Work:Relief Ratio, 1:3 $\dfrac{}{C} \dfrac{(\quad)}{3 \times C}$

Training Time 440 yds: $\dfrac{}{B}/4 = \dfrac{}{} - 4 = \dfrac{}{D}$

Work:Relief Ratio, 1:2 $\dfrac{}{D} \dfrac{(\quad)}{2 \times D}$

Set 1   4 × 440 at $\dfrac{}{D} \dfrac{(\quad)}{2 \times D}$ = 1 mile

Set 2   4 × 220 at $\dfrac{}{C} \dfrac{(\quad)}{3 \times C}$ = ½ mile

Intervals and sets different in combination from the above may be used. The only requirement is that total distance of the work intervals be 1½ to 2 miles.

The relief interval between sets above should be 4:22.

The total time for the above work-out would be slightly under 30 minutes.

Table A–10a may be used to outline a personal interval training prescription.

For more comprehensive information on interval training and an extensive coverage of specific interval training prescriptions, see reference 2 below.

REFERENCES

1. Cumming, G.: Stroke volume during recovery from supine bicycle exercise. J. Appl. Physiol. *32*:575, 1972.
2. Fox, E. L., and Mathews, D. K.: *Interval Training*. Philadelphia, W. B. Saunders Co., 1974.
3. Mathews, D. K., and Fox, E. L.: *The Physiological Basis of Physical Education and Athletics*. Philadelphia, W. B. Saunders Co., 1976.
4. Wilt, F.: Training for Competitive Running. *In* H. B. Falls (ed.), *Exercise Physiology*. New York, Academic Press, 1968.

Appendix A–11

Test Your Flexibility

Flexibility is defined as the range of motion about a joint, and is very important from a quality of movement viewpoint and as a safeguard against injury. Although flexibility is specific to body areas and muscle groups, it will be useful to measure the flexibility of at least one body area—the posterior leg muscles (hamstrings) and the low back. Lack of flexibility in one or both of these areas has been shown to be clinically related to "low back syndrome" and other types of musculoskeletal dysfunction. Coupled with weak abdominal muscles, it is one of the most significant health problems. The test apparatus should be placed against a solid object such as a wall or post so that it will not shift during the measurement.

Procedure:
1. Persons being tested sit with both legs straight in front of them.
2. They place the soles of the feet against a box, board, bench, or

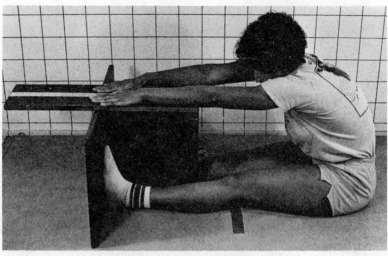

Figure A–11 a. Sit and reach test.

Table A-11a. PERCENTILE NORMS FOR SIT AND REACH
(YOUNG ADULTS)

Percentile	Males	Females
100	15.5	15.0
90	13.4	13.0
80	12.0	12.0
70	10.5	10.5
60	10.0	10.0
50	9.0	8.5
40	8.5	8.0
30	7.5	7.5
20	6.0	6.5
10	5.0	5.0
0	1.0	1.0

Scores are in inches. Based on a test procedure where 9 inches is at the level of the soles of the feet. Based on data from Manitoba Dept. of Education: *Manitoba Physical Fitness Performance Test Manual and Fitness Objectives.* Winnipeg, Manitoba, Canada, Manitoba Dept. of Education, 1977.

other flat surface, as shown in Figure A-11a. A yardstick scale has been placed on the board so that the 9-inch mark is level with the edge of the board, i.e., the soles of the feet.

3. Persons being tested *slowly* bend forward four times to see how far down on the scale they can reach. On the fourth slow reach, the position is held for 1 second and the score in inches is read from the scale. Individuals should not forcefully bounce into position. The knees *cannot* be flexed: they must be kept extended throughout the reach.

4. An apparatus similar to that in Figure A-11a can be constructed easily by attaching a yardstick to the top of a bench that is 12 to 16 inches high.

5. Compare your recorded score with the percentile norms presented in Table A-11a.

6. From the norms, determine if your flexibility generally is below average, average, or above average. What is your percentile?

7. Suggest specific stretching exercises that can be used to increase the flexibility of the hamstring area.

8. What are other body areas that commonly exhibit flexibility problems?

9. If the above apparatus cannot be made available, a quick estimate of flexibility can be obtained by sitting on the floor, feet against a wall, as in Figure A-11a. *Slowly* bend forward with the *knees straight.* See which of the body parts below you can hold to the wall for 1 second after bobbing forward *slowly* three times. The following is a rough approximation to the inch scale norms.

Heel of hand:	about 15 inches.
Knuckles of fist:	about 11 inches.
Fingertips of extended hand:	about 9 inches.
Lacks about 2 inches touching fingertips:	about 7 inches.
Lacks about 4 inches touching fingertips:	about 5 inches.

Appendix A–12

Rating of Perceived Exertion

In Chapter 7, p. 193, we emphasized the importance of attending to bodily sensations, i.e., "reading" your body during exercise, as a precaution against both the excessive stress of anaerobic work during the initial training sessions and the stress of extreme environmental conditions such as high heat and humidity. Borg's rating of perceived exertion (RPE) scale (Fig. 7–4) was presented as one method of assessing the subjective estimate of exercise intensity, based on its previously observed relationship with physiological correlates of *actual* exercise stress. In Borg's model, the similarity between perceived exercise intensity, as determined by RPE, and actual metabolic intensity, as determined by heart rate, is given by RPE × 10 = HR at any given work load. The following laboratory experience is designed to allow you to determine the ability of this model to describe your individual perceptions of exercise stress.

This lab requires that students work in pairs. One will exercise while the other serves as the recorder. Use the worksheet provided in Figure A–12a to record RPE and heart rate at each of the work intensities outlined. For information about determining the suggested running intensities, refer to Appendix A–9, Table A–9a. Follow the instructions in Appendix A–9 for carrying out the walks and runs to be used for obtaining the rating of perceived exertion. This laboratory experiment and the one in Appendix A–9 may be conveniently combined.

As you are exercising at each intensity, you should estimate how hard you *feel* the work is: i.e., rate the degree of perceived exertion you feel. This perceived exertion includes the total amount of exertion and physical fatigue you experience, and should be the combination of all sensations and feelings of physical stress, effort, and fatigue. Don't concern yourself with any one factor, such as leg discomfort or shortness of breath, but try to concentrate on your *total, inner* feeling of over-all exertion. Try to estimate as honestly and objectively as possible. Don't underestimate the degree of exertion you feel, but don't overestimate it either; just try to estimate as accurately as possible. When you rate your work intensity, you should do so by giving the numerical value on Borg's scale (Fig. 7-4) that best represents your evaluation of your perceived exertion at that moment.

Always rate and record RPE *before* heart rate. Exercise at each intensity, as indicated in Table A-9a. During the last few seconds of each 440-yard lap of the track, choose an RPE value from Borg's scale. The number you choose should be your best estimate of how intense the exercise actually is. Report this number to your recorder so that it may be marked in the appropriate space on the work sheet. *Immediately* after you have rated your perceived exertion and have stopped exercising, locate your radial or temporal pulse (see p. 151). Have the

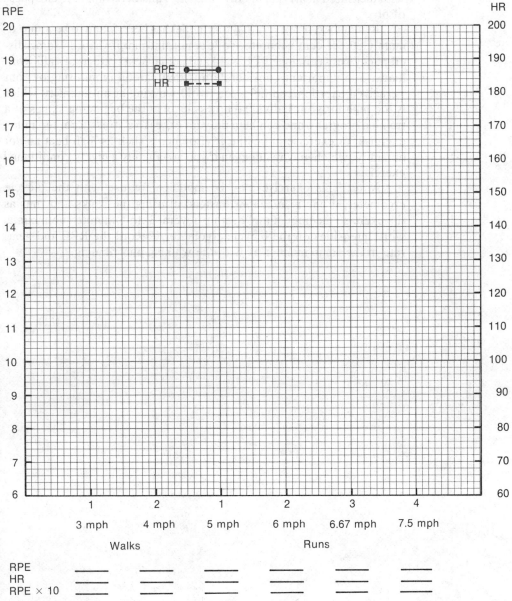

Figure A-12 a. Graph for recording perceived exertion and heart rate responses to graded intensities of exercise.

recorder time a 15-second period during which you count the number of times the heart beats. Multiply the number of beats counted during the 15 seconds by four to obtain a heart rate per minute. Record this number on the worksheet in its appropriate space.

After you have completed all the work levels and have recorded RPE and heart rate for each exercise intensity, connect each RPE point with a straight line, and each heart rate point with a straight line, so that you have one plot each for both RPE and heart rate. Compare the slopes of the two lines. How similar are they? They should be reasonably close. As another way to view your personal results with Borg's model, multiply your RPE by ten at each work level. Compare this new plot with measured heart rate at each intensity, and determine the closeness of fit.

Remember, however, that this model has been found to be approximately 80 per cent accurate, so it is not unusual if there is some discrepancy between your RPE × 10 and actual heart rate at certain work loads. The important consideration is that careful monitoring of your perceived exertion can help you avoid working at an intensity which is too high for your individual fitness level at the beginning stages of a training program, and can help prevent excessive stress from too much exercise, or exercise in hostile environments such as high heat and/or humidity, which may result even if you are already a highly conditioned exerciser.

Note: This exercise may be modified for use with the bicycle ergometer, if one is available. Instead of using the walks and runs as the exercise medium, simply set up several 3- to 5-minute submaximal work intensities on the bicycle ergometer. Record the RPE and heart rate in the same manner as with the walking and running.

Appendix A–13

Self-Motivation Assessment and Determination of Likely Adherence to Exercise

As mentioned in Chapter 7, p. 189, the beneficial effects of regular participation in vigorous physical activity are well established from the standpoint of physiological and psychological wellness. However, roughly 50 per cent of those individuals who begin an exercise program subsequently quit. This drop-out phenomenon possibly might be reduced if those prone to drop out were aware of their tendency toward or probability of adhering. Since self-motivation and body composition have been found to be strong influences in the decision to adhere or drop out in exercise programs, the following laboratory experience is designed to provide a rough estimate of your individual tendency toward exercise adherence.

First, read each of the statements below, and circle the number beneath the letter corresponding to the alternative that best describes how characteristic the statement is when applied to you. The alternatives are:

A. *extremely un*characteristic of me.
B. *somewhat un*characteristic of me.
C. neither characteristic nor uncharacteristic of me.
D. *somewhat characteristic* of me.
E. *extremely characteristic* of me.

Please be sure to answer every item, and try to be as honest and accurate as possible in your responses. No one but you will know your score.

SELF-MOTIVATION ASSESSMENT SCALE*

A B C D E

5 ④ 3 2 1   1. I get discouraged easily.

5 ④ 3 2 1   2. I don't work any harder than I have to.

1 ② 3 4 5   3. I seldom if ever let myself down.

5 4 3 ② 1   4. I'm just not the goal-setting type.

1 2 3 4 ⑤   5. I'm good at keeping promises, especially the ones I make to myself.

5 4 3 2 ①   6. I don't impose much structure on my activities.

1 2 ③ 4 5   7. I have a very hard-driving, aggressive personality.

To obtain your self-motivation score, simply add together the seven numbers you circled above. If this total summated score is equal to or less than *24,* you are probably drop-out prone. The lower your self-motivation score, the more likely it is that you may eventually discontinue a regular exercise program.

An additional prediction of your likelihood of adhering can be determined by using the percentage of your body weight which is fat. Body fat is discussed in Chapter 8 and can be estimated by using Appendix A–16. If your body fat is estimated to be equal to or more than *19 per cent* (men) or *25 per cent* (women), you are probably drop-out prone. In this case, the higher your percentage of body fat, the more likely you are eventually to stop exercising.

A low self-motivation score combined with high body fat is even more suggestive that, for you, adherence to exercise is probably a more difficult goal to attain than it is for many other people. However, if your scores indicate that you are a drop-out candidate, view them as an incentive to remain active, not as a self-fulfilling prophecy to quit. That is, be aware of your drop-out tendency and try to overcome it; don't stop exercising just because your score *suggests* that eventually you will stop.

Remember that self-motivation and body composition have been found to predict with only 80 per cent accuracy whether or not you may adhere or drop out. Some individuals who are highly self-motivated and who are quite lean *do drop out,* whereas others who have generally low self-motivation and relatively high body fat *do adhere.* View your results with some caution, as they neither insure that you will stay with an exercise program, nor indicate that you definitely will discontinue. There are many factors, both personal and situational, which influence the decison to lead a physically active lifestyle as opposed to a sedentary one, and self-motivation and body composition represent only two of them.

Appendix A–14

Benson's Relaxation Response

A major thrust of this text has centered around exercise and its effectiveness in adapting to, or coping with, stress. Specifically, vigorous physical activity has been shown to be quite useful in managing tension and anxiety—prevalent health problems in our society. In this regard, it was pointed out in Chapter 7, p. 200, that exercise not only offers an opportunity for distraction from an anxiety-provoking situation or thought and an important change in arousal, but also has an inherent relaxation effect on both neuromuscular tension and peripheral blood pressure—two important correlates of anxiety. However, it was noted also that certain meditational practices, or even simple rest, or just taking "time out," appear to offer equally effective alternatives for anxiety reduction. The usefulness of these auxiliary techniques in the management of stress appears quite obvious in instances where an injury may prevent exercise, or in the case of the over-stressed or "stale" exerciser who needs temporarily to abstain from exercise or reduce exercise activity below the level necessary to manage tension or anxiety resulting from life stressors. Also, some individuals simply do not enjoy exercising. Consequently, the following laboratory experience is designed to introduce an alternative for stress management based on Benson's Relaxation Response, which was introduced in Chapter 7, p. 199. Remember, this technique is based on the following ingredients: (1) a quiet environment; (2) a mental symbol (mantra), such as a word or phrase repeated in a rhythmical cadence; (3) a passive attitude, i.e., diffuse concentration with no attention to any single thought; and (4) a comfortable, stationary position.

Find a quiet, isolated area and then simply follow the instructions below:

1. *Sit quietly* in a comfortable position.
2. *Close* your eyes.
3. Thoroughly *relax* all your *muscles*. Begin at your feet and

continue up to your face. Keep them relaxed throughout the entire session.

4. *Breathe* through your nose and become aware of your breathing. As you breathe out, say the word "ONE" silently to yourself (you may substitute another word or phrase of your preference). For example, breathe IN . . . OUT, "ONE"; IN . . . OUT, "ONE"; etc. Breathe easily and naturally.

5. *Continue* for 10 to 20 minutes. You may open your eyes to check the time, but do not use an alarm (the alarm would be arousing to the RAS and would work against the objective of relaxation). When you finish, sit quietly for several minutes, at first with eyes closed and later with eyes open. Do not stand up for a few minutes.

6. Do not worry about whether you are successful in achieving a deep level of relaxation. Maintain a *passive* attitude and permit relaxation to occur at its own pace. When distracting thoughts occur, try to ignore them by not dwelling on them, and return to repeating "ONE." With practice, the response should come with little effort. Practice the technique once or twice daily, but not within two hours after any meal, since the digestive processes appear to interfere with the attainment of the Relaxation Response.

The above instructions are a slight modification of those appearing in Benson, H.: *The Relaxation Response*. New York, Morrow, 1975.

Appendix A–15

Basal Metabolic Rate (BMR) Plus Activity Increment

BMR represents the energy needs of the body at complete rest in a fasting state, i.e., the energy necessary to sustain life. In Chapter 8 many factors affecting BMR were briefly discussed, such as age, sex, body surface area, amount of muscle mass, amount of sleep, climate, state of nutrition, illness, and function of the endocrine glands. Since the primary determinants of how many kcal the body needs are BMR and exercise, the following procedure will allow you more closely to estimate your daily caloric needs.

1. Determine your ideal or desired weight in kilograms (simply divide your weight in lbs by 2.2 to obtain kilograms). If needed, use Tables 8–2 and 8–3 or Appendix A–16 for an estimate of ideal weight.
2. Determine BMR estimate based on appropriate sex:
   Male = 1.0 kcal per kg of ideal body weight per hour × 24 hours.
   Female = 0.9 kcal per kg of ideal body weight per hour × 24 hours.
3. Subtract 0.1 kcal per kg of ideal body weight per hours of sleep.
4. Add activity increment from below:

| | Kcal per day | |
Amount of Activity	Men	Women
Sedentary or light	225	225
Moderate	750	500
Heavy	1500	1000
Very Heavy	2500	—

DESCRIPTION OF CATEGORIES

Sedentary or Light—Sedentary persons expend few kcal/day. Most of their time is spent in a seated position, mostly on mental activity that has little influence on caloric consumption. Lightly active individuals also sit, walk, and stand throughout the day.

Table A–15a. EXAMPLE ESTIMATES FOR BMR PLUS ACTIVITY INCREMENT FOR EACH LEVEL OF ACTIVITY*

	Reference Man				Reference Woman		
Step 1: Ideal Weight	70 kg				58 kg		
Step 2: BMR Estimate	$1 \times 70 \times 24 = 1680$				$.9 \times 58 \times 24 = 1252.8$		
Step 3: Sleep Adjustment (subtract 0.1/kg per hour of sleep)	$.1 \times 70 \times 8 = -56$ subtotal $\overline{1624}$				$.1 \times 58 \times 8 = -46.4$ subtotal $\overline{1206.4}$		
Step 4: Activity Increment	Light	Moderate	Heavy	Very Heavy	Light	Moderate	Heavy
	225	750	1500	2500	225	500	1000
Subtotal	1849	2374	3124	4124	1431.4	1706.4	2206.4
Step 5: Specific Dynamic Action (add 10%)	185	237	312	412	143	171	221
Step 6: Estimated Total Needs	2034	2611	3436	4536	1574.4	1877.4	2427.4

*Adapted from Krause, M. V., and Hunscher, M. A.: *Food, Nutrition, and Diet Therapy*, 5th ed. Philadelphia, W. B. Saunders Co., 1972, pp. 37–38.

Moderate—These individuals spend little time sitting, but engage in little vigorous activity. They are continually active in such tasks as standing, walking, bending, lifting light objects, etc.

Heavy—These persons are constantly active, and participate in some vigorous activity. They may spend considerable hours at difficult physical labor or many hours in active sport-type activities. Appendix A–17 may be used to aid in the estimate of physical activity needs.

5. Add specific dynamic action (10 per cent of basal needs plus activity increment). Since different foods affect metabolism differently, 10 per cent is the estimated rise for the average person's mixed diet. For primarily carbohydrate diets, this should be lowered to 5 per cent; for high-protein diets, it should be 15 per cent.

6. The sum of the above five steps equals the estimate of your 24-hour caloric requirement.

Sample problems for the reference man and reference woman at varying levels of activity are presented in Table A–15a. Compare your estimates with those of the reference person of your sex. Are they the same or do they differ? Why should you expect them to differ?

What dietary changes would a change in activity level produce for you? You can work out your BMR plus activity increment for each activity level to answer this question.

REFERENCE

Krause, M. V., and Hunscher, M. A.: *Food, Nutrition and Diet Therapy*, 5th ed. Philadelphia, W. B. Saunders Co., 1972.

Appendix A–16

Methods for Estimating Body Fatness

PERCENTAGE STANDARD WEIGHT. Use the following procedures to estimate your percentage of ideal weight.
1. Use the procedures in Table 8–3, p. 216, to determine an estimate of frame size.
2. Apply the indoor clothing correction: if shoes are worn, add 1 inch in height for men and 2 inches in height for women. Use this corrected height and your frame size for the appropriate chart value.
3. Use the chart for ideal weight in Table 8–2, p. 214, to get the ideal estimate.
4. Divide your weight in lbs by the value determined in step 3, and multiply by 100 to get your percentage of ideal weight.
5. Most individuals should fall within 10 per cent of the standard, i.e., have a percentage ideal weight between 90 and 110. Values above 100 per cent indicate a tendency toward overweight, and values below 100 a tendency toward underweight. Remember that persons with a heavy musculature will be *overweight when they may not be overfat.*

RELATIVE WEIGHT. Relative weight is an expression of the ratio of one's actual weight to one's expected (predicted) weight, based on a consideration of height and basic skeletal framework. The following measures are needed:
1. Height without shoes (in inches).
2. Weight without shoes and wearing gym clothes (in lbs).
3. Biacromial diameter (shoulder width) in inches: the distance between the most lateral margins of the acromial processes of the scapulae, with the subject standing erect but with shoulders relaxed. The measurement should be taken from the rear (Fig. A–16a). The acromial processes can be felt by palpation as a ridge at the lateral border of the shoulder. The measurement may be taken with a

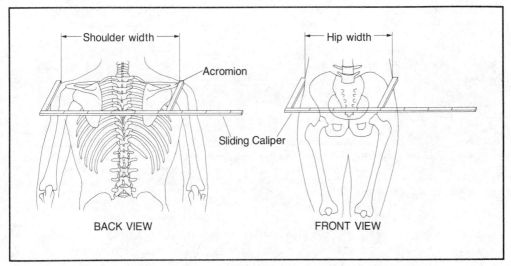

Figure A–16 a. Measurement locations for shoulder and hip width.

sliding or obstetrical calipers. These calipers may be improvised (Fig. A–16b).

4. Bi-iliac diameter (hip width) in inches: the width of the pelvic girdle as measured at the greatest distance between the lateral margins of the iliac crests (lateral points of the hips). The measurement may be taken with a sliding, obstetrical, or improvised caliper, with strong pressure to minimize the soft tissue included.

After the above measures are obtained, predicted weight is determined by working out a regression equation of the following form:

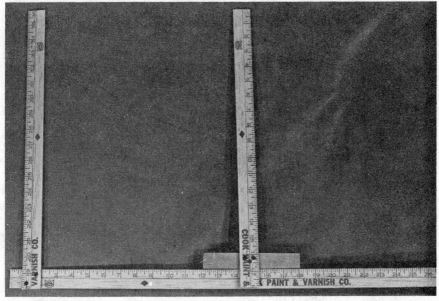

Figure A–16 b. Improvised calipers for measuring shoulder and hip width.

Table A–16a. CONVERSION FACTORS TO DETERMINE PREDICTED BODY WEIGHT*

| | | Males | | | | Females | | |
| | | Shoulder | Hip | | | Shoulder | Hip | |
Age	Ht	Width	Width	Constant	Ht	Width	Width	Constant
	(a)	(b)	(c)		(a)	(b)	(c)	
15–16	0.66	8.27	17.78	217.21	0.84	7.66	15.75	199.14
17–19	2.62	10.34	11.24	314.73	1.45	9.28	10.85	207.68
20+	1.84	7.10	6.09	145.07	1.12	8.94	9.28	168.01

Note: Since skeletal growth is virtually complete at age 20, the 20+ age-group conversion factors can be used for all ages above 20. Equations for younger ages may be found in the footnote below.

*Adapted from Montoye, H. J. (ed.): *An Introduction to Measurement in Physical Education,* Vol. II. Indianapolis, Phi Epsilon Kappa, 1970.

Predicted weight = a(Ht) + b(shoulder width) + c(hip width) − constant; where a, b, c, and the constant are obtained from Table A–16 *a.*

For example, suppose a man who is 19 years old has the following current measurements:

Body weight 175 lbs
Body height 70 inches
Biacromial width 14 inches
Bi-iliac width 13 inches

Predicted weight = (70)(2.62) + (14)(10.34) + (13)(11.24) − 314.73
                 = 159.42 lbs

$$\text{Relative weight} = \frac{\text{Actual weight}}{\text{Predicted weight}} \times 100 =$$

For the example: $\dfrac{175}{159.42} \times 100 = 109.8$

This means our young man is 9.8 per cent above desirable weight. From a health standpoint, anyone who is more than 15 per cent above desirable weight should reduce body fat.

The difference between actual weight and predicted weight gives the actual number of pounds above desirable weight. This may serve as a target figure in a weight reduction program.

The relative weight procedure has an advantage over the percentage standard weight shown above in that it provides a better estimate of frame size.

SKINFOLD MEASUREMENTS (Estimation of Percentage Body Fat). This is the most satisfactory procedure in this Appendix, since it provides a more valid estimate of actual body fat.

To estimate the percentage body fat from skinfold equations, follow the procedures outlined below. You will need a pair of skinfold calipers.

A. Decide on the measurement sites (Fig. A–16c, d, e, and f). All measurements are made on the right side of the body.
    Females
    1. Suprailiac—a vertical skinfold over the iliac crest (point of hip) in the midaxillary (armpit) line.
    2. Triceps—a vertical skinfold on the back of the arm, halfway

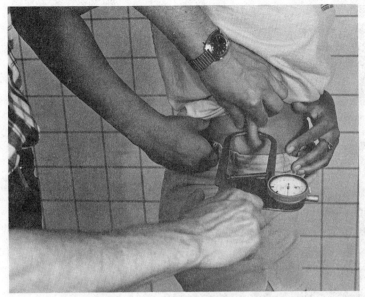

Figure A–16 c. Suprailiac skinfold measurement.

between the acromion and the rear point (olecranon process) of the elbow joint with arm hanging relaxed at side.

Males

1. Thigh—a vertical skinfold in the anterior midline of the thigh, halfway between the inguinal ligament (where hip joint bends in front) and the top of the patella (kneecap).
2. Subscapular—running downward and diagonally lateral in the natural fold of the skin from the inferior angle (lower corner) of the scapula (shoulder blade).

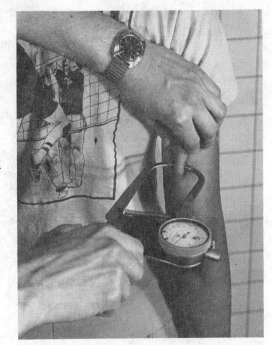

Figure A–16 d. Triceps skinfold measurement.

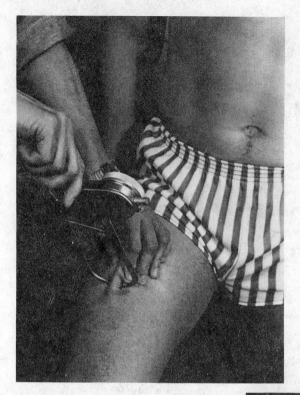

Figure A–16 e. Thigh skinfold measurement.

Figure A–16 f. Subscapular skinfold measurement.

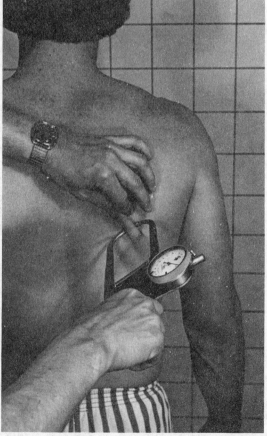

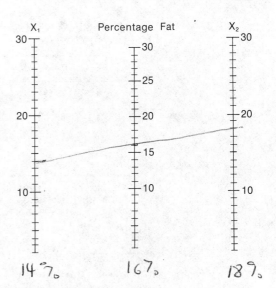

Figure A–16 g. Nomogram for calculating percentage body fat from thigh (X_1) and subscapular (X_2) skinfold thicknesses (mm) in young adult males. Connect X_1 and X_2 with a ruler or other straight edge. Read percentage fat from middle column. (Adapted from Sloan, A. W., and de V. Weir, J. B.: Nomograms for the prediction of body density and total body fat from skinfold measurements. J. Appl. Physiol. *28*:221, 1970.)

14 %   16 %   18 %

B. For the best results, the person doing the skinfold measurements should be well practiced. Practice taking measurements until you get within ±2 mm consistency.
C. Grasp the skinfold between the thumb and forefinger about 1 cm from the caliper placement. Place the calipers on the fold and release the fingers slightly so that most of the pressure is on the calipers, not the fingers. Take the average of three measurements at each site. *Note* that numerous measurements at the same site may unduly compress the skinfold and result in an underestimate of body fat.
D. The percentage fat may be calculated from Figure A–16g for males and A–16h for females.
E. The average percentage fat for college males is about 10 to 15, for females about 20 to 25. *Desirable* fat in the male is no more than 10 to 12 per cent; the *desirable* level for the female is no more than 17 to 19 per cent.

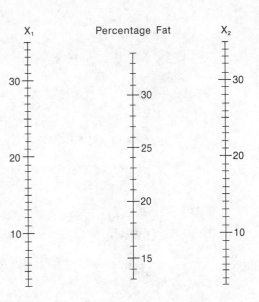

Figure A–16 h. Nomogram for calculating percentage body fat from suprailiac (X_1) and triceps (X_2) skinfold thicknesses (mm) in young adult females. Connect X_1 and X_2 with a ruler or other straight edge. Read percentage of fat from middle column. (Adapted from Sloan, A. W., and de V. Weir, J. B.: Nomograms for the prediction of body density and total body fat from skinfold measurements. J. Appl. Physiol. *28*:221, 1970.)

Table A–16b. PERCENTILE NORMS (YOUNG ADULTS)
FOR SUM OF TRICEPS AND SUBSCAPULAR SKINFOLDS (mm)*

Percentile	Males	Females
95	9	14
90	10	17
75	12	20
50	15	27
25	22	37
10	32	48
5	41	59

*Based on data from Johnston, F. E., Hamill, P. V. V., and Lemeshow, S.: Skinfold thickness of youths 12–17 years. *In U.S. Vital and Health Statistics,* Series 11, No. 132. Washington, D.C., U.S. Dept. of HEW, 1974.

PERCENTILE NORMS FOR SKINFOLD MEASURES.   If you desire to compare yourself with norms, follow the procedures outlined below.
1.   Males and females both use the sum of the triceps and subscapular skinfolds in millimeters, as described previously.
2.   Compare your skinfold sum to the value in Table A–16b for your percentile rank compared with other young adults.

CALCULATION OF "IDEAL" OR DESIRABLE BODY WEIGHT.
Use the worksheet below to calculate your desirable body weight. Make a subjective estimation of your ideal body weight *before* completing the exercise.

$$\text{Fat wt} = \underset{\text{B. wt}}{\underline{\hspace{2cm}}} \times \underset{\text{\% fat}}{\underline{\hspace{2cm}}} = \underline{\hspace{2cm}} \text{ lbs of fat in B. wt}$$

$$\text{Fat-free wt} = \underset{\text{B. wt}}{\underline{\hspace{2cm}}} - \underset{\text{F. wt}}{\underline{\hspace{2cm}}} = \underline{\hspace{2cm}} \text{ lbs}$$

$$\text{Optimum fat wt} = \underset{\text{ideal \%}}{\underline{\hspace{2cm}}} \times \underset{\text{F. F. wt}}{\underline{\hspace{2cm}}} = \underline{\hspace{2cm}} \text{ lbs}$$

$$\text{Optimum B. wt} = \underset{\text{F. F. wt}}{\underline{\hspace{2cm}}} + \underset{\text{opt. F. wt}}{\underline{\hspace{2cm}}} = \underline{\hspace{2cm}} \text{ lbs}$$

Your subjective estimate of ideal weight = \underline{\hspace{2cm}} lbs.

Notations:
   B. wt is body weight to nearest pound.
   % fat is % total body fat.
   F. wt is fat weight.
   F. F. wt is fat-free weight.
   Opt. B. wt is optimal body weight (ideal weight).
   Opt. F. wt is optimal fat weight.

How does your subjective estimate of ideal body weight compare with the scientific estimate? Do you need to reduce body fat?

SKINFOLD ESTIMATE OF BODY FAT PERCENTAGE FOR OLDER ADULTS.   The nomograms presented above for estimating body fat percentage are applicable to young adults up to about age 25. Because body fat percentage increases and lean body mass decreases in older adults, differences in age should be considered. The two equations below may be used for obtaining estimates of body fat percentage in adults over age 25.

Males:
Equation A–16(1):

$$\text{Body Density (BD)} = 1.10938 - 0.0008267\ (S) + 0.0000016\ (S^2) - 0.0002574\ (A)$$

where S = Sum of thigh, abdomen, and chest skinfolds;
    A = Age, years

Females:
Equation A–16(2):

$$\text{Body Density (BD)} = 1.0994921 - 0.0009929\ (S) + 0.0000023\ (S^2) - 0.0001392\ (A)$$

where S = Sum of triceps, thigh, and suprailiac skinfolds

For Both Males and Females:

$$\%\ \text{Body Fat} = \left(\frac{4.950}{\text{BD}} - 4.500\right) \times 100$$

The reader should note that abdominal and chest skinfolds are needed for the above equations. These were not shown in Figure A–16c to *f*. Their locations are outlined on the illustration in Figure A–16i. The chest skinfold is taken over the lateral border of the pectoralis major running *diagonally* in the natural fold of the skin. The abdominal skinfold is a *horizontal* fold just to the right of the umbilicus.

SKINFOLD CALIPERS. Best results on skinfold measurements will be obtained when calipers with a constant pressure of 10 gm/mm² are used. Most body composition researchers use either the Lange or the Harpenden caliper. These are very accurate but relatively expensive, $100.00+. Recently, several inexpensive skinfold calipers have become available, at a price range under $20.00. Recent studies at Southwest Missouri State University and Wisconsin State University at LaCrosse have shown that, for screening body fat, these calipers give results that are nearly as accurate as the more expensive calipers. Figure A–16j shows some inexpensive calipers in comparison with the Harpenden caliper. Their sources are listed below.
Lange caliper (not pictured): Cambridge Scientific Industries, 18 Poplar Street, Cambridge, MD.
Harpenden caliper: Quinton Instrument Co., 2121 Terry Avenue, Seattle, WA 98121.

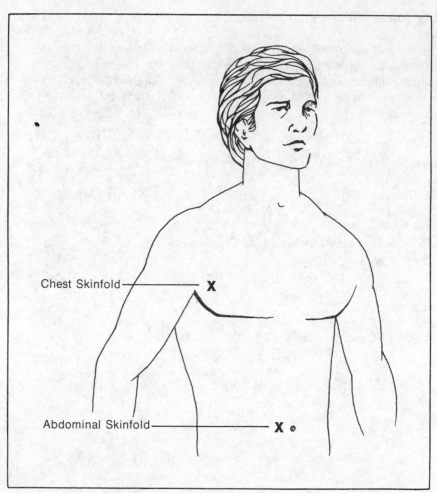

Figure A–16 *i*. Locations for chest and abdominal skinfold measurements. See text for instructions on how to take the measurements.

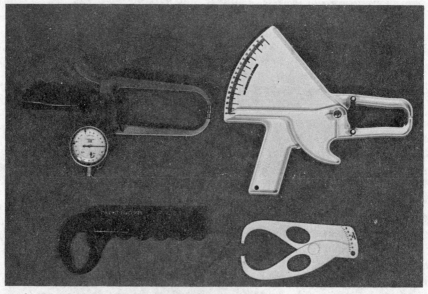

Figure A–16 *j*. Several skinfold calipers are pictured. *Upper left:* Harpenden caliper; *upper right:* Slim Guide; *lower left:* Fat-O-Meter; *lower right:* Physique Meter.

Fat-O-Meter: Health and Education Services, 2442 Irving Park Rd., Chicago, IL 60618.

Physique Meter: Dr. H. Co., P.O. Box 266, Chesterfield, MO 63017.

Slim Guide: P.O. Box 299, Alexandria, IN 46001.

REFERENCES

1. Behnke, A. R., and Wilmore, J. H.: *Evaluation and Regulation of Body Build and Composition*. Englewood Cliffs, N.J., Prentice-Hall, 1974.
2. Jackson, A. J., and Pollock, M. L.: Generalized equations for predicting body density of men. Br. J. Nutr. *40*:497, 1978.
3. Jackson, A. J., Pollock, M. L., and Ward, A.: Generalized equations for predicting body density and percent body fat of women. Med. Sci. Sports *12*: In press, 1980.
4. Montoye, H. J. (ed.): *An Introduction to Measurement in Physical Education,* Vol. II. Indianapolis, Phi Epsilon Kappa, 1970.
5. Sloan, A. W., and de V. Weir, J. B.: Nomograms for prediction of body density and total body fat from skinfold measurements. J. Appl. Physiol. *28*:221, 1970.

Appendix A–17

How Active Are You?

A. Record your daily activity for a period of one week. Try to make it a typical week with no special efforts involved. Write down approximately how much time is spent in sleeping, sitting, walking, and various work and sports activities. Record the time of the day.

B. Take the activity charts in Table A–17a and Table 8–4 and determine how many kcal are spent on each of these activities that is above sedentary.

C. On the average, how many kcal per day do you consume in household, recreational, and sports activities?

D. What changes in body weight would the above difference make in a month's time? a year? (Hint: 3500 kcal = one lb of fat.)

E. If you develop the goal of using an extra 300 to 500 kcal per day, as recommended for weight control, use Table A–17a to work out a week of desired activity at your body weight, choosing activities that you enjoy or think you will enjoy participating in.

Table A–17a. ENERGY EXPENDITURE IN HOUSEHOLD, RECREATIONAL, AND SPORT ACTIVIES (CALORIES/MIN)*

Activity	kg 50 lbs 110	53 117	56 123	59 130	62 137	65 143	68 150	71 157	74 163	77 170	80 176	83 183	86 190	89 196	92 203	95 209	98 216
Badminton	4.9	5.1	5.4	5.7	6.0	6.3	6.6	6.9	7.2	7.5	7.8	8.1	8.3	8.6	8.9	9.2	9.5
Basketball	6.9	7.3	7.7	8.1	8.6	9.0	9.4	9.8	10.2	10.6	11.0	11.5	11.9	12.3	12.7	13.1	13.5
Canoeing (leisure)	2.2	2.3	2.5	2.6	2.7	2.9	3.0	3.1	3.3	3.4	3.5	3.7	3.8	3.9	4.0	4.2	4.3
Housework	2.7	2.9	3.1	3.3	3.5	3.7	3.9	4.1	4.3	4.5	4.7	4.8	5.0	5.2	5.4	5.6	5.8
Cycling: 5.5 mph	3.2	3.4	3.6	3.8	4.0	4.2	4.4	4.6	4.8	5.0	5.1	5.3	5.5	5.7	5.9	6.1	6.3
9.4 mph	5.0	5.3	5.6	5.9	6.2	6.5	6.8	7.1	7.4	7.7	8.0	8.3	8.6	8.9	9.2	9.5	9.8
Dancing: ballroom	2.6	2.7	2.9	3.0	3.2	3.3	3.5	3.6	3.8	3.9	4.1	4.2	4.4	4.5	4.7	4.8	5.0
disco	5.2	5.5	5.8	6.1	6.4	6.7	7.0	7.3	7.6	7.9	8.2	8.5	8.9	9.2	9.5	9.8	10.1
square	4.2	4.4	4.6	4.9	5.1	5.4	5.6	5.9	6.1	6.4	6.6	6.9	7.1	7.4	7.6	7.9	8.1
Farm work:																	
driving tractor	1.9	2.0	2.1	2.2	2.3	2.4	2.5	2.6	2.7	2.8	3.0	3.1	3.2	3.3	3.4	3.5	3.6
feeding cattle	4.3	4.5	4.8	5.0	5.3	5.5	5.8	6.0	6.3	6.5	6.8	7.1	7.3	7.6	7.8	8.1	8.3
forking straw bales	6.9	7.3	7.7	8.1	8.6	9.0	9.4	9.8	10.2	10.6	11.0	11.5	11.9	12.3	12.7	13.1	13.5
shoveling grain	4.3	4.5	4.8	5.0	5.3	5.5	5.8	6.0	6.3	6.5	6.8	7.1	7.3	7.6	7.8	8.1	8.3
Fishing	3.1	3.3	3.5	3.7	3.8	4.0	4.2	4.4	4.6	4.8	5.0	5.1	5.3	5.5	5.7	5.9	6.1
Gardening:																	
digging	6.3	6.7	7.1	7.4	7.8	8.2	8.6	8.9	9.3	9.7	10.1	10.5	10.8	11.2	11.6	12.0	12.3
mowing	5.6	5.9	6.3	6.6	6.9	7.3	7.6	8.0	8.3	8.6	9.0	9.3	9.6	10.0	10.3	10.6	11.0
raking	2.7	2.9	3.0	3.2	3.3	3.5	3.7	3.8	4.0	4.2	4.3	4.5	4.6	4.8	5.0	5.1	5.3
Golf	4.3	4.5	4.8	5.0	5.3	5.5	5.8	6.0	6.3	6.5	6.8	7.1	7.3	7.6	7.8	8.1	8.3
Machine tooling	3.0	3.1	3.3	3.5	3.7	3.8	4.0	4.2	4.4	4.5	4.7	4.9	5.1	5.2	5.4	5.6	5.8
House painting:																	
outside	3.9	4.1	4.3	4.5	4.8	5.0	5.2	5.5	5.7	5.9	6.2	6.4	6.6	6.9	7.1	7.3	7.5
inside	1.7	1.8	1.9	2.0	2.1	2.2	2.3	2.4	2.5	2.6	2.7	2.8	2.9	3.0	3.1	3.2	3.3
Skiing (cross-country)	5.6	5.9	6.2	6.5	6.9	7.2	7.5	7.9	8.2	8.5	8.9	9.2	9.5	9.9	10.2	10.5	10.9
Swimming (most strokes, moderate speed)	7.6	8.0	8.5	8.9	9.4	9.8	10.3	10.8	11.2	11.6	12.1	12.5	13.0	13.5	13.9	14.3	14.7
Tennis	5.5	5.8	6.1	6.4	6.8	7.1	7.4	7.7	8.1	8.4	8.7	9.0	9.4	9.7	10.0	10.4	10.7
Volleyball	2.5	2.7	2.8	3.0	3.1	3.3	3.4	3.6	3.7	3.9	4.0	4.2	4.3	4.5	4.6	4.8	4.9
Weight-training	5.4	5.7	6.1	6.4	6.7	7.0	7.4	7.7	8.0	8.3	8.7	9.0	9.3	9.6	10.0	10.3	10.6

*Adapted from Katch, F. I., and W. D. McArdle: *Nutrition, Weight Control, and Exercise.* Boston, Houghton Mifflin Co., 1977. (For energy expenditure in other work and sport activities, consult the above reference *or* Banister, E. W., and Brown, S. R.: The Relative Energy Requirements of Physical Activity. *In* H. B. Falls (ed.), *Exercise Physiology.* New York, Academic Press, 1968.)

Appendix A–18

Analysis of Diet

A. Record everything you eat or drink for a full week (an absolute minimum of three days is essential). Do not rely on memory: keep a small note pad or card and pencil with you and record what was consumed, how much, and when. Try not to alter your diet during this period; eat as normally as you can.

B. Use Appendices C and D* and try to estimate the number of Calories consumed at each meal on each day.

C. Use Table 8–1 and check to see if you have eaten properly each day from the four basic food groups.

D. With the results of the above, try to answer the following questions concerning your diet.

    1. On how many days in the seven did you eat properly from the four basic food groups? Which group do you tend to omit? to overeat in? You may want to analyze each meal to determine if you have difficulty with poor adherence at any one meal, e.g., breakfast.

    2. What was the average number of kcal consumed per day?

    3. On the average how many kcal did you consume at breakfast, at lunch, at dinner, for snacks?

---

*Appendices C and D present only a limited number of foods, and may not contain all the items in your diet. The most extensive and authoritative listing of nutritional value of foods is: Nutritive Value of Foods, Washington, D.C., Home and Garden Bulletin No. 72. Agricultural Research Service, U.S. Dept. of Agriculture, 1977. This booklet is for sale by the Superintendent of Documents, U.S. Government Printing Office, Washington, DC 20402, price $1.05. Order Stock No. 001-000-03667-0. The reader is encouraged to obtain a copy as a personal reference. Other good references are:

1. Briggs, G. M., and Calloway, D. H.: *Bogert's Nutrition and Physical Fitness.* Philadelphia, W. B. Saunders Co., 1979.
2. Krause, M. V., and Hunscher, M. A.: *Food, Nutrition, and Diet Therapy.* Philadelphia, W. B. Saunders Co., 1972. ("Nutritive Value of Foods," noted above, is reprinted in this text.)
3. Netzer, C. T.: *The Brand-Name Calorie Counter.* New York, The Dell Publishing Co., 1969.

4. When is your greatest problem time for eating kcal? During what hours of the day do you eat more of your kcal?

5. Recall your BMR Plus Activity Increment from Appendix A-15; how does your average kcal per day consumption compare to that estimate?

6. On the basis of this record, what specific recommendations can you make regarding your current eating habits?

7. Make two lists: (1) foods of which I need to eat less; and (2) foods of which I need to eat more.

8. List your problem eating times of the day, and suggest low caloric, nutritious snacks that you could make available at these times.

Appendix A-19

Reduction of Dietary Fat (Suggestions For)

GOOD DIETARY HABITS INCLUDE REDUCING THE LEVEL OF FATS

A. Study the food charts in Table 3-2 and Appendices C and D, and make lists of foods that are (1) high in fat and (2) low in fat.

B. Take the list of foods that are high in fat, and separate it into two separate lists: (1) foods high in saturated fat; and (2) foods high in unsaturated fat. These two sets of lists will acquaint you with approximate levels of fats in various foods and where to find this type of information (see C, 10 below).

C. Make a list of specific food changes which you can make in your diet that will insure the following dietary principles. These principles have been highly recommended for the average adult American.

  1. The total caloric intake should be adjusted to achieve or maintain a desirable body weight.

  2. Replace simple sugars with complex carbohydrates. Simple sugars should constitute only 15 per cent of the calories; complex carbohydrates should constitute about 40 to 45 per cent.

  3. Decrease the amount of salt in the diet.

  4. Increase the consumption of fruits and vegetables.

  5. Your dietary goals should be to reduce the level of fat in your diet from the current approximately 40 to 45 per cent fat to 30 per cent.

  6. You should limit the amount of saturated fat to about 10 per cent of your daily calories. The rest of your fat should be unsaturated (about 20 per cent of total calories).

  7. Decrease dietary cholesterol from the American average of 600 mg to 300 mg daily.

  8. Substitute nonfat milk for whole milk.

9. Decrease the consumption of meat, and increase consumption of fish and poultry.
10. Eat fewer foods that are high in saturated fat and cholesterol. Reduce your consumption of the following specific foods:
    a. Fatty cuts of pork, lamb, and beef, including most luncheon meats such as frankfurters, sausage, bacon, salami, and liverwurst.
    b. Fat-rich dairy products such as cheese, butter, whole milk, cream, and ice cream.
    c. Most commercially prepared baked goods, including cakes, pastry, cream pies, sweet rolls, donuts, muffins, and cookies.
    d. Egg yolks, fish roe, organ meats such as brains, kidney, and liver and sweetbreads.
    e. Products made from an unspecified vegetable fat or shortening. For example, coconut oil, a saturated vegetable oil, is often used in nondairy coffee lighteners, frozen puddings and whip cream substitutes, frozen cakes and pastry, crackers, snack chips, and cookies.
    f. Foods that have been hydrogenated or partially hydrogenated for a longer shelf life. For example, most peanut butter contains normally unsaturated peanut oil, but most manufacturers hydrogenate the oil so that it will not rise to the top of the jar and will not need refrigeration.
11. Replace some of the saturated fat with polyunsaturated oils; these oils should be used in cooking and salad dressing for their cholesterol-lowering effect. Food sources include the following:
    a. Safflower oil, corn oil, and cottonseed-soybean blend oil.
    b. Margarines listing one of these oils, in liquid form, as the first ingredient.
    c. Mayonnaise.
    d. Nuts and seeds such as walnuts, soy nuts, and sunflower seeds.
    e. Fish.
12. Choose a diet that is varied and includes adequate amounts of all known essential nutrients. Keep servings moderate-to-small in size to achieve or maintain desirable body weight. The following daily food pattern is recommended for the American adult:
    a. Two servings of fish, poultry, veal, lean meat, or legumes. One serving equals 3 to 4 ounces of cooked fish, poultry, meat, or liquids. Limit egg yolks to two per week.
    b. Two or more cups of skim milk, low-fat milk, buttermilk, or yogurt made from skim milk. Cheeses made from skimmed or partially skimmed milk such as skim milk cottage cheese, farmer's, ricotta, and mozarella cheese also may be used.
    c. At least four servings of whole grain or enriched bread and cereals. The amount varies with how many calories you can afford. One serving equals one slice of bread,

½ cup of cooked pasta or cooked cereal, or one cup of cold cereal.

d. Two to four tablespoons of polyunsaturated oil, margarine, or mayonnaise. The amount varies with how many calories you can afford.

e. At least four servings of vegetables and fruits. One serving should be a source of vitamin C, such as citrus fruit or juice, and one serving should be a source of vitamin A, consisting of such dark green leafy or deep yellow vegetables as spinach and carrots. Deep yellow fruits such as apricots, cantaloupe, mango, and papaya also provide vitamin A.

The above is adapted from:

1. Arlis, R., et al.: Nutrition: principles of dietary modification. Preventive Med. *3*:412, 1974.

2. Mayer, J.: Dietary goals for the United States. Family Health *10(11)*:39, 1978.

Appendix B

Sources of Vitamins and Minerals

Vitamin A. Important to growth of children, healthy skin, and vision. Lack of vitamin A shows dry, crusty eyelids and reddening of the eyeballs, poor night-time vision, skin problems.

Liver: beef, calf, and pork
Sweet potatoes
Cantaloupe
Dark green leafy
   vegetables: spinach,
   kale, chard, broccoli,
   turnip greens,
   beet greens, and
   mustard greens

Other yellow vegetables,
   such as carrots, winter
   squash, and pumpkin
Apricots
Tomatoes
Egg yolk
Butter or fortified
   margarine
Milk and cheese

Vitamin B Group—Thiamine. Important to growth, good appetite, digestion of fats and carbohydrates, and healthy nerves. Lack of thiamine leads to malnutrition, poor appetite, nervousness, and irritability.

Lean pork: fresh or cured
Dry peas, beans, and nuts
Liver: pork, calf, and beef
Other vegetables:
   green peas, potatoes

Enriched, restored and
   whole grain bread, flour,
   and cereals
Poultry and fish
Other meats: lamb, beef,
   and veal
Milk
Eggs

Vitamin B Group—Riboflavin. Important to growth, good vision, and metabolism.

Lack of riboflavin leads to poor growth and burning eyes that are sensitive to light.

Milk, milk products
Liver: calf, pork, beef, chicken
Lean pork, veal, lamb, and beef
Salmon
Eggs
Enriched, restored and whole grain bread, flour, and cereals
Green leafy vegetables, such as spinach, broccoli

Vitamin B Group—Niacin. Important to the body's use of protein. Lack of niacin leads to pellagra, which has the following symptoms: rough or inflamed skin; nervousness; mental depression; and intestinal problems.

Liver: pork, calf, chicken, beef
Fish, such as tuna and salmon
Lean pork, veal, and beef
Poultry
Green peas and lima beans
Enriched, restored and whole grain bread, flour, and cereals
White potatoes
Eggs
Peanuts and peanut butter
Almonds

Vitamin C. Important to the body's ability to maintain cellular integrity and heal wounds.

Lack of vitamin C results in scurvy, a disease which in advanced stages is characterized by tender, bleeding gums; joints that are weak, swollen, painful; and bleeding from other areas of the body.

Oranges, lemons, grapefruit, and tangerines
Strawberries and pineapple
Tomatoes
Cauliflower
Cantaloupe
Cabbage (raw)
Broccoli and kale
Turnip greens, mustard greens, and collards
Potatoes, sweet and white
Green pepper

Vitamin D—The Sunshine Vitamin. Important to healthy bones and teeth.

Lack of vitamin D results in poor bone growth and structure.

Sunshine
Fortified milk
Egg yolks
Liver

Mineral—Calcium. Important to bones and teeth.

Lack of calcium results in poor bone growth and possibly rickets, which is a disease characterized by skeletal deformity.

Milk, and milk products
Cheese
Dishes or foods prepared with milk and cheese
Dried peas and beans
Salmon, crab, clams
Mustard greens, turnip greens, broccoli, and collards
Enriched breads made with milk or dry milk solids, or containing calcium-based yeast foods

Mineral—Iron.   Important to hemoglobin in the red blood cells.
Lack of iron results in anemia, which is characterized by low levels of
oxygen-carrying hemoglobin in the blood.

Liver: pork, calf, beef	Enriched, restored and
Lean beef, pork, and lamb	whole grain bread, flour,
Dried beans	and cereals
Prunes and other dried	Leafy green vegetables
fruits	Oysters and other
Eggs	shellfish

Mineral—Iodine.   Important to thyroxine, an energy-regulating hormone produced by the thyroid gland.
Insufficient iodine results in an enlarged thyroid gland, goiter, and
sluggish behavior.

      Iodized salt
      Seafoods
      Foods grown on iodine-rich soils near the seashore

Appendix C

The Exchange List Diets*

This appendix is organized in the following manner. Part A contains the seven exchange lists. They are to be used in connection with *each* of the diets that follow in Part B. Diets with approximately 1200, 1500, 2000, 2200, and 2500 Calories are presented. The foods allowed in each diet should be selected from the seven exchange lists in Part A. *Foods in the same list are interchangeable* because, in the quantities specified, they provide approximately the same amount of carbohydrate, protein, and fat. For example, when a menu calls for one bread exchange, any item in List 4 may be used in the amount stated. If two bread exchanges are allowed, double the specified amount, or use a single exchange of *two* foods in List 4.

A. The Exchange Lists

List 1, Allowed as Desired (need not be measured)
Seasonings: Cinnamon, celery salt, garlic, garlic salt, lemon, mustard, mint, nutmeg, parsley, pepper, saccharin and other sugarless sweeteners, spices, vanilla, and vinegar.
Other Foods: Coffee or tea (without sugar or cream), fat-free broth, bouillon, unflavored gelatin, rennet tablets, sour or dill pickles, cranberries (without sugar), rhubarb (without sugar).

Vegetables: Group A—insignificant carbohydrate or calories. You may eat as much as desired of the raw vegetable. If cooked vegetable is eaten, limit amount to one cup.

Asparagus	Cauliflower
Broccoli	Celery
Brussels sprouts	Chicory
Cabbage	Cucumbers

---

*The diets and exchange lists are supplied through courtesy and permission of Eli Lilly and Company, Indianapolis, Indiana.

Eggplant	Peppers, green
Escarole	or red
Greens: beet, chard, collard,	Radishes
dandelion, kale, mustard, spinach,	Sauerkraut
turnip	String beans
Lettuce	Summer squash
Mushrooms	Tomatoes
Okra	Watercress

List 2, Vegetable Exchanges
Each portion supplies approximately 7 gm of carbohydrate and 2 gm of protein, or 36 Calories.

Vegetables: *Group B*—one serving equals ½ cup, or 100 gm.

Beets	Pumpkin
Carrots	Rutabagas
Onions	Squash, winter
Peas, green	Turnips

List 3, Fruit Exchanges (fresh, dried, or canned without sugar)
Each portion supplies approximately 10 gm of carbohydrate, or 40 Calories.

	Household Measurement	Weight of Portion
Apple	1 small (2″ diam.)	80 gm
Applesauce	½ cup	100 gm
Apricots, fresh	2 med	100 gm
Apricots, dried	4 halves	20 gm
Banana	½ small	50 gm
Berries	1 cup	150 gm
Blueberries	⅔ cup	100 gm
Cantaloupe	¼ (6″ diam.)	200 gm
Cherries	10 large	75 gm
Dates	2	15 gm
Figs, fresh	2 large	50 gm
Figs, dried	1 small	15 gm
Grapefruit	½ small	125 gm
Grapefruit juice	½ cup	100 gm
Grapes	12	75 gm
Grape juice	¼ cup	60 gm
Honeydew melon	⅛ (7″)	150 gm
Mango	½ small	70 gm
Orange	1 small	100 gm
Orange juice	½ cup	100 gm
Papaya	⅓ med	100 gm
Peach	1 med	100 gm

	Household Measurement	Weight of Portion
Pear	1 small	100 gm
Pineapple	½ cup	80 gm
Pineapple juice	⅓ cup	80 gm
Plums	2 med	100 gm
Prunes, dried	2	25 gm
Raisins	2 tbsp	15 gm
Tangerine	1 large	100 gm
Watermelon	1 cup	175 gm

List 4, Bread Exchanges
Each portion supplies approximately 15 gm of carbohydrate and 2 gm of protein, or 68 Calories.

	Household Measurement	Weight of Portion
Bread	1 slice	25 gm
Biscuit, roll	1 (2″ diam.)	35 gm
Muffin	1 (2″ diam.)	35 gm
Cornbread	1½″ cube	35 gm
Flour	2½ tbsp	20 gm
Cereal, cooked	½ cup	100 gm
Cereal, dry (flakes or puffed)	¾ cup	20 gm
Rice or grits, cooked	½ cup	100 gm
Spaghetti, noodles, etc.	½ cup	100 gm
Crackers, graham	2	20 gm
Crackers, oyster	20 (½ cup)	20 gm
Crackers, saltine	5	20 gm
Crackers, soda	3	20 gm
Crackers, round	6–8	20 gm
Vegetables		
Beans (lima, navy, etc.), dry, cooked	½ cup	90 gm
Peas (split peas, etc.), dry, cooked	½ cup	90 gm
Baked beans, no pork	¼ cup	50 gm
Corn	⅓ cup	80 gm
Parsnips	⅔ cup	125 gm
Potato, white, baked or boiled	1 (2″ diam.)	100 gm
Potatoes, white, mashed	½ cup	100 gm
Potatoes, sweet, or yams	¼ cup	50 gm
Sponge cake, plain	1½″ cube	25 gm
Ice cream (omit 2 fat exchanges)	½ cup	70 gm

List 5, Meat Exchanges
Each portion supplies approximately 7 gm of protein and 5 gm of fat, or 73 Calories (30 gm = 1 oz).

	Household Measurement	Weight of Portion
Meat and poultry (beef, lamb, pork, liver, chicken, etc.) (med. fat)	1 slice (3″ × 2″ × ⅛″)	30 gm
Cold cuts	1 slice (4½″ sq., ⅛″ thick)	45 gm
Frankfurter	1 (8–9 per lb)	50 gm
Codfish, mackerel, etc.	1 slice (2″ × 2″ × 1″)	30 gm
Salmon, tuna, crab	¼ cup	30 gm
Oysters, shrimp, clams	5 small	45 gm
Sardines	3 med	30 gm
Cheese, cheddar, American	1 slice (3½″ × 1½″ × ¼″)	30 gm
Cheese, cottage	¼ cup	45 gm
Egg	1	50 gm
Peanut butter	2 tbsp	30 gm

Limit peanut butter to one exchange per day unless allowance is made for carbohydrate in the diet plan.

List 6, Fat Exchanges

Each portion supplies approximately 5 gm of fat, or 45 Calories.

	Household Measurement	Weight of Portion
Butter or margarine	1 tsp	5 gm
Bacon, crisp	1 slice	10 gm
Cream, light	2 tbsp	30 gm
Cream, heavy	1 tbsp	15 gm
Cream cheese	1 tbsp	15 gm
French dressing	1 tbsp	15 gm
Mayonnaise	1 tsp	5 gm
Oil or cooking fat	1 tsp	5 gm
Nuts	6 small	10 gm
Olives	5 small	50 gm
Avocado	⅛ (4″ diameter)	25 gm

List 7, Milk Exchanges

Each portion supplies approximately 12 gm of carbohydrate, 8 gm of protein, and 10 gm of fat, or 170 Calories.*

	Household Measurement	Weight of Portion
Milk, whole	1 cup	240 gm
Milk, evaporated	½ cup	120 gm
Milk, powdered	¼ cup	35 gm
Buttermilk	1 cup	240 gm

*Skimmed milk eliminates the fat and about 90 Calories.

B. The Menu Guides

1200 Calories
(approximately)

carbohydrate	145 gm
protein	65 gm
fat	35 gm

BREAKFAST

1 fruit exchange (List 3)
1 bread exchange (List 4)
1 meat exchange (List 5)
1 milk (skimmed) exchange (List 7)
Coffee or tea (any amount)

LUNCH

2 meat exchanges (List 5)
2 bread exchanges (List 4)
Vegetable(s) as desired (List 1)
1 fruit exchange (List 3)
1 vegetable exchange (List 2)
1 milk (skimmed) exchange (List 7)
1 fat exchange (List 6)
Coffee or tea (any amount)

DINNER

2 meat exchanges (List 5)
2 bread exchanges (List 4)
Vegetable(s) as desired (List 1)
1 vegetable exchange (List 2)
1 fruit exchange (List 3)
1 fat exchange (List 6)
Coffee or tea (any amount)

1500 Calories
(approximately)

carbohydrate	180 gm
protein	75 gm
fat	55 gm

BREAKFAST

1 fruit exchange (List 3)
2 bread exchanges (List 4)
1 meat exchange (List 5)
1 milk (skimmed) exchange (List 7)
1 fat exchange (List 6)
Coffee or tea (any amount)

LUNCH

2 meat exchanges (List 5)
2 bread exchanges (List 4)
Vegetable(s) as desired (List 1)
1 fruit exchange (List 3)
1 vegetable exchange (List 2)
1 milk exchange (List 7)
1 fat exchange (List 6)
Coffee or tea (any amount)

DINNER

2 meat exchanges (List 5)
2 bread exchanges (List 4)
Vegetable(s) as desired (List 1)
2 vegetable exchanges (List 2)
2 fruit exchanges (List 3)
½ milk exchange (List 7)
1 fat exchange (List 6)
Coffee or tea (any amount)

2000 Calories (approximately)	carbohydrate	260 gm
	protein	105 gm
	fat	60 gm

BREAKFAST

2 fruit exchanges (List 3)
3 bread exchanges (List 4)
2 meat exchanges (List 5)
1 milk (skimmed) exchange (List 7)
2 fat exchanges (List 6)
Coffee or tea (any amount)

LUNCH

2 meat exchanges (List 5)
2 bread exchanges (List 4)
Vegetable(s) as desired (List 1)
2 vegetable exchanges (List 2)
2 fruit exchanges (List 3)
1 milk exchange (List 7)
1 fat exchange (List 6)
Coffee or tea (any amount)

DINNER

3 meat exchanges (List 5)
3 bread exchanges (List 4)
Vegetable(s) as desired (List 1)
2 vegetable exchanges (List 2)
2 fruit exchanges (List 3)
1½ milk (skimmed) exchanges
  (List 7)
1 fat exchange (List 6)
Coffee or tea (any amount)

2200 Calories (approximately)	carbohydrate	320 gm
	protein	95 gm
	fat	60 gm

BREAKFAST

3 fruit exchanges (List 3)
3½ bread exchanges (List 4)
2 meat exchanges (List 5)
1 milk exchange (List 7)
1 fat exchange (List 6)
Coffee or tea (any amount)

LUNCH

2 meat exchanges (List 5)
4 bread exchanges (List 4)
Vegetable(s) as desired (List 1)
2 fruit exchanges (List 3)
1 vegetable exchange (List 2)
1 milk (skimmed) exchange (List 7)
1 fat exchange (List 6)
Coffee or tea (any amount)

DINNER

2 meat exchanges (List 5)
4 bread exchanges (List 4)
Vegetable(s) as desired (List 1)
2 vegetable exchanges (List 2)
2 fruit exchanges (List 3)
1 milk (skimmed) exchange (List 7)
2 fat exchanges (List 6)
Coffee or tea (any amount)

2500 Calories	carbohydrate	305 gm
(approximately)	protein	115 gm
	fat	85 gm

BREAKFAST

3 fruit exchanges (List 3)
4 bread exchanges (List 4)
3 meat exchanges (List 5)
1 milk exchange (List 7)
2 fat exchanges (List 6)
Coffee or tea (any amount)

LUNCH

2 meat exchanges (List 5)
4 bread exchanges (List 4)
Vegetable(s) as desired (List 1)
2 fruit exchanges (List 3)
1 vegetable exchange (List 2)
1 milk (skimmed) exchange (List 7)
2 fat exchanges (List 6)
Coffee or tea (any amount)

DINNER

3 meat exchanges (List 5)
4 bread exchanges (List 4)
Vegetable(s) as desired (List 1)
2 vegetable exchanges (List 2)
2 fruit exchanges (List 3)
1 milk exchange (List 7)
2 fat exchanges (List 6)
Coffee or tea (any amount)

Note: The original exchange list diets allow approximately 40 per cent of the total caloric intake as fat. Most recent dietary goal recommendations by epidemiologists and nutritionists are that fat be restricted to no more than 30 per cent of total caloric intake (Figure 3–6 and Appendix A–19). The diets in this appendix have been modified slightly to reflect that goal.

C. Some Useful Equivalents by Volume and Weight

1 cup (237 milliliters)	8 fluid oz ½ pint 16 tablespoons
2 tablespoons (30 milliliters)	1 fluid oz
1 tablespoon (15 milliliters)	3 teaspoons
1 lb butter or margarine	4 sticks 2 cups
1 lb	453.6 gm
1 oz	28.35 gm
3½ oz	100 gm

Appendix D

Caloric and Nutritional Values of Fast Foods

	Wt (gm)	kcal	Pro* (gm)	Carb** (gm)	Fat (gm)	Chol† (mg)
BURGER CHEF						
Big Shef	186	542	23	35	34	—
Cheeseburger	104	304	14	24	17	—
Double Cheeseburger	145	434	24	24	26	—
French Fries	68	187	3	25	9	—
Hamburger, Regular	91	258	11	24	13	—
Mariner Platter	373	680	32	85	24	—
Rancher Platter	316	640	30	44	38	—
Shake	305	326	11	47	11	—
Skipper's Treat	179	604	21	47	37	—
Super Shef	252	600	29	39	37	—
BURGER KING						
Cheeseburger	—	305	17	29	13	—
Hamburger	—	252	14	29	9	—
Whopper	—	606	29	51	32	—
French Fries	—	214	3	28	10	—
Vanilla Shake	—	332	11	50	11	—
Whaler	—	486	18	64	46	—
Hot Dog	—	291	11	23	17	—

*Protein.
**Carbohydrate.
†Cholesterol.

Adapted from Young, E. A., Brennan, E. H., and Irving, G. L. (guest eds.): Perspectives on Fast Foods. Public Health Currents, 19(1), 1979, published by Ross Laboratories, Columbus, Ohio 43216.
Note: Fast foods tend to be:
1. high in calories;
2. low in vitamin A;
3. low in fiber;
4. high in sodium;
5. adequate in protein;
6. high in cost compared to a comparable product made at home.
Note: Blanks in columns indicate information not available.

	Wt (gm)	kcal	Pro* (gm)	Carb** (gm)	Fat (gm)	Chol† (mg)
DAIRY QUEEN						
Big Brazier Deluxe	213	470	28	36	24	—
Big Brazier Regular	184	457	27	37	23	—
Big Brazier w/Cheese	213	553	32	38	30	—
Brazier w/Cheese	121	318	18	30	14	—
Brazier Cheese Dog	113	330	15	24	19	—
Brazier Chili Dog	128	330	13	25	20	—
Brazier Dog	99	273	11	23	15	—
Brazier French Fries, 2.5 oz	71	200	2	25	10	—
Brazier French Fries, 4.0 oz	113	320	3	40	16	—
Brazier Onion Rings	85	300	6	33	17	—
Brazier Regular	106	260	13	28	9	—
Fish Sandwich	170	400	20	41	17	—
Fish Sandwich w/Cheese	177	440	24	39	21	—
Super Brazier	298	783	53	35	48	—
Super Brazier Dog	182	518	20	41	30	—
Super Brazier Dog w/Cheese	203	593	26	43	36	—
Super Brazier Chili Dog	210	555	23	42	33	—
Banana Split	383	540	10	91	15	—
Buster Bar	149	390	10	37	22	—
DQ Chocolate Dipped Cone, sm	78	150	3	20	7	—
DQ Chocolate Dipped Cone, med	156	300	7	40	13	—
DQ Chocolate Dipped Cone, lg	234	450	10	58	20	—
DQ Chocolate Malt, sm	241	340	10	51	11	—
DQ Chocolate Malt, med	418	600	15	89	20	—
DQ Chocolate Malt, lg	588	840	22	125	28	—
DQ Chocolate Sundae, sm	106	170	4	30	4	—
DQ Chocolate Sundae, med	184	300	6	53	7	—
DQ Chocolate Sundae, lg	248	400	9	71	9	—
DQ Cone, sm	71	110	3	18	3	—
DQ Cone, med	142	230	6	35	7	—
DQ Cone, lg	213	340	10	52	10	—
Dairy Queen Parfait	284	460	10	81	11	—
Dilly Bar	85	240	4	22	15	—
DQ Float	397	330	6	59	8	—
DQ Freeze	397	520	11	89	13	—
DQ Sandwich	60	140	3	24	4	—
Fiesta Sundae	269	570	9	84	22	—
Hot Fudge Brownie Delight	266	570	11	83	22	—
Mr. Misty Float	404	440	6	85	8	—
Mr. Misty Freeze	411	500	10	87	12	—
KENTUCKY FRIED CHICKEN						
Individual Pieces						
(Original Recipe)						
Drumstick	54	136	14	2	8	73
Keel	96	283	25	6	13	90
Rib	82	241	19	8	15	97
Thigh	97	276	20	12	19	147
Wing	45	151	11	4	10	70
9 Pieces	652	1892	152	59	116	864
LONG JOHN SILVER'S						
Breaded Oysters, 6 pc	—	460	14	58	19	—
Breaded Clams, 5 oz	—	465	13	46	25	—
Chicken Planks, 4 pc	—	458	27	35	23	—
Cole Slaw, 4 oz	—	138	1	16	8	—
Corn on Cob, 1 pc	—	174	5	29	4	—

*Protein.
**Carbohydrate.
†Cholesterol.

	Wt (gm)	kcal	Pro* (gm)	Carb** (gm)	Fat (gm)	Chol† (mg)
Fish w/Batter, 2 pc	—	318	19	19	19	—
Fish w/Batter, 3 pc	—	477	28	28	28	—
Fryes, 3 oz	—	275	4	32	15	—
Hush Puppies, 3 pc	—	153	1	20	7	—
Ocean Scallops, 6 pc	—	257	10	27	12	—
Peg Leg w/Batter, 5 pc	—	514	25	30	33	—
Shrimp w/Batter, 6 pc	—	269	9	31	13	—
Treasure Chest						
2 pc Fish, 2 Peg Legs	—	467	25	27	29	—
McDONALD'S						
Egg McMuffin	132	352	18	26	20	192
English Muffin, Buttered	62	186	6	28	6	12
Hot Cakes, w/Butter & Syrup	206	472	8	89	9	36
Sausage (Pork)	48	184	9	tr	17	43
Scrambled Eggs	77	162	12	2	12	301
Big Mac	187	541	26	39	31	75
Cheeseburger	114	306	16	31	13	41
Filet O Fish	131	402	15	34	23	43
French Fries	69	211	3	26	11	10
Hamburger	99	257	13	30	9	26
Quarter Pounder	164	418	26	33	21	69
Quarter Pounder w/Cheese	193	518	31	34	29	96
Apple Pie	91	300	2	31	19	14
Cherry Pie	92	298	2	33	18	14
McDonaldland Cookies	63	294	4	45	11	9
Chocolate Shake	289	364	11	60	9	29
Strawberry Shake	293	345	10	57	9	30
Vanilla Shake	289	323	10	52	8	29
PIZZA HUT						
Thin 'N Crispy‡						
Beef§	—	490	29	51	19	—
Pork§	—	520	27	51	23	—
Cheese	—	450	25	54	15	—
Pepperoni	—	430	23	45	17	—
Supreme	—	510	27	51	21	—
Thick 'N Chewy‡						
Beef§	—	620	38	73	20	—
Pork§	—	640	36	71	23	—
Cheese	—	560	34	71	14	—
Pepperoni	—	560	31	68	18	—
Supreme	—	640	36	74	22	—
TACO BELL						
Bean Burrito	166	343	11	48	12	—
Beef Burrito	184	466	30	37	21	—
Beefy Tostada	184	291	19	21	15	—
Bellbeefer	123	221	15	23	7	—
Bellbeefer w/Cheese	137	278	19	23	12	—
Burrito Supreme	225	457	21	43	22	—
Combination Burrito	175	404	21	43	16	—
Enchirito	207	454	25	42	21	—
Pintos 'N Cheese	158	168	11	21	5	—
Taco	83	186	15	14	8	—
Tostada	138	179	9	25	6	—

*Protein.
**Carbohydrate.
†Cholesterol.
‡Based on a serving size of ½ of a 10-inch pizza (3 slices).
§Topping mixture of ingredient.

	Wt (gm)	kcal	Pro* (gm)	Carb** (gm)	Fat (gm)	Chol† (mg)
BEVERAGES						
Coffee, 6 oz	180	2	tr	tr	tr	—
Tea, 6 oz	180	2	tr	—	tr	—
Orange Juice, 6 oz	183	82	1	20	tr	—
Chocolate Milk, 8 oz	250	213	9	28	9	—
Skim Milk, 8 oz	245	88	9	13	tr	—
Whole Milk, 8 oz	244	159	9	12	9	27
Coca-Cola, 8 oz	246	96	0	24	0	—
Fanta Ginger Ale, 8 oz	244	84	0	21	0	—
Fanta Grape, 8 oz	247	114	0	29	0	—
Fanta Orange, 8 oz	248	117	0	30	0	—
Fanta Root Beer, 8 oz	246	103	0	27	0	—
Mr. Pibb, 8 oz	245	93	0	25	0	—
Mr. Pibb Without Sugar, 8 oz	237	1	0	tr	0	—
Sprite, 8 oz	245	95	0	24	0	—
Sprite Without Sugar, 8 oz	237	3	0	0	0	—
Tab, 8 oz	237	tr	0	tr	0	—
Fresca, 8 oz	237	2	0	0	0	—

*Protein.
**Carbohydrate.
†Cholesterol.

Glossary

ABDUCTION: A movement away from anatomical position in the side plane. See Figure 2–4.

ABSOLUTE MUSCULAR ENDURANCE: The number of repetitions that can be performed by a muscle group at a specified workload, e.g., 50 lbs.

ADDUCTION: The return movement from abduction in which the body part is moved back toward the midline of the body. See Figure 2–4.

ADENOSINE-TRIPHOSPHATE (ATP): A complex chemical compound formed with the energy released through the degradation of food substances and stored in all cells, particularly muscles. The cell derives its energy from the breakdown of this compound.

ADIPOSE: Cells and tissues that contain the body's fat.

AEROBIC: A term used in referring to metabolism. Aerobic metabolism requires oxygen to complete the energy transformation process.

AEROBIC POWER: Synonomous with maximal oxygen consumption. The maximal rate at which aerobic metabolism can be carried on within the body.

AFFERENT NEURONS: Sensory neurons that carry information into the central nervous system.

ANAEROBIC: A term used in referring to metabolism. Anaerobic metabolism (splitting of ATP and glycolysis) can occur without the use of oxygen.

ANATOMICAL POSITION: The reference body position from which all movements are described. See Figure 2–3.

ANDROGENS: The male sex hormones, primarily testosterone from the testes.

ANGINA PECTORIS: Chest pain, usually caused by low oxygen supply to the myocardium. Generally precipitated by physical effort or emotional stimulation.

ANTERIOR SURFACES OF THE BODY: Those surfaces on the front side while one is standing in anatomical position. See Figure 2–3.

ANTIGRAVITY MUSCLES: Generally, the large extensor muscles of the body that counteract the tendency for the bony skeletal framework to collapse with the pull of gravity. See Figure 2–5.

ANXIETY: An emotional condition characterized by feelings of tension and apprehension and increased activity of the autonomic nervous system.

AORTA: The main artery leading into the systemic circulation. It arises from the left ventricle of the heart.

AROUSAL (CENTRAL): An increase in the complexity of neural organization manifested by desynchronization of electrical recordings made from the brain; a state of activation of the cerebral cortex which is regulated by the RAS.

ARTERIOSCLEROSIS: Loss of elasticity in arteries. "Hardening of arteries."

ARTERIOVENOUS (A-V) OXYGEN DIFFERENCE: The difference in oxygen concentration between the arterial and venous blood.

ATHEROSCLEROSIS: Narrowing of the lumen (inside diameter) of arteries. Usually caused by fatty deposits on their walls.

ATRIUM (pl. ATRIA): Upper chambers of the heart which receive blood from the pulmonary and systemic circuits.

ATROPHY: A term usually applied to muscle tissue, meaning decrease in size or function.

AXON: The long, cable-like part of a neuron that projects from the cell body to the synapse. See Figure 2–10.

BALLISTIC STRETCHES: Bouncing-type stretches in which a sudden pull is placed on the muscle at the end of the range of joint motion.

BASAL GANGLIA: A group of nuclei in the brain that perform a key role in planning and initiating movements.

BASAL METABOLIC RATE (BMR): The energy needs of the body at complete rest in a fasting state, i.e., the energy necessary to sustain life.

BLOOD PRESSURE: The pressure exerted on the walls of blood vessels by the blood as it flows through them.

BLOOD PRESSURE (MEAN): Systolic pressure + diastolic pressure/2. The arithmetical average of the systolic and diastolic pressures.

BODY COMPOSITION: The relative percentages of fat and fat-free body weight. Usually referred to as percentage body fat and lean body weight.

BODY FAT PERCENTAGE: The percentage of a person's total weight that is fat tissue.

CALORIE: See Kilocalorie.

CARBOHYDRATE: One of the three basic energy nutrients.

CARDIAC OUTPUT: The volume of blood pumped from the heart per minute.

CARDIORESPIRATORY: Refers to interaction between the respiratory and circulatory systems in delivery of oxygen to the body tissues.

CARDIOVASCULAR: A term pertaining to the heart and blood vessels.

CARDIOVASCULAR FUNCTION: The relative level of functional capacity within the heart and circulatory system.

CATECHOLAMINES: A group of chemical substances, including epinephrine and norepinephrine, manufactured by the adrenal gland and secreted during the stress response.

CENTRAL NERVOUS SYSTEM: A division of the nervous system containing the brain and the spinal cord. The other division is the peripheral nervous system. See Figure 2–8.

CEREBELLUM: A part of the brain that plays an important role in planning and controlling movements.

CHOLESTEROL: A blood alcohol similar to fat.

COLLATERAL CIRCULATION: The passage of blood through smaller adjoining vessels when a main vessel is blocked. Also, the development of additional capillary networks. See Figure 5–18.

CONCENTRIC CONTRACTION: A normal isotonic contraction in which the muscle shortens as it contracts against a load. See Figure 4–3.

CONNECTIVE TISSUE: Fibrous tissue used for connection of bones, muscle to bone, and support of internal body organs.

CONSCIOUSNESS ALTERATION: A change in arousal of the central nervous system.

CONTRACTION (MUSCLE): The development of tension within muscle fibers. The fibers attempt to shorten.

COPING STRATEGY: A behavioral pattern or cognitive style that facilitates adaptation to environmental stressors.

CORONARY ARTERIES: Arteries that carry blood to the heart muscle.

CORONARY CIRCULATION: Circulation within the heart muscle itself.

CORONARY HEART DISEASE: A common name for coronary atherosclerosis, which is a condition in which blood flow is restricted through a coronary artery by the thickening of the arterial wall by deposits of a fat-like substance.

CORONARY OCCLUSION: Blockage of one of the coronary blood vessels leading to the heart muscle.

CORONARY RISK FACTORS: Identified factors which have been associated with higher incidences of coronary heart disease.

DEHYDRATION: Lower-than-normal body water.

DEPRESSION: Feelings of helplessness, hopelessness, inadequacy, or sadness, sometimes overwhelmingly accompanied by a general lowering of psychophysical activity.

DIASTOLIC BLOOD PRESSURE: The blood pressure when the heart is relaxed between beats.

DISSOCIATION: A perceptual or cognitive strategy for coping with stress (e.g., exercise), in which bodily sensations are ignored by selectively directing attention elsewhere.

ECCENTRIC CONTRACTION: An antigravity contraction in which the muscle is contracting but gradually lengthening. This contraction lets the weights down slowly after they have been lifted. See Figure 4–3.

EFFERENT NEURON: Motor neurons or fibers carrying information from the central nervous system to the muscles or glands.

ELECTROCARDIOGRAM (EKG or ECG): A graphic record of the electrical activity of the heart.

ELECTROLYTE: A substance that ionizes in solution, such as salt (NaCl) and sugar, and is capable of conducting an electrical impulse.

ENDURANCE: One's relative ability to continue exercising at a given rate or intensity.

ENERGY OF THE BODY: Expressed in Calories, and defined as the force or power that enables the body to carry on life-sustaining or physical activity.

EPIDEMIOLOGY: The field of science dealing with the relationships of the various factors that determine disease processes in a population.

EPINEPHRINE: Also called adrenaline; a hormone secreted by the medulla of the adrenal gland. Its general effects are to mobilize the body systems to cope with an emergency or a stressful situation. Specifically, it stimulates production of sugar from the liver, increases heart rate, facilitates muscle contraction, and inhibits digestion. Predominantly responsive to psychological stressors.

ERGOGENIC: Any substance or phenomenon that enhances the functional ability to perform physical work, e.g., exercise.

ERGONOMICS: The science relating to man and his work, embodying the anatomical, physiological, psychological, and mechanical principles affecting efficient use of human energy.

ESSENTIAL HYPERTENSION: Hypertension with undiagnosed cause.

EXHAUSTION: Extreme fatigue; specifically, the limiting condition when a body system(s) ceases to respond to a stimulus. The final stage of Selye's general adaptation syndrome.

EXTENSION: The return movement of a body part from flexion back toward anatomical position. Joint angles increase, and body parts generally move toward the back surfaces of the body. See Figure 2–4.

FAT: One of the three basic energy nutrients.

FLEXIBILITY: The degree of normal extensibility or range of motion within the various joints of the body.

FLEXION: A movement from anatomical position in which the joint angle gets smaller.

GLOTTIS: A small amount of tissue that covers the trachea (windpipe) while food and water are swallowed. The glottis prevents food, water, etc., from entering the trachea.

GLUCOSE INTOLERANCE: Inability of the liver to take up and store large quantities of glucose. Blood sugar remains high after taking glucose, even in a fasting state.

GOLGI TENDON ORGAN: A proprioceptor located in the muscle tendon. It is sensitive to stretch or muscle load.

HEALTH-RELATED FITNESS: Positive aspects of physiological and psychological functioning that appear to protect the individual against degenerative diseases such as coronary heart disease, obesity, musculoskeletal disorders, and mental stress.

HEART VOLUME: Basic size of the heart expressed in a volume measure (ml).

HEAT STRESS: Any situation wherein the body has difficulty dissipating the heat that accumulates within it as a result of metabolism.

HEAT STROKE: Failure of the body to regulate its temperature. It is characterized by high internal body temperature; hot, dry skin (usually flushed); and sometimes, delirium or unconsciousness. It can be fatal.

HEMOGLOBIN: The oxygen-carrying red pigment of the red blood cell.

HIGH BLOOD PRESSURE: See Hypertension.

HUMIDITY: Pertaining to the moisture in the air. Relative humidity is the ratio of water vapor in the atmosphere to the amount of water vapor required to saturate the atmosphere at the same temperature.

HYPERLIPEMIA: An excess of fat or lipids in the blood.

HYPERTENSION: Chronic elevation of blood pressure above normal levels.

HYPERTROPHY: A term usually applied to muscle tissue, meaning increased size.

HYPOKINETIC DISEASE: Diseases caused by low levels of energy expenditure, e.g., heart disease, obesity, etc.

HYPOXIA: Low oxygen content or tension.

INFARCTION: See Myocardial Infarction.

ISCHEMIA: A local, usually temporary, deficiency of blood to some body part.

ISOKINETIC EXERCISE: A type of resistive exercise in which a special training device controls the limb speed and allows a person to exert maximal force throughout the range of joint motion.

ISOMETRIC CONTRACTION: A contraction in which the limb does not move because it cannot overcome the resistance. See Figure 4–3.

ISOTONIC CONTRACTION: A contraction in which the resistance is overcome and the limb moves. See Figure 4–3.

JOINT: Connecting point between two adjacent body segments; e.g., the forearm and upper arm are connected at the elbow joint.

KILOCALORIE: The basic unit of energy measurement in nutrition and exercise. The amount of heat necessary to raise the temperature of 1 liter of water 1 degree Centigrade. Also written as Calorie. A calorie is 1/1000 of a Calorie or kcalorie.

KILOGRAM-METER: A unit of work. The force of 1 kilogram acting through a distance of 1 meter. At normal acceleration of gravity, it is equivalent to 1 kilopond-meter.

LACTIC ACID (LACTATE): A fatiguing metabolic product resulting from the incomplete breakdown of sugars in the cell. The lactic acid system manufactures ATP when glucose (sugar) is broken down to lactic acid. High-intensity physical efforts requiring ½ to 3 minutes' duration draw energy primarily from this system.

LEAN BODY MASS: The fat-free proportion of the total body weight.

LIGAMENTS: Connective tissue that connects bones together.

LIPEMIA: See Hyperlipemia.

LIPID: See Fat.

LIPOPROTEIN: A complex of fat and protein molecules.

LITER: The basic unit of volume in the metric system. It is the equivalent of 1.0567 quarts liquid measure.

MANTRA: A word or phrase repeated in a chant-like manner in conjunction with certain meditational techniques.

MAXIMAL HEART RATE: The maximum rate at which the heart beats when stressed to a maximum level; decreases with advancing age in the adult.

MAXIMAL OXYGEN CONSUMPTION: Maximal volume of oxygen that can be taken into the body, delivered by the lungs and circulation to the cells, and used for metabolism per minute.

MEDITATION: A state of contemplation or reflection which may include relaxation to quiescence in an attempt to counteract stress.

METABOLISM: A general term to designate all chemical changes that occur to substances within the body.

MILLILITER (ml): A metric unit of volume that is 1/1000 of a liter.

MINERALS: Inorganic substances needed by the body in various amounts.

MOTIVATION: A term generally employed to describe phenomena involved with the operation of incentives, drives, or needs, and which result in goal-directed behavior.

MOTOR CORTEX: The area just in front of the central sulcus in the brain which controls some motor pathways. See Figure 2–16.

MOTOR NEURON: A type of neuron that carries impulses from the central nervous system to effector organs such as muscles.

MOTOR UNIT: The motor neuron plus all the muscle fibers it innervates. See Figure 2–13.

MUSCLE ENDURANCE: The ability of a muscle group to make repeated contractions against a defined load. The emphasis here is *how many* repetitions.

MUSCLE FIBER: The same as a muscle cell. A long cell containing the life-sustaining properties of all cells plus the special contraction mechanism to shorten.

MUSCLE SPINDLE: A proprioceptor located in muscle which responds to stretch and has reflexive connections in the spinal cord. See Figure 2–11.

MUSCLE STRENGTH: The ability of a muscle group to contract against a resistance, i.e., how much weight a person can lift or how much tension can be exerted.

MYOCARDIAL INFARCTION: A term generally used to denote a heart attack or damage resulting therefrom.

MYOCARDIUM: The heart muscle.

NEURON: The functional cell of the nervous system which is specialized in receiving and sending neural impulses. See Figure 2–10.

NEUROSIS: Any of a variety of relatively mild mental disorders primarily characterized by anxiety and a tendency to dwell on anxiety-provoking thoughts; emotional instability. A neurosis does not exhibit the gross distortion or misinterpretation of reality or the personality disorganization that typifies psychotic disorders.

NOREPINEPHRINE: A hormone secreted by the adrenal medulla, and formed at sympathetic nerve endings, which functions as a neurotransmitter and produces body reactions characteristic of emotional excitement. Predominantly responsive to physiological stressors, e.g., exercise.

NORMOTENSION: Blood pressure within the normal range for age and sex.

OBESITY: A condition wherein the body has a greater-than-desirable or -essential amount of body fat.

OSMOSIS: The diffusion through a semipermeable membrane of a solvent such as water from a lower to a more concentrated solution.

OVERWEIGHT: A condition in which the individual weighs more than average for age, height, and skeletal framework. May be due to obesity and/or heavy muscle development.

OXIDATION: The "burning" of food substances within the body in the presence of oxygen. The energy bound in them is released so that it can be stored in other forms, especially ATP.

OXYGEN CONSUMPTION: The volume of oxygen per minute taken into the body, delivered by the lungs and circulation to the cells, and used for metabolic activity.

PARTIAL PRESSURE: The pressure exerted by a gas in proportion to its percentage or concentration in a gas volume; i.e., if oxygen is 20 per cent of a gas mixture, it will exert 20 per cent of the total pressure.

PERCEIVED EXERTION (RPE): A verbalizable subjective estimate of actual metabolic work. Effort sense; a psychophysical judgment of the intensity of muscular and cardiovascular exercise.

PERCEPTION: The process of obtaining information about the environment (either internal or external) through the senses.

PERFORMANCE-RELATED FITNESS: Positive aspects of physiological and psychological functioning that aid in sports participation and performance (speed, power, etc.).

PERIPHERAL NERVOUS SYSTEM: A division of the nervous system containing the cranial (head) and spinal nerves; everything except the brain and spinal cord of the central nervous system. See Figure 2–9.

PHYSIQUE: Basic body type or build.

PHOSPHOCREATINE (PC): A chemical compound stored in muscle. Its breakdown aids in the manufacture of ATP.

PLACEBO: An innocuous substance or phenomenon that produces no real treatment effects, but which does result in artificial changes in biological function or performance owing to the recipient's belief in its effectiveness.

POLYUNSATURATED FAT: A fat that can absorb a significant amount of additional hydrogen. These fats usually are liquids at room temperature and of vegetable origin.

PRESSURE GRADIENT: The difference in pressure of gas from one body compartment to another. Because of activity of the gas molecules, they will tend to move by diffusion from the area of higher pressure to the area of lower pressure.

PROPRIOCEPTORS: A class of sensory receptors that respond to movement and body position.

PROTEIN: One of the three basic energy nutrients.

PSYCHOLOGICAL STATE: A temporary, transitory, fluctuating emotional or cognitive condition which is quite sensitive to situational influence, but also may be somewhat dependent on more stable characteristics of the individual.

PSYCHOLOGICAL TRAIT: A relatively stable and enduring disposition to behave or respond somewhat independent of situational influence. May be genetically influenced or acquired through learning.

PSYCHOMOTOR RETARDATION: A reduction in effective functioning of the neuromuscular system to include decreases in the expression of strength, endurance, coordination of movement, or reaction time.

PSYCHOSIS: Any abnormal or pathological mental disorder that tends to constitute a disease and which interferes seriously with the usual functions of life.

PSYCHOTHERAPY: Psychological treatment of mental disorders without the use of physical or pharmacological (chemical) methods.

PULMONARY CIRCULATION: The blood vessel circuit associated with circulation of the blood through the lungs.

RECIPROCAL INNERVATION: A principle of the nervous system whereby the antagonist muscle group is relaxed as the agonist muscle group contracts. It functions to prevent co-contraction of agonist and antagonist muscle groups, but can be overcome by messages from the brain.

REFERENCE MAN: A standard man 22 years old who weighs 154 lbs and is used as a nutrition reference for body size.

REFERENCE WOMAN: A standard woman 22 years old who weighs 128 lbs and is used as a nutrition reference for body size.

REFLEX: An involuntary, hard-wired neural response. The response is wired into the spinal cord instead of being planned by the brain.

RELATIVE HUMIDITY: See Humidity.

RELATIVE MUSCULAR ENDURANCE: The number of repetitions that can be performed by a muscle group at a given percentage of its maximal strength.

RELATIVE WEIGHT: The ratio of actual weight to predicted or desirable weight. Usually multiplied by 100. Values above 100 represent overweight, and those below 100 underweight, according to the norm.

REPETITION MAXIMUM (RM): The maximal amount of weight that can be lifted a specified number of times, i.e., 1 RM, 6 RM, 10 RM, etc.

SAID PRINCIPLE (Specific Adaptations to Imposed Demands): In order to obtain results from an exercise program, the demands must be sufficient to force adaptation, and the adaptation that occurs will be specific to the type of training performed.

SARCOMERE: The contractile unit of the muscle fiber containing the thick and thin filaments. See Figures 2–6 and 2–7.

SATURATED FAT: A fat which is not capable of absorbing any more hydrogen. These usually are solid fats of animal origin.

SECONDARY HYPERTENSION: Hypertension *with* diagnosed cause.

SEDENTARY: Describes a lifestyle that contains very little or no vigorous physical activity.

SENSORY: A term that refers to information about the environment going into the nervous system. Sensory fibers often are referred to as afferent fibers.

SERUM: The liquid portion of the blood.

SPOT REDUCE: An exercise myth in which fat patterning is lost from selected body areas.

STATIC STRETCHES: Stretches which are held in a stretched position for a period of time; no bouncing occurs.

STRENGTH: The relative capacity of a muscle or muscle group for exerting force against some external resistance.

STRETCH REFLEX: A muscle spindle reflex that counteracts stretch placed on the muscle. See Figure 2–14.

STROKE: A cerebrovascular accident in which the blood supply to the brain is blocked. It may result from a clot in an artery or a rupture in a blood vessel.

STROKE VOLUME: Volume of blood pumped from the heart with each beat.

SYNAPSE: A functional contact between neurons, or between neurons and muscles.

SYSTEMIC CIRCULATION: The division of the total circulation that receives blood from the left side of the heart; includes circulation to all tissues except the lungs.

SYSTOLIC BLOOD PRESSURE: The pressure during the heart's contraction phase.

TENDONS: Connective tissue that connects muscles to bone.

TENSION: Also referred to as hyperponesis; a state of exaggerated neuromuscular reactivity that may accompany anxiety and feelings of uneasiness and apprehension.

TESTOSTERONE: A sex hormone found in both males and females, but in much higher concentrations in the male. It is associated with increased hypertrophy of muscle tissue.

THROMBOSIS: The development or presence of a blood clot in the circulatory system.

"TIME-OUT" THERAPY: Any treatment that makes use of distraction from situations or thoughts that may precipitate a mental disorder such as anxiety or depression.

TRIGLYCERIDES: Fat particles circulating in the blood.

VALSALVA PHENOMENON: Occurs when an individual lifts heavy weights with a closed glottis (while holding the breath). Holding the breath produces increased pressure in the chest area and hinders the return of blood to the heart, causing an increase in blood pressure.

VENTRICLES: Lower chambers of the heart that pump blood into the systemic and pulmonary circuits.

VERTEBRAL COLUMN: The backbone, formed by many small vertebrae stacked on top of each other.

VESTIBULAR APPARATUS: The balance receptors of the inner ear. Consists of three different proprioceptors that signal acceleration, deceleration, and position of the head.

VIGOR (PSYCHIC): Feelings of enthusiasm, energy, and high spirits.

VITAMINS: Organic substances needed in small amounts for specific body functions.

WARM-DOWN: A gradual cooling of the body after an exercise bout by a continuation of exercise at a very low rate.

WARM-UP: Activation of physiological systems and elevation of body temperature by prior exercise.

WATT: A unit of power (work done per unit of time). One watt is equivalent to about 6 kilogram-meters/minute.

WIND CHILL: Effective temperature usually used in colder weather. Takes into consideration the heat-removing effect of cold air movement.

WOLFF'S LAW: States that the internal architecture and external shape of bones are altered by stresses applied to them. This is a specific example of the SAID principle.

Index

Page numbers in italics refer to illustrations. Page numbers followed by the letter *t* refer to tables.